Taijiquan Theory

of Dr. Yang, Jwing-Ming

The Root of Taijiquan

YMAA Publication Center
Wolfeboro, NH USA

YMAA Publication Center
Main Office:
    PO Box 480
    Wolfeboro, NH, 03894
    800-669-8892 • info@ymaa.com • www.ymaa.com

20200217

ISBN-13: 978-0-940871-43-4   ISBN-10: 0-940871-43-2
Edited by James O'Leary
Cover design by Tony Chee

Publisher's Cataloging in Publication

(Prepared by Quality Books Inc.)

Yang, Jwing-Ming, 1946-
    Taijiquan theory of Dr. Yang, Jwing-Ming : the root
of taijiquan.— 1st ed.
    p. cm
    Includes bibliographical references and index.
    LCCN: 2003103098
    ISBN: 0-940871-43-2

    1. Tai chi I. Title.

GV504.Y374 2003   613.7'148
                QBI03-200240

Anatomy drawings copyright ©1994 by TechPool Studios Corp. USA, 1463 Warrensville
Center Road, Cleveland, OH 44121

Disclaimer:
The authors and publisher of this material are NOT RESPONSIBLE in any manner whatsoever for
any injury which may occur through reading or following the instructions in this manual.
The activities, physical or otherwise, described in this material may be too strenuous or dangerous
for some people, and the reader(s) should consult a physician before engaging in them.

Printed in USA.

Contents

Romanization of Chinese Words

This book uses the Pinyin romanization system of Chinese to English. Pinyin is standard in the People's Republic of China, and in several world organizations, including the United Nations. Pinyin, which was introduced in China in the 1950's, replaces the Wade-Giles and Yale systems. In some cases, the more popular spelling of a word may be used for clarity.

Some common conversions:

Pinyin	Also Spelled As	Pronunciation
Qi	Chi	chē
Qigong	Chi Kung	chē kǔng
Qin Na	Chin Na	chǐn nǎ
Jin	Jing	jǐn
Gongfu	Kung Fu	gōng foo
Taijiquan	Tai Chi Chuan	tī jē chüén

For more information, please refer to *The People's Republic of China: Administrative Atlas, The Reform of the Chinese Written Language,* or a contemporary manual of style.

About the Author

Dr. Yang, Jwing-Ming, Ph.D. 楊俊敏博士

Dr. Yang, Jwing-Ming was born on August 11th, 1946, in *Xinzhu Xian* (新竹縣), *Taiwan* (台灣), Republic of China (中華民國). He started his *Wushu* (武術) (*Gongfu* or *Kung Fu,* 功夫) training at the age of fifteen under the *Shaolin* White Crane (*Bai He,* 少林白鶴) Master Cheng, Gin-Gsao (曾金灶) (1911-1976). Master Cheng originally learned *Taizuquan* (太祖拳) from his grandfather when he was a child. When Master Cheng was fifteen years old, he started learning White Crane from Master Jin, Shao-Feng (金紹峰), and followed him for twenty-three years until Master Jin's death.

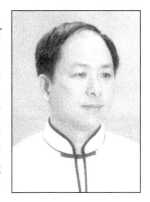

In thirteen years of study (1961-1974) under Master Cheng, Dr. Yang became an expert in the White Crane Style of Chinese martial arts, which includes both the use of barehands and of various weapons such as saber, staff, spear, trident, two short rods, and many other weapons. With the same master he also studied White Crane *Qigong* (氣功), *Qin Na* (or *Chin Na,* 擒拿), *Tui Na* (推拿) and *Dian Xue* massages (點穴按摩), and herbal treatment.

At the age of sixteen, Dr. Yang began the study of *Yang Style Taijiquan* (楊氏太極拳) under Master Kao Tao (高濤). After learning from Master Kao, Dr. Yang continued his study and research of *Taijiquan* with several masters and senior practitioners such as Master Li, Mao-Ching (李茂清) and Mr. Wilson Chen (陳威伸) in *Taipei* (台北). Master Li learned his *Taijiquan* from the well-known Master Han, Ching-Tang (韓慶堂), and Mr. Chen learned his *Taijiquan* from Master Zhang, Xiang-San (張祥三). Dr. Yang has mastered the *Taiji* barehand sequence, pushing hands, the two-man fighting sequence, *Taiji* sword, *Taiji* saber, and *Taiji Qigong.*

When Dr. Yang was eighteen years old he entered Tamkang College (淡江學院) in *Taipei Xian* (台北縣) to study Physics. In college he began the study of traditional *Shaolin* Long Fist (*Changquan* or *Chang Chuan,* 少林長拳) with Master Li, Mao-Ching at the Tamkang College Guoshu Club (淡江國術社) (1964-1968), and eventually became an assistant instructor under Master Li. In 1971 he completed his M.S. degree in Physics at the National Taiwan University (台灣大學), and then served in the Chinese Air Force from 1971 to 1972. In the service, Dr. Yang taught Physics at the Junior Academy of the Chinese Air Force (空軍幼校) while also teaching *Wushu*. After being honorably discharged in 1972, he returned to Tamkang College to teach Physics and resumed study under Master Li, Mao-Ching. From Master Li, Dr. Yang learned Northern Style *Wushu*, which includes both barehand (especially kicking) techniques and numerous weapons.

In 1974, Dr. Yang came to the United States to study Mechanical Engineering at Purdue University. At the request of a few students, Dr. Yang began to teach *Gong-fu* (*Kung Fu*), which resulted in the foundation of the Purdue University Chinese Kung Fu Research Club in the spring of 1975. While at Purdue, Dr. Yang also taught college-credited courses in *Taijiquan*. In May of 1978 he was awarded a Ph.D. in Mechanical Engineering by Purdue.

In 1980, Dr. Yang moved to Houston to work for Texas Instruments. While in Houston he founded Yang's Shaolin Kung Fu Academy. The Academy was eventually taken over by his disciple Mr. Jeffery Bolt after Dr. Yang moved to Boston in 1982. Dr. Yang founded Yang's Martial Arts Academy (YMAA) in Boston on October 1, 1982.

In January of 1984 he gave up his engineering career to devote more time to research, writing, and teaching. In March of 1986 he purchased property in the Jamaica Plain area of Boston to be used as the headquarters of the new organization, Yang's Martial Arts Association (YMAA). The organization has continued to expand, and, as of July 1st 1989, YMAA has become just one division of Yang's Oriental Arts Association, Inc. (YOAA, Inc.).

In summary, Dr. Yang has been involved in Chinese *Wushu* since 1961. During this time, he has spent thirteen years learning *Shaolin* White Crane (*Bai He*), *Shaolin* Long Fist (*Changquan*), and *Taijiquan*. Dr. Yang has more than thirty-three years of instructional experience: seven years in Taiwan, five years at Purdue University, two years in Houston, Texas, and nineteen years in Boston, Massachusetts.

In addition, Dr. Yang has also been invited to offer seminars around the world to share his knowledge of Chinese martial arts and *Qigong*. The countries he has visited include Argentina, Austria, Barbados, Belgium, Bermuda, Botswana, Canada, Chile, England, France, Germany, Holland, Hungary, Ireland, Italy, Latvia, Mexico, Poland, Portugal, Saudi Arabia, Spain, South Africa, Switzerland, and Venezuela.

Since 1986, YMAA has become an international organization, which currently includes 54 schools located in Argentina, Belgium, Canada, Chile, England, France, Holland, Hungary, Iran, Ireland, Italy, Poland, Portugal, South Africa, Venezuela and the United States. Many of Dr. Yang's books and videotapes have been translated into languages such as French, Italian, Spanish, Polish, Czech, Bulgarian, Russian, Hungarian, and Persian.

Dr. Yang has published twenty-nine other volumes on the martial arts and *Qigong*:

1. *Shaolin Chin Na*; Unique Publications, Inc., 1980.
2. *Shaolin Long Fist Kung Fu*; Unique Publications, Inc., 1981.
3. *Yang Style Tai Chi Chuan*; Unique Publications, Inc., 1981.
4. *Introduction to Ancient Chinese Weapons*; Unique Publications, Inc., 1985.
5. *Qigong for Health and Martial Arts*; YMAA Publication Center, 1985.
6. *Northern Shaolin Sword*; YMAA Publication Center, 1985.
7. *Tai Chi Theory and Martial Power*; YMAA Publication Center, 1986.
8. *Tai Chi Chuan Martial Applications;* YMAA Publication Center, 1986.
9. *Analysis of Shaolin Chin Na*; YMAA Publication Center, 1987.
10. *Eight Simple Qigong Exercises for Health*; YMAA Publication Center, 1988.
11. *The Root of Chinese Qigong—The Secrets of Qigong Training*; YMAA Publication Center, 1989.
12. *Muscle/Tendon Changing and Marrow/Brain Washing Chi Kung—The Secret of Youth*; YMAA Publication Center, 1989.
13. *The Essence of Taiji Qigong—Health and Martial Arts*; YMAA Publication Center, 1990.
14. *Qigong for Arthritis*; YMAA Publication Center, 1991.
15. *Chinese Qigong Massage—General Massage*; YMAA Publication Center, 1992.
16. *How to Defend Yourself*; YMAA Publication Center, 1992.
17. *Baguazhang—Emei Baguazhang*; YMAA Publication Center, 1994.
18. *Comprehensive Applications of Shaolin Chin Na—The Practical Defense of Chinese Seizing Arts*; YMAA Publication Center, 1995.
19. *Taiji Chin Na—The Seizing Art of Taijiquan*; YMAA Publication Center, 1995.
20. *The Essence of Shaolin White Crane*; YMAA Publication Center, 1996.
21. *Back Pain—Chinese Qigong for Healing and Prevention*; YMAA Publication Center, 1997.
22. *Ancient Chinese Weapons*; YMAA Publication Center, 1999.
23. *Taijiquan—Classical Yang Style*; YMAA Publication Center, 1999.
24. *Tai Chi Secrets of Ancient Masters*; YMAA Publication Center, 1999.
25. *Taiji Sword—Classical Yang Style*; YMAA Publication Center, 1999.
26. *Tai Chi Secrets of Wŭ and Li Styles*; YMAA Publication Center, 2001.
27. *Tai Chi Secrets of Yang Style*; YMAA Publication Center, 2001.
28. *Tai Chi Secrets of Wu Style*; YMAA Publication Center, 2002.
29. *Xingyiquan—Theory, Applications, Fighting Tactics, and Spirit*; YMAA Publication Center, 2002.

Dr. Yang has also produced the following videotapes:

1. *Yang Style Tai Chi Chuan and Its Applications*; YMAA Publication Center, 1984.
2. *Shaolin Long Fist Kung Fu—Lien Bu Chuan and Its Applications*; YMAA Publication Center, 1985.
3. *Shaolin Long Fist Kung Fu—Gung Li Chuan and Its Applications*; YMAA Publication Center, 1986.

4. *Shaolin Chin Na*; YMAA Publication Center, 1987.

5. *Wai Dan Chi Kung, Vol. 1— The Eight Pieces of Brocade*; YMAA Publication Center, 1987.

6. *The Essence of Tai Chi Chi Kung*; YMAA Publication Center, 1990.

7. *Qigong for Arthritis*; YMAA Publication Center, 1991.

8. *Qigong Massage—Self Massage*; YMAA Publication Center, 1992.

9. *Qigong Massage—With a Partner*; YMAA Publication Center, 1992.

10. *Defend Yourself 1—Unarmed Attack*; YMAA Publication Center, 1992.

11. *Defend Yourself 2—Knife Attack*; YMAA Publication Center, 1992.

12. *Comprehensive Applications of Shaolin Chin Na 1*; YMAA Publication Center, 1995.

13. *Comprehensive Applications of Shaolin Chin Na 2*; YMAA Publication Center, 1995.

14. *Shaolin Long Fist Kung Fu—Yi Lu Mai Fu & Er Lu Mai Fu*; YMAA Publication Center, 1995.

15. *Shaolin Long Fist Kung Fu—Shi Zi Tang*; YMAA Publication Center, 1995.

16. *Taiji Chin Na*; YMAA Publication Center, 1995.

17. *Emei Baguazhang—1; Basic Training, Qigong, Eight Palms, and Applications*; YMAA Publication Center, 1995.

18. *Emei Baguazhang—2; Swimming Body Baguazhang and Its Applications*; YMAA Publication Center, 1995.

19. *Emei Baguazhang—3; Bagua Deer Hook Sword and Its Applications;* YMAA Publication Center, 1995.

20. *Xingyiquan—12 Animal Patterns and Their Applications;* YMAA Publication Center, 1995.

21. *24 and 48 Simplified Taijiquan*; YMAA Publication Center, 1995.

22. *White Crane Hard Qigong*; YMAA Publication Center, 1997.

23. *White Crane Soft Qigong*; YMAA Publication Center, 1997.

24. *Xiao Hu Yan—Intermediate Level Long Fist Sequence*; YMAA Publication Center, 1997.

25. *Back Pain—Chinese Qigong for Healing and Prevention*; YMAA Publication Center, 1997.

26. *Scientific Foundation of Chinese Qigong*; YMAA Publication Center, 1997.

27. *Taijiquan—Classical Yang Style*; YMAA Publication Center, 1999.

28. *Taiji Sword—Classical Yang Style*; YMAA Publication Center, 1999.

29. *Chin Na in Depth—1*; YMAA Publication Center, 2000.

30. *Chin Na in Depth—2*; YMAA Publication Center, 2000.

31. *San Cai Jian & Its Applications*; YMAA Publication Center, 2000.

32. *Kun Wu Jian & Its Applications*; YMAA Publication Center, 2000.

33. *Qi Men Jian & Its Applications*; YMAA Publication Center, 2000.

34. *Chin Na in Depth—3*; YMAA Publication Center, 2001.

35. *Chin Na in Depth—4*; YMAA Publication Center, 2001.

36. *Chin Na in Depth—5*; YMAA Publication Center, 2001.

37. *Chin Na in Depth—6*; YMAA Publication Center, 2001.

38. *12 Routines Tan Tui*; YMAA Publication Center, 2001.

39. *Chin Na in Depth—7*; YMAA Publication Center, 2002.

40. *Chin Na in Depth—8*; YMAA Publication Center, 2002.
41. *Chin Na in Depth—9*; YMAA Publication Center, 2002.
42. *Chin Na in Depth—10*; YMAA Publication Center, 2002.
43. *Chin Na in Depth—11*; YMAA Publication Center, 2002.
44. *Chin Na in Depth—12*; YMAA Publication Center, 2002.
45. *Shaolin White Crane Gongfu—1*; YMAA Publication Center, 2002.
46. *Shaolin White Crane Gongfu—2*; YMAA Publication Center, 2002.

前言
李茂清老師

"知其源則流易測，得其本則枝葉易探"。童年受書于家君於燭下，釋「易經」之為書也。「易經」傳自上古，是記「祀」與「戎」（祭祀鬼神與治國安邦）之大事。

在「伏羲氏」未劃八卦之前，人類部落社會，是以葛藤結繩記事，用繩打結成不同的形狀和數量，標記憶其不同的事件。傳「伏羲」為一部落社會之首長，其仰觀天的日月星辰之像，俯察地理山川水紋（流）之形狀，覽河洛而悟劃八種不同的符號，以此符號來替代用繩打結之記事之方法。

「伏羲」其一劃而分天地（陰陽），亦是文字始生之始。天地運轉，陰陽更替，而萬物因之而生（無陰不生，無陽不長），萬物而人為靈，此「天地人」稱「三才」之定位本源。

「伏羲」劃一長橫「—」代表天（陽），再劃兩短橫「– –」代表地（陰），又再加一橫「—」代表萬物（人）。依此構想劃成的符號是：☰、☱、☲、☳、☴、☵、☶、☷。傳此為「伏羲氏」始成之八卦（組）符號，後之人稱為八卦，即是八卦之起源。

以此符號替代了上古用繩打結記事方法之精意，演進到後的「商朝」時，有其「西伯侯」依「伏羲氏」創劃的八組符號，再兩組（個）相疊成六十四組不同的組合符號，以記更多更繁雜（複）的事物，後之人稱其謂「周文王」六十四卦（仍簡稱八卦），增加了更多的文字記更詳細之事物，構成「易經」一書之起源。「易經」有「太極」二字，謂「大極生兩儀」（陰陽）。「太極」為道，兩儀為陰陽。陰陽一道也而萬物生焉。萬物負陰抱陽，無一不有太極，也無一不有兩儀。

「太極」為人所用，遠取六合（宇宙）之外，近取自身之中，無暫瞬息，微於動靜（呼吸），精神（氣）之運，心術（氣體）之喘動，與四時（季）合其序，人類養性（生）其學須知此本源也。

「太極」之始，陰陽未分（兩儀未生），為純然氣體，此為元極之始。無生之生，賴氣流體之運轉不息，因而道心凝靜（固），太極始成形（型）焉。「太極」動則生陽，靜則生陰。天地更替，因之四時成序，萬物生生不息。

人之生命，受于中（精）氣，「太極」謂之元氣。「天命之謂性」，「性」即人之元氣。元氣儲于人體之腎內，謂先天之氣，「肺、胃」儲後天自然之空氣，（中醫謂二步氣）即上述，萬物賴氣而生存。「氣」之運轉無瞬息之停，日月往來無一時之失。天地自然成序，其度不乖，萬物依時而繁衍。古者六藝，弦歌之外，不廢武事。

今之五育，科術爾昌，人體康壯為一切幸福之重心。中華民族數千年來之所以能鑄造悠久宏偉之文化，端賴人心均衡發展之仁人先賢們堅苦卓絕中，奮鬥鍛鍊累積之經驗，推展于後世人中。

新竹俊敏博士，學貫中西，禮仁之士也。教讀之暇，將其數十年之教研心得，編著〝楊俊敏博士之太極拳理論〟一書，內容精懇，旨在啟勵運動，發揚太極技藝，導源清流，清敬其為人，更欽其用心，學研者亦當知此序也。

中華國術進修會
研究委員
　　李茂清敬識
　　西元二零零零十二月冬至日

Foreword

Grandmaster Li, Mao-Ching 李茂清老師

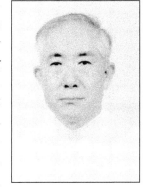

"Knowing its origin, then the flow can be gauged effortlessly; cognizing its root, then its branches and leaves can be explored easily." When I was a child, I was educated by my father under the candle light. The book used was *Yi Jing* (易經) (i.e., *The Book of Change*). *Yi Jing* was passed down from ancient times and it was used to record the important events of "Si" (祀) (i.e., worship the ghosts and deities) and "Rong" (戎) (i.e., ruling and martial affairs of the countries).

Before "Fu Xi" (伏羲) (i.e., first ruler of China) (2852-2737 B.C.) created Bagua (八卦) (i.e., Eight Trigrams), all Chinese used kudzu vine and rope knots to record events. Rope was tied up with different shapes and numbers of knots to record different affairs. It was said that "Fu Xi" was the chief of a society at the time. He looked up to see the repeating phenomenon of the sun, moon, and stars in the sky, looked down to inspect the geographic structure and landscape of the mountains and the rivers, looked at the basin between the Yellow River and Ruo River (河洛) and so enlightened he created eight different symbols which were used to replace the rope knots in recording affairs.

"Fu Xi" drew a long line, —— , to represent heaven (i.e., Yang, 陽), and two short lines, – – , to represent earth (i.e., Yin, 陰), and added a long line, —— , that is used to represent millions of objects (including humanity). From these conceptions, the symbols are constructed as: ☰ , ☷ , ☲ , ☵ , ☳ ☶ , ☱ , ☴ . This is what is known as Fu Xi's eight compositions of symbols, later called "Bagua" (八卦) (i.e., Eight Trigrams). This is the origin of the Eight Trigrams.

Later in the Chinese Shang Dynasty (商朝) (1766-1122 B.C.), "Xi Bo Hou" (西伯侯) (i.e., Marquis Xi Bo) used two sets of Fu Xi's Eight Trigrams and overlapped them to create sixty-four different sets of symbols. These could therefore record more complicated events and objects. Later, these were called "King Zhou's Sixty-Four Trigrams (周文王六十四卦) (still commonly called Eight Trigrams). This had thus increased the possibility in recording more matters in a detailed manner. Thereupon, the book *Yi Jing* (易經) (*Book of Changes*) was originated. There are two references to "Taiji" (太極) in *Yi Jing*, saying that "Taiji produces two polarities" (太極生兩儀) (i.e., Yin and Yang). Also "Taiji" is the "Dao" (道) and with two polarities of Yin and Yang, millions of objects are generated. Millions of objects carry Yin and embrace Yang, therefore, there is no place without Taiji and there is no place without "Two Polarities" (Liang Yi, 兩儀).

The philosophy of Taiji (i.e., Dao) was applied to study humanity. From afar, we take those transcendent six harmonies (Liu He, 六合) (i.e., universe or heaven); in close, we adopt what has been demonstrated in our bodies. There is no pause, (the Dao is) manifested in the movements and calmness (i.e., breathing), Jing and Shen (Qi) (精神) is thus transported, the inner mind (drawing in Qi) is thus in the actions. Anyone who is learning how to cultivate their human nature (for living), must know all of these origins.

Before "Taiji" began to act, Yin and Yang were not discriminated (i.e., two polarities were not yet generated) and there was a pure energy state. This is the beginning state of "Yuan Ji" (元極) (i.e., Wuji state, no extremity) (無極). In this state, there was no separation between living things, and all relied on the Qi's circulation ceaselessly. Subsequently, the core of "Dao" (i.e., Taiji) was condensed and calmed (i.e., formalized), and this resulted in the formation of the "Taiji" state. When "Taiji" moved, then Yang was produced and when it was calm, Yin was yielded. Heaven and Earth mutually replaced each other (i.e., Yin and Yang are exchangeable). Finally, four seasons were ordered and millions of lives have been born and continue to be born ceaselessly.

Human life begins with the receiving of (essence) Qi (Jing Qi, 精氣) (i.e., Qi produced from original essence), Taiji calls it "original Qi" (Yuan Qi, 元氣). This Qi is manifested from the heavenly mandate (i.e., nature) and is called "human nature" (Xing, 性). The original Qi is stored in the kidneys and is called "pre-heaven Qi" (Xian Tian Qi, 先天氣), while the lungs and stomach produce and store the "post-heaven Qi" (Hou Tian Qi, 後天氣) (Chinese medicine calls this the 'two layers of Qi'). There is no moment of cessation in Qi's transportation, the sun and the moon's cyclings have not missed even a moment. Consequently, millions of lives are propagating, and the six arts (Liu Yi, 六藝) (including music and martial arts) have been developed.

Today, there are five educations (Wu Yu, 五育) and science has flourished. Humanity's health and strength have become an important center for happiness. The level of Chinese culture which has been amassed through long thousands of years is being passed down by those ancient people who tried so hard to accumulate it.

Dr. Yang, Jwing-Ming from Xinzhu county (新竹縣) has mastered his cultures both in Asia and the West. He is a polite and kind gentleman. He has, during leisure time, between teaching and studying, summarized his experience and understanding in his more than thirty years of teaching and research, and has compiled them here under the title *Taijiquan Theory of Dr. Yang, Jwing-Ming*. The contents are profound and sincere. His intention is to publicize the exercises and promote the skills of Taijiquan so Taijiquan practitioners can be led onto the correct path. I respect his personality and more admire his intention.

Chinese Guoshu Promoting Association
Research Member
Li, Mao-Ching
December, 2000

前言
劉振寰將軍

我初識楊博士於一九九零年在溫恰斯特鎮 The Taste of China Tournament. 短期相處，得知他適退出高科技工作行列，轉而從事中國武術之推廣，以其淵博的學識及純熟的英文，著書立說，闡發至為精詳，令我深為驚喜與欽佩。及至去歲冬季，有幾位美籍學生，先後以楊博士所撰〝楊氏太極拳〞一書示我，並徵求意見。經數度拜讀後，深以該書圖文並茂，資料充實，釋義正確，實為難得的佳作。在心儀之下，更願本同好之誼，與楊博士彼此切磋，交換教學心得。是以坦率指出在〝太極舊論〞諸篇中有幾處似有商榷之餘地；同時多年來，對王宗岳〝太極論〞中「我順人背謂之『粘』或『沾』字」，以為若改為『輾』子則音近意義更為明確，且可與後文「活似車輪」之句相呼應。乃不揣淺陋，逕函楊博士詢以是否可提供意見以作參考。回信表示歡迎。經數次書信往返，楊博士廣徵博引，認為原著無誤。至此我等雖未得到共識，終以見仁見智而暫告中止討論。

爾後，楊博士寄來新作〝楊俊敏博士之太極拳理論〞初稿，囑我過目並作序言。因我雖從鄭師曼青習拳多年，惟目的只在強身，其後亦曾致力推手，亦僅力求體會以柔克剛之妙趣，所得淺薄。對楊博士要求為大作寫序實感惶恐，難以應命，懇切辭謝不敏。惟楊博士仍以「義不容辭」堅請。我雖感力有未逮，不得綜述這段經歷以應之。

數讀來稿，察其立論透澈，而對道家修身養性之道理，釋義精闢。採分篇論述，說明詳盡，使科學者研究領略，可謂全備矣。誠為不可多得之佳構。竊以太極之理論源於易經，而剛柔之說出自老子，若能就此加以發揮，即可與本稿所引孫子兵法各篇相媲美。區區之見謹供參考。

再者，我國固有太極拳之論述，多循道家傳統論說，對於西方人士頗有難解之困惑。楊博士能以現代科學化慣用詞句加以解說，對太極拳之推廣並發楊光大必大有助益也。是以不揣固陋以此為序。期共勉之。

劉愚謹識
西元二零零零・元月

Foreword

Grandmaster Abraham Liu 劉振寰將軍

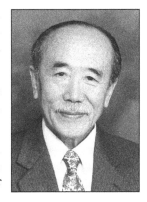

I first made Dr. Yang's acquaintance at **The Taste of China** Tournament (Winchester, Virginia) in 1990. Shortly after we became friends, I became aware that he had recently resigned his position as a high-tech engineer, and began to place all his efforts into the publicizing of the art of Chinese Wushu (武術). With his both vast and profound knowledge and fluency with the English language, Dr. Yang has written numerous books and articles, in which his descriptions and explanations are both detailed and refined. This made me very surprised and impressed. It was not until the winter of last year, that several of my American students showed me Dr. Yang's book, *Yang Style Taijiquan* and asked my opinion about it. After reading it a few times, I fully realized the depth of the body of text and illustrations. The material was quite substantial and the explanations were precise and accurate. It is very hard to find a written work of this quality. I felt deeply that, because of the nature of our common interests, Dr. Yang and I would be able to learn from each other by discussing the knowledge we had gained from our teaching experience. Therefore, other than highly recommending to my students to read his books, I also frankly pointed out to him that there were a few places in some classics of the *Old Taiji Thesis* that needed to be discussed. At the same time, I brought up my thoughts, from the last few years concerning the sentence, "I flow with the opponent('s coming force) (我順人背) is called Zhan (粘) (sticking) or Zhan (沾) (attaching)" from Wang, Zong-Yue's *Taiji Thesis*. I believe that if the word is changed into Zhan (輾) (i.e., half-rotating) then not only would the sound be nearly the same, but its meaning would make more sense. In addition, it would correspond better to the later text about "alive as a cart wheel" (活似車輪). I humbly wrote to Dr. Yang and asked for his opinion on my thoughts and hoped that he could offer me some support. The reply was welcome. Throughout the exchange, Dr. Yang explained his perspective and cited examples as to why he believed that the original writing was no mistake. Ultimately, though we did not come to an agreement about this word, we decided to temporarily discontinue our discussions, agreeing that the interpretation of this word should depend on the individual's understanding and the actual situation when applied.

Later, Dr. Yang mailed me the draft of this new book, *Taijiquan Theory of Dr. Yang, Jwing-Ming,* asking me to review it and to write a foreword. Although I have studied Taijiquan with Grandmaster Cheng, Man-Ching (鄭曼青) for many years, my initial motivation was only the strengthening of my body. Later, I also made a great effort in engaging Pushing Hands training. I was attracted to the theory and applications of "using the soft to conquer the hard" (以柔克剛). My understanding is still shallow and superficial, and it is for this reason that I was very nervous and daunted by Dr. Yang's request. Subsequently, I sincerely declined his request with thanks. However Dr. Yang, using the word "obligatory" (義不容辭), insisted that I should write this foreword. And though I feel that I am unable to fulfill this obligation, I cannot help but describe these past events as the foreword.

After reading the draft several times, I concluded that the theory discussed inside is very deep and clear. The explanation of the Daoist theory on the cultivation of human nature is especially refined. The explanation was divided into several parts and is detailed and complete. With regard to scientifically-minded practitioners, this book can be a complete guideline for their comprehension. The quality of its structuring is a rarity. Since the theory of Taiji originated from the *Yi Jing* (易經) (i.e., *Book of Change*) and the philosophy of soft and hard came from *Lao Zi* (老子) (i.e., *Dao De Jing*, 道德經), I personally believe that, should Dr. Yang use this as a foundation and develop it further, he will be able to draw a comparison to the theoretical essence of *Sun's Tactics of War* (孫子兵法) which is discussed in this book. This is only my personal suggestion for his consideration.

In general, Chinese theoretical discussions of traditional Taijiquan frequently follow the theory of Daoism. This is very confusing to Westerners. Because Dr. Yang is able to use scientific terms and knowledge to interpret and explain the traditional theory, he will greatly help the understanding and the development of Taijiquan. Therefore I do not hesitate to write this foreword with my poor knowledge. I hope we (all Taijiquan practitioners) will be able to learn from each other in the future.

Liu, Yu
January, 2000

Preface

In the last seven centuries many songs and poems have been composed about Taijiquan. These have played a major role in preserving the knowledge and wisdom of the masters, although in many cases the identity of the authors and the dates of origin have been lost. From these songs and poems, Taijiquan practitioners have had a guideline or a map which continues to lead them to the correct path of practice.

Most of these documents were considered secrets in every Taijiquan style. It was not until the last few decades that these secrets were gradually revealed to the general public. In the last 20 years, I have translated and made commentary on many of these documents. They include the songs and poems written by unknown authors, Yang's family (楊), Wu's family (吳), Li's family (李), Wǔ and Li's family (武・李), and Chen's family (陳). However, after I translated these documents, I realized that none of these families has revealed all aspects of Taijiquan theory and training. I believe that there are several reasons for this:

1. Many of the secrets were passed down orally. Normally, these oral secrets would not be written down, to prevent them from being revealed to outside people. Because of this, many of the top key secrets were not passed down through writing.

2. Those masters who wrote down the secrets drew from their individual understanding of the art. Some of them specialized in some subjects but were unfamiliar with others.

3. Part of the writings passed down are still hidden and have not been revealed to the general public yet.

I have been practicing Chinese martial arts since 1962 and have accumulated an abundant level of experience and understanding from learning, practicing, teaching, lecturing, translating, and writing. The styles with which I am most familiar are Shaolin Southern White Crane (少林南白鶴拳), Yang Style Taijiquan (楊氏太極拳), and Shaolin Long Fist (少林長拳). Taijiquan is considered to be an internal style (soft style) (Ruan Quan, 軟拳), White Crane is an internal-external style (soft-hard style) (Ruan Ying Quan, 軟硬拳), while Long Fist is classified as an external style (hard style) (Ying Quan, 硬拳). Due to this wide range of study and practice, I believe I am able to comprehend the entire scale of Chinese martial arts, both theory and training, to a profound level.

Since Southern White Crane is a soft-hard (internal and external) style of Chinese martial arts, by itself it covers a broad range of theory and practice. Since the

Dao (theory) (道) of the arts remains the same, the soft aspect (internal aspect) of Southern White Crane can easily be applied into Taijiquan.

Based on my personal background and understanding, I have tried my best to compile the Taijiquan theory and practice concepts in this book. I have attempted to make this effort as complete as possible even though I know it is difficult to fulfill this goal. Therefore, I hope those Taijiquan masters who are open-minded will continue to share their knowledge with the general public through writing and teaching, to make this art more complete and perfect. In order to make this book more complete with the growth of my own knowledge and experience in the future, I will at times revise it and continue to share my experiences with the readers.

When you read this book, you should keep your mind open, and make your judgement from a logical and scientific point of view. In fact, you should also always question any information you obtain regardless of its source. This is because the information you are obtaining is only the author's or teacher's personal interpretation and opinion. You must compile the information you have obtained, and ponder and test it carefully and critically. Only after you have comprehended the information can you say you have gained the knowledge.

This book is structured with a translation of a passage from one of the songs and poems, followed by the original Chinese text, and then any interpretation of the passage. Chinese text has been included because often, when a Chinese sentence has been translated into English, part of the actual meaning or feeling can be lost. In addition, this book is intended to be published in China.

With great appreciation for General Abraham Liu's suggestion (see foreword), I added the theory of Taiji and Yin-Yang from *Yi Jing* (易經) (i.e., *Book of Change*) and the concept of "using softness to conquer the hardness" (以柔克剛) from Lao Zi's Dao De Jing (老子・道德經). The reason for this is simply because these two ancient books are the original philosophies of these two concepts, and the foundation of Taijiquan.

Acknowledgments

Thanks to Tim Comrie for his photography and typesetting. Thanks to Grandmaster Li, Mao-Ching (李茂清) and Grandmaster Abraham Liu (劉振寰), for their Forewords. Thanks to Erik Elsemans, Jeff Rosen, Mark Klein, Ira Krepchin, Corlius Birkill, Jeff Pratt, Susan Bullowa, and Chris Hartgrove for proofing the manuscript and contributing many valuable suggestions and discussions. Thank to Mr. Vadas Mihaly for general assistance. Thanks to Tony Richard Chee for the cover design. Special thanks to the editor, James C. O'Leary.

PART I

General Concepts of
Taijiquan 太極拳概論

1. About Taiji 太極說

Changes; Great Biography said: "The ancestor surnamed Bao-Xi had become the king of heaven and earth. (He) looked up to see the phenomenal (changes) of the heavens, looked down to observe the (natural) rules (i.e., patterns) of the earth, watched the (instinctive) behaviors of birds and animals and how they were situated with (i.e., related to) the earth. Near, (he) observed the (changes) of things around him and far, (he) observed the (repeating patterns of) objects, then (he) created the 'Eight Trigrams.' This was thus used to understand the virtue of the divine (i.e., natural spirit or natural rules) and also thus used to resemble (i.e., classify, pattern, or understand) the behaviors of millions of objects (i.e., lives)." From this, (we) can see that the creation of the 'Eight Trigrams' was based on the ceaselessly repeating cycles of great nature, following the instinctive behaviors of the million objects (i.e., lives) between heaven and earth.

《易·大傳》曰：〝古者包義氏之王天下也。仰則觀象於天，俯則觀法於地。觀鳥獸之文，與地之宜，近取諸身，遠取諸物。於是始作八卦，所以通神明之德，所以類萬物之情。〞由是可知八卦之作乃始於大自然循環不已之理，遵天地萬物之情。

The quotation in this paragraph is from the "Great Biography" section of *The Book of Changes*. Bao-Xi (包義) was the ancient ruler in China (2852-2737 B.C.). After he observed the cyclical patterns of nature and the instinctive behavior of animals, he created the "Eight Trigrams" (Bagua, 八卦). From the "Eight Trigrams," natural cyclical patterns can be classified, traced, and predicted. Since animals and humans are part of nature, the "Eight Trigrams" can also be used to interpret an event and predict its possible consequences in the future.

Changes; Series Diction said: "(In) changes, there is Taiji. This therefore, produces Liangyi (i.e., Two Polarities), Liangyi generates Sixiang (i.e., Four Phases), and Sixiang bears Bagua (i.e., Eight Trigrams). (From) Bagua, good or bad luck can be defined (i.e., calculated or predicted). (From) good or bad luck, the great accomplishment can be achieved." It again said: *"What is Liangyi (i.e., Two Polarities)? (It is) one Yin and one Yang."* Lao Zi, Chapter 24 also said: *"Dao generates one, one produces two, two yields three, and three yields millions of objects."* From this (we) can see that it is due to the natural rules of Taiji, that Wuji (i.e., no extremity) evolves into Yin and Yang Two Polarities. From Yin and Yang's generation Two Polarities, the Four Phases are generated, and subsequently, from Yin and Yang's generation of the Four Phases, the Eight Trigrams are formalized. From this (we) can figure out that *"One Yin and one Yang is called Dao."* This also means that the *"Book of Changes"* is the (book which describes) the consistent natural laws that apply to the universe and the human body. From interaction of Yin and Yang, millions of objects are generated. From the variations of Yin and Yang, millions of affairs are communicative (i.e., exchangeable). Therefore, Changes; Series Diction also said: *"To close means Kun and to open means Qian, one closes and one opens means variations. To and fro exchange from each other ceaselessly means communicative (i.e., exchangeable)."* What is Kun? It is Yin. What is Qian? It is Yang.

《易・系辭》曰：〝易有太極，是生兩儀。兩儀生四象，四象生八卦，八卦定吉凶，吉凶生大業。〞又曰〝兩儀者，一陰一陽也。〞《老子・四十二章》亦曰：〝道生一，一生二，二生三，三生萬物。〞如是可知，因自然太極之理，無極衍化生為陰陽兩儀。由兩儀之陰陽衍化，四象而生。再由四象陰陽之衍化，八卦而成。由此可推，〝一陰一陽謂之道，〞亦即易經即宇宙人身互古一致之律。由陰陽之交媾，萬物生。由陰陽之變，萬事通。因之，《易・系辭》又曰：〝闔戶謂之坤，辟戶謂之乾，一闔一辟謂之變，往來不窮謂之通。〞坤者，陰也；乾者，陽也。

Changes; Series Diction (易・系辭) was written by Zhou Wen Wang (周文王), the first ruler of the Zhou Dynasty (周朝) (1122-255 B.C.). He wrote an interpretation for *The Book of Changes*. In his book, he clearly pointed out that because of the existence of Taiji (太極) (i.e., Grand Ultimate), there are changes in the universe. Taiji is an invisible force or power which makes the Wuji (無極) (i.e., No Extremity) divide into Two Polarities (i.e., Yin and Yang) and also from Two Polarities return back to the Wuji state. Moreover, due to the existence of the Taiji, Two Polarities can again be divided into Four Phases and from Four Phases into Eight Trigrams. The explanation of this kind of natural derivation has also been found in Lao Zi's *Dao De Jing* (老子・道德經). *Dao De Jing* (道德經) has also commonly been called "Lao Zi" (老子) in Chinese society. Lao Zi explained that due to the existence of Dao, one is created. In addition, one can create two, and then three, and so on until millions of objects exist. From this, we can see that Taiji is the same as Dao. That is why it is said: "What is Taiji? It is the Dao" (何謂太極？道也。).

Furthermore, from Yin and Yang's mutual interaction and exchange, millions of objects can be differentiated. For example, the soil interacts with water and sunshine, to produce growing plants. It is a study of the need of animals to consume other life in order to survive. Finally, animals die and return to the soil. All of these natural cycles are due to the natural exchanges and interaction of Yin and Yang.

What is Wuji? It means the insubstantial emptiness or an infinitesimal point of space, not big or small (i.e., no dimension), no Yin nor Yang. Through Taiji's pivotal action, Yin and Yang two Polarities are divided. Thus, the Yin-Yang symbol is formalized. This symbol can then be again distinguished as Yang Yin-Yang symbol and Yin Yin-Yang symbol depending on how the four phases of Yin and Yang are demonstrated (e.g., four seasons) through cycling. For example, if we demonstrate it with our right hand, the clockwise direction of cycling is classified as Yang symbol while the counterclockwise direction of cycling is classified as Yin. However, if we demonstrate it with our left hand, then everything is reversed. This is simply because generally our right hand is classified as Yang while left hand is classified as Yin.

無極者乃空空虛虛者或為太空之一小微點，無大無小，無陰無陽。由太極之動機陰陽兩儀因之分別。由之，陰陽圖現。根據陰陽如何運轉而演化成四象之方向，此陰陽圖可再區分為陽陰陽圖與陰陰陽圖。譬如我等以右手例，右旋為陽，左旋為陰。然而，如我等以左手為例，則一切反向矣。亦即左旋為陽，右旋為陰。這是因為一般而言，右手為陽，左手為陰也。

Wuji (無極) is a state of emptiness or simply a single point in space (Figure 1). There is no discrimination and there are no polarities (or poles). According to *Yi Jing* (i.e., Book of Change), originally the universe was in a Wuji state. Later, due to the pivotal action of Taiji (Figure 2), Two Polarities (Liang Yi, 兩儀) (i.e., Yin and Yang) were discriminated (Figure 3). However, we should understand that Yin and Yang are not definite (or absolute) but relative according to specifically defined rules. From these rules, Four Phases (Si Xiang, 四象) are again derived. From different perspectives, the Yin-Yang two polarities can again be divided into Yin and Yang. For

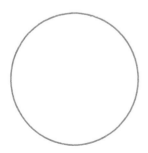

Figure 1. Wuji State

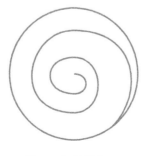

Figure 2. Taiji State

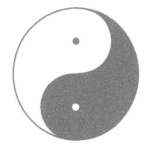

Figure 3. Yin-Yang State (Two Poles or Polarities)

example, if you use your right hand to follow the Yin and Yang pattern, the clockwise cycling belongs to Yang while the counterclockwise cycling belongs to Yin (Figure 4). Generally speaking, your right hand action is classified as Yang and your left hand action is classified as Yin. From this rule, the Yin-Yang cycling will be completely reversed if you use your left hand (Figure 5). These general rules are applied in Taijiquan and also in other internal styles such as Baguazhang.

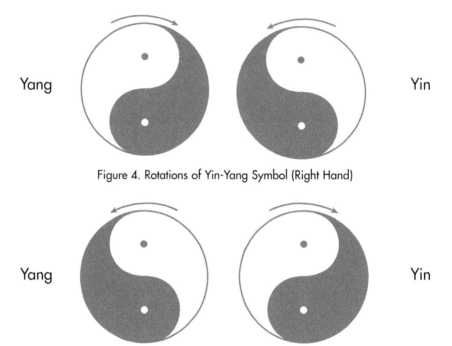

Yang   Yin

Figure 4. Rotations of Yin-Yang Symbol (Right Hand)

Yang   Yin

Figure 5. Rotations of Yin-Yang Symbol (Left Hand)

The above saying is talking about the Yin-Yang's derivation in two dimensions. When this Yin-Yang derivation is manifested in three dimensions, then right spiral to advance forward is classified as Yang while left spiral to withdraw is classified as Yin. Similarly, the manifestation of the left hand is reversed. From this, we can see that (if we are) able to comprehend the theory of great nature's Yin-Yang spiral derivation, then (we) will be able to comprehend the function of the Dao and use this Dao to understand the theory of ceaseless recycling of millions of lives in nature, furthermore, to trace back the origin of our human and physical life. The purpose of learning Taijiquan is to aim for the comprehension of Taiji and Yin-Yang so (we) are able to reach the Dao, therefore, (allows us) to protect (our body), strengthen (our body), and enjoy longevity. Furthermore, by nourishing and cultivating (our) human nature, (we are) able to reach the final goal of unification of heaven and human spirit.

以上所言為陰陽圖在二度空間中之演化。當此陰陽圖在
三度空間演化時，再以右手為例，右螺旋形而進者為陽，
左螺旋形而退者為陰。同理，左手反之。此為太空中無
窮生機變化之理，萬物賴之而衍生和轉化。因之，能理
解此大自然陰陽螺旋變化之理，即能通乎道機並利用此
道機去瞭解自然萬物生息不已之理，並可追朔己身性命
之來由。習太極拳之的，乃求此太極陰陽之理解，以臻
保身、強身、長生之道，並由養性、修性晉而達天人合
一之地也。

From the above discussion, you can see that there are some specific rules that apply when you manifest the Yin-Yang polarities into two dimensions. However, we exist in a universe of at least three dimensions. Therefore, the concept of two polarities should be adapted to three dimensions so we can comprehend the natural Dao thoroughly. Once you add the third dimension to the Yin and Yang symbols, you can see that the energy patterns and derivation are spiral actions. When the nature loses its balance, the energy manifests in spirals and millions of lives are influenced, or even are created. All of these manifestations can be seen from galaxies in space, to tornados and other storms, to the formation of sea shells, and even the tiny, twisted strands of our DNA (Figure 6).

From the above discussion, you can see that when Yin-Yang is manifested in two dimensions in Taijiquan, it is an action of coiling, and when it is acting in three dimensions, it is a spiraling maneuver. If you use your right hand to generate this spiral motion, then the clockwise and forward motion is classified as Yang while the counterclockwise and backward motion is classified as Yin (Figure 7). If you use your left hand, since the left is classified as Yin, all directions are reversed (Figure 8). This is a method to practice the basic skills in Taijiquan for changing from insubstantial to substantial and back again. All action in Taijiquan originates from the Real Dan Tian (a point, center of gravity), where

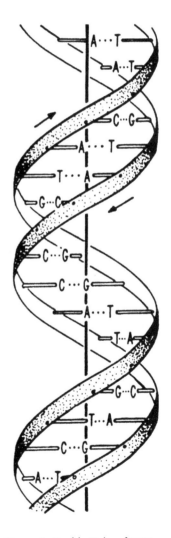

Figure 6. Double Helix of DNA

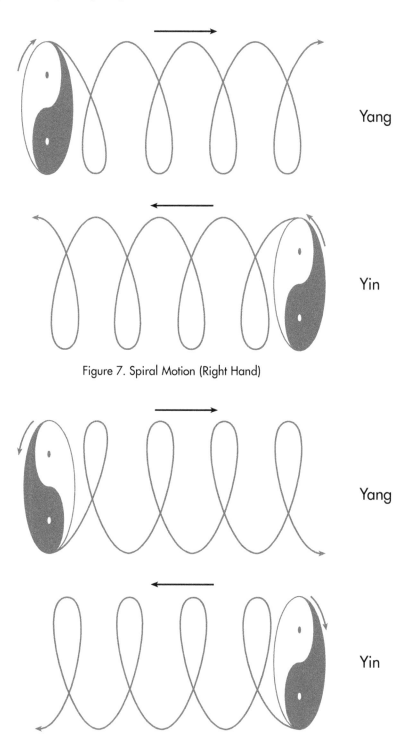

Yang

Yin

Figure 7. Spiral Motion (Right Hand)

Yang

Yin

Figure 8. Spiral Motion (Left Hand)

the Wuji is located. From this Wuji center, through Taiji (i.e., mind) the Qi is led, Yin and Yang spiraling actions are initiated, and Taijiquan movements are derived.

Taijiquan is an internal style of martial arts that was created in the Daoist monastery of the Wudang mountain, Hubei Province (湖北・武當山). Taijiquan's creation was based on the above philosophies of Taiji and Yin-Yang. It is believed that from understanding the theory of Taiji and Yin-Yang, we will be able to trace back the origin of our lives. Also, through this understanding, we will be able to train our bodies correctly, to maintain our health and strength of our physical and mental bodies, and gain longevity. Since Daoists are monks, the final goal of their spiritual cultivation is to reunite with the natural spirit (Tian Ren He Yi, 天人合一) (i.e., the state of Wuji). In order to reach this goal, they must cultivate their human nature and nourish it (i.e., discipline their temperament).

2. The Meaning of Taiji in Taijiquan 太極在太極拳中之義

> *Wang, Zong-Yue said: "What is Taiji? It is generated from Wuji, and is a pivotal function of movement and stillness. It is the mother of Yin and Yang. When it moves it divides. At rest it reunites." From this, it is known that Taiji is not Wuji, and is also not Yin and Yang. Instead an inclination of the natural pivotal function which makes the Wuji derive into Yin and Yang also makes the Yin and Yang reunite into the state of Wuji. This natural pivotal function of movement and stillness is called the 'Dao' or the 'rule' of great nature.*

王宗岳云：〝太極者，無極而生，動靜之機，陰陽之母也。動之則分，靜之則合。〞由此可知太極並非無極，亦非陰陽，而是自然之機驅使無極演化為陰陽或陰陽復合為無極之勢。此自然動靜之機，即所謂道或大自然之理。

Wang, Zong-Yue was a renowned Taijiquan master who was born in Shan-You, Shanxi Province (山右，山西省), during Chinese Qing Qian Long period (1736-1796 A.D.) (清乾隆). Taiji (太極) can be translated as "Grand Ultimate," or "Grand Extremity," and Wuji (無極) is translated as "Without Ultimate," "Without Limit," or "No Extremity." Wuji can also mean "No Opposition." This means Wuji is uniform and undifferentiated, a point in space or at the center of your physical, mental and energetic bodies. For example, at the beginning of the universe, there was no differentiation, and this state was called Wuji. Then it began its separation into complimentary opposites, called Yin (陰) and Yang (陽). From the interaction of Yin and Yang, all things are created and grow.

You should understand that even though the theory of Taiji (太極) originated from the *Yi Jing* (易經) (*The Book of Changes*) and has been studied and practiced for more than four thousand years in China, its applications in martial arts were

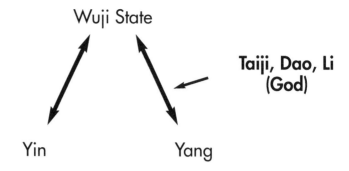

Figure 9. The Pivotal Action of Taiji (Dao)

probably not started until several thousand years later. When Taiji theory was adopted into the applications of martial arts and became a style, it was called Taijiquan (i.e., The Fist of Taiji) (太極拳). Therefore, if we wish to understand the real meaning of Taijiquan, the first task is to comprehend the meaning of Taiji.

From Wang, Zong-Yue's statement, it is clear that Taiji is neither Wuji nor Yin-Yang, but is between them. It is the pivotal force or energy which makes the Wuji state divide into the Yin and Yang (i.e., two polarities) and also causes the Yin-Yang to reunite to the state of Wuji (Figure 9). This natural pivotal force, energy, or function is called "Taiji" (太極), "Dao" (道) (i.e., natural way), or "Li" (理) (i.e., natural rules) of nature.

> *When Yin and Yang are divided, the Two Polarities are established. From Two Polarities, the Four Phases are generated. From Four Phases, the Eight Trigrams (Bagua) are produced. Again, from the Eight Trigrams, Sixty-Four trigrams are derived, and this pattern continues to divide until unlimited (variations) are produced. Yin and Yang's mutual interaction and correspondence, there are produced thousands of interchanges and millions of derivations, (consequently), millions of objects (i.e., lives) are born. (When) all of this is traced back to its origin, there is nothing but the theory of Yin and Yang. Therefore, those who practice Taijiquan must know Yin and Yang. If (one) wishes to know Yin and Yang, (he/she) must know the meaning of Taiji. If (one) wishes to know the meaning of Taiji, (he/she) must first comprehend the Dao and the real meaning of how Yin and Yang are derived from the Wuji state and also how Yin and Yang return to the Wuji state.*

陰陽分而兩儀生，由兩儀而生四象，再由四象而生八卦，由八卦再生六十四卦。由此推論，以至無窮。由陰陽之互感互應，千變萬化，萬物衍生。歸其宗，僅陰陽之理而已矣。因此習太極者，必知陰陽。欲知陰陽，必知太極之義，要知太極之義，必先領悟無極演變至陰陽與陰陽返歸回無極之道與真諦。

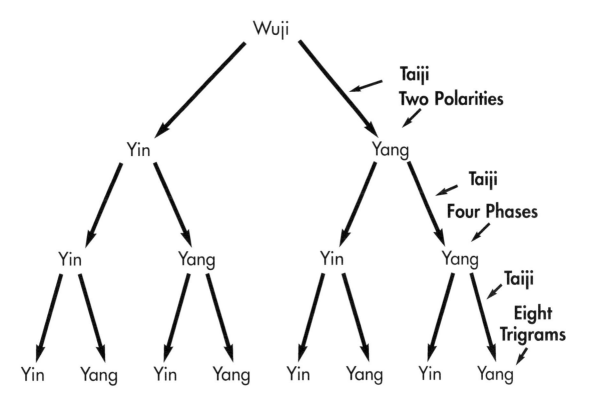

Figure 10. The Continuous Derivations of Yin and Yang due to Taiji's Pivotal Actions

Yin and Yang, two polarities, originate from Wuji through Taiji's action or function. From these two polarities, again through Taiji's action, four phases are derived. With the same theory, the variations continue until there are unlimited changes in the universe (Figure 10). From Yin and Yang's mutual interaction, millions of lives are born. From this, you can see that all life and all things are produced from the mutual interaction of Yin and Yang through the mediating function of Taiji. Therefore, if you are interested in learning Taijiquan, you must understand Yin and Yang, and their relationship with Taiji. Without knowing the theory and the Dao, your Taijiquan practice will be limited to the external forms and movements. In this case, you will have lost the real meaning of practicing Taijiquan.

> *Before the action of Taijiquan movement, the Xin (i.e., emotional mind) is peaceful and the Qi is harmonious, the Xin and Yi (wisdom mind) are at the (Real) Dan Tian and the Qi stays in its residence. This is the state of extreme calmness and is the state of Wuji. However, when the Xin and Yi begin to act, the Qi's circulation begins, the physical body's movement is thus initiated, and the Yin and Yang accordingly divides. From this (we) can see that Xin and Yi are what is called Taiji in Taijiquan. That means the Dao of Taijiquan is the Dao of Xin and Yi (i.e., minds).*

太極拳起勢在未動之前，心平氣和，心意在丹田，氣守
於舍，此極靜之態，是為無極。然者，當心動意動，氣
由之引發，身體而動，陰陽始分。由此可知心意在太極
拳中即所謂太極也。亦即太極拳之道即心意之道也。

The Wuji state exists inside each of us. It is the state from which all creative impulses grow. Taiji is generated out of Wuji and is the mother of Yin and Yang. Thus, Taiji is the cause of the Yin and Yang division, and is itself neither Wuji nor Yin and Yang, but the cause of the separation of Yin and Yang. In this sense it is a part of the divine aspect of the Dao.

All objects, ideas, spirits, etc. can be classified as either Yin or Yang. Taijiquan was created according to this theory. In the beginning posture of the Taijiquan sequence, the mind is calm and empty, and the weight is evenly distributed on both feet. This state is Wuji. When your mind starts to lead the body into the posture of Grasp Sparrow's Tail (攬雀尾), internal (Yin) and external (Yang) aspects of Taijiquan features start to be discriminated. Moreover, the hands and feet are differentiated into insubstantial (Yin) and substantial (Yang). This is the state of Two Polarities. Through interaction of substantial (Yang) and insubstantial (Yin), all of Taijiquan's fighting strategies and techniques are generated. From this, you can see that the Taiji (i.e., the Dao) in Taijiquan is actually the mind. It is the mind that makes the body move and divides the Wuji state into Yin and Yang two polarities. We can conclude from this that Taijiquan is actually a martial art of the mind (i.e., Taiji).

Though a human body is bonded between the heaven and the earth, (its) Xin and Yi are able to reach (anywhere) unlimitedly in the universe without being restricted by time and space. From Xin and Yi, the Yin and Yang are initiated and (continue to) move into unlimited variations. This is the theory of millions of divisions and creations of Taiji. Therefore, those who practice Taijiquan must begin from the (training of) Xin and Yi.

人身雖束於天地之間，然心意可達無窮於宇宙，並不為
時間、空間所限。由心意，陰陽生而演變分化無窮。此
為太極萬象衍生創造之理。因此，學太極者，必須從心
意著手。

Though our physical bodies are restricted by our three-dimensional reality, our minds are free to travel and reach anywhere in the universe, unrestricted by time, or even beyond this universe (i.e., the mind is Grand Ultimate). All human creations, from shovels to airplanes, arose first in our imaginations. From our thoughts, new ideas are created. It is the same for Taijiquan. It was created from the mind, and its creation will continue without an end. Since it is an active, living, and creative art, Taijiquan is a product of spiritual enlightenment and an understanding of life.

Xin (i.e., emotional mind) and Yi (i.e., wisdom mind) are contained internally, which belongs to Yin. The movements (actions) of Taijiquan are manifested externally, which belongs to Yang. When the functions of Xin and Yi are applied to our spiritual feeling, they direct us into the correct Dao of cultivating our human nature, through efforts toward strengthening the mind, raise up the spirit, and comprehend the real meaning of human life, and from this, further to comprehend the meaning and relationship among humans, between humans and objects around us, and also to search for the truth of nature in heaven and earth. When the function of Xin and Yi is applied to our physical body, it is the great Dao of cultivating the physical life for self-defense, nourishing the physical life, and strengthening the physical body. This is the foundation for extending our lives and establishing a firm root of health.

心意者，內含也，陰也。太極動作，外顯也，陽也。心意活動於己身之精神內感，即強心、提神、領悟人生之養性正道。由之去瞭解人與人、人與事物關係之真諦並尋求天地自然之真理。心意活動於己身物理之造化，即防身、養生、與強身之修命大道。此為延命立基之本。

As mentioned earlier, Xin and Yi are the Taiji in Taijiquan. This internal thinking is Yin. When this Yin is manifested externally, then Yang is demonstrated. When Xin and Yi are acting on internal spiritual feeling, it serves to cultivate our human temperaments and helps us to understand the meaning of our lives. When Xin and Yi are acting and manifested externally, it promotes physical health and self-defense. Therefore, when we practice Taijiquan, we should cultivate both our spiritual beings (Yin) and train our physical bodies (Yang).

Taijiquan originated from the Daoist family. Its ultimate goal is to reach enlightenment and so as to achieve the Dao of unification between heaven and human. Therefore, the final goal of practicing Taijiquan is to reach the unified harmonious Wuji world (i.e., state) of the heaven and human. From practicing Taijiquan, (we are able) to further comprehend the meaning of human life and the universe.

太極拳始於道家，其終的在通乎神明以臻天人合一之道。
因而太極拳之終的亦即在於天人合一大合諧之無極世界，
由習太極拳而領悟人生宇宙之理也。

Taijiquan was created in the religious (Daoist) school of Qigong. The goal of Daoist cultivation is to reach enlightenment, to unify the human spirit with the natural spirit. This is the Wuji harmonious state. To reach this destination, the first step is to appreciate the meaning of life and to understand natural truth.

3. Taijiquan Yin-Yang Illustrations 太極拳陰陽圖解

Two Polarities 兩儀	Four Phases 四象	Eight Trigrams 八卦	Sixteen Trigrams A&B 十六卦

Hard/Hard (Yang)—Qian-Peng
硬中帶硬〔陽〕－乾－掤
Hard/Soft (Yin)—Xun-Cai
硬中帶軟〔陰〕－巽－採

Hard (Yang)
硬〔陽〕

Soft/Hard (Yang)—Li-An
軟中帶硬〔陽〕－離－按
Soft/Soft (Yin)—Zhen-Lie
軟中帶軟〔陰〕－震－挒

Soft (Yin)
軟〔陰〕

Actions (Yang)
執行〔陽〕

External Gong (Yang)
外功〔陽〕

Offense/Offense (Yang)—Dui-Zhou
攻中帶攻〔陽〕－兌－肘
Offense/Defense (Yin)—Kan-Ji
攻中帶守〔陰〕－坎－擠

Offense (Yang)
攻〔陽〕

Defense/Offense (Yang)—Gen-Kao
守中帶攻〔陽〕－艮－靠
Defense/Defense (Yin)—Kun-Lu
守中帶守〔陰〕－坤－攦

Defense (Yin)
守〔陰〕

Strategies (Yin)
戰略〔陰〕

Taijiquan
太極拳

Flesh, Skin (Yang)—Qian-Baihui **C**
肌、膚〔陽〕－乾－百會
Tendon, Ligament (Yin)—Xun-Tiantu **D**
筋、腱〔陰〕－巽－天突

G/C Vessels
M/T Changing (Yang)
易筋〔陽〕

Bone (Yang)—Li-Mingmen **E**
骨〔陽〕－－－離－命門
Marrow (Yin)—Zhen-Jiuwei **F**
髓〔陰〕－－－震－鳩尾

Thrusting Vessel
M/B Washing (Yin)
洗髓〔陰〕

Moving (Yang)
動〔陽〕

Internal Gong (Yin)
內功〔陰〕

Xin (Yang)-Dui—Yintang **G**
心〔陽〕－－－兌－印堂
Body (Yin)—Kan-Yinjiao **E**
身〔陰〕－－－坎－陰交

Girdle Vessel (Yang)
帶脈〔陽〕
〔膚息〕

Spirit (Yang)—Gen-Lingtai **F**
神〔陽〕－－－艮－靈台
Yi (Yin)—Kun-Huiyin
意〔陰〕－－－坤－會陰

Embryo Wuji (Yin)
胎息·無極息〔陰〕
〔洗髓〕

Calmness (Yin)
靜〔陰〕

A. External Bagua (i.e., Eight Trigrams) manifestation follows Zhang, San-Feng's statement in his Taijiquan Classic. When Taijiquan externally manifests, the Eight Trigrams evolve out of the Two Polarities. There can be many versions of external actions that correspond to different phases of the Eight Trigrams. When you reach the Eight Trigrams stage of derivations, your movements and awareness are complex and alive. Many possibilities exist depending on how the mind responds to the situation. Remember, mind is the Taiji of Taijiquan. When this mind is manifested, the result is physical action.

B. Internal Bagua originates from the author's understanding and opinion.

C. Baihui (Gv-20) (百會) and Huiyin (Co-1) (會陰) belong to the Thrusting Vessel (Chong Mai, 衝脈) (Figure 11). Baihui is Extreme Yang and is the meeting point of the entire body's Yang. Baihui manifests spirit (Shen, 神). Shen is generally classified as Yang and is called Yang-Shen (陽神). The Huiyin stores water and belongs to Yin. The Huiyin is commonly called "Sea Bottom" (Haidi, 海底) or "Yin Water" (Yin Shui, 陰水). It is the meeting point of the four Yin vessels and is therefore Extreme Yin.

D. Tiantu (Co-22) (天突 is where manifested sounds originate. The two sounds "Hen" "Ha" govern the Jin's manifestation (Figure 12). Tiantu is Yin while the sound manifestation is Yang.

E. Mingmen (Gv-4) (命門) (Yang) and Yinjiao (Co-7) 陰交) (Yin) are two main gates which are the Qi exits from the Real Dan Tian (i.e., center of gravity). Mingmen belongs to the Governing Vessel (Du Mai, 督脈) while Yinjiao belongs to the Conception Vessel (Ren Mai, 任脈) (Figure 13). From these two gates the Qi can either be manifested externally and used to strengthen the Girdle Vessel (Dai Mai, 帶脈) (i.e., Guardian Qi, Wei Qi, 衛氣) or led inward to be stored at the Real Dan Tian (Wuji Breathing, 無極息).

F. Lingtai (Gv-10) (靈台) and Jiuwei (Co-15) (鳩尾) are two main gates which connect the Xin (心) (i.e., heart, emotional mind) (Figure 13). Emotional mind is the motor force while Yi (意) is the steering wheel.

G. Yintang (M-HN-3) (印堂) (i.e., The third eye) is the manifestation of physical strength. When the sense of enemy is strong, the Qi manifestation is strong (Figure 12).

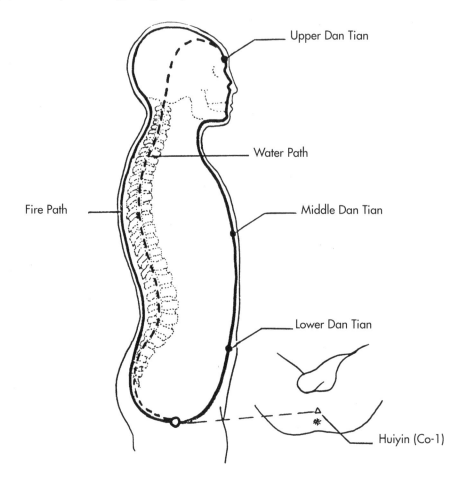

Figure 11. Baihui (Gv-20) and Huiyin (Co-1) Cavities

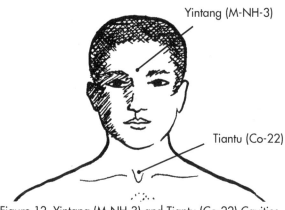

Figure 12. Yintang (M-NH-3) and Tiantu (Co-22) Cavities

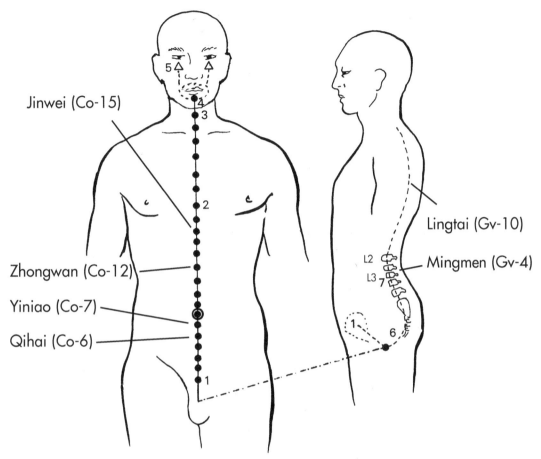

Jinwei (Co-15)

Zhongwan (Co-12)

Yiniao (Co-7)

Qihai (Co-6)

Lingtai (Gv-10)

Mingmen (Gv-4)

Figure 13. Yinjiao (Co-7), Mingmen (Gv-4), Jiuwei (Co-15), and Lingtai (Gv-4) Cavities

Explanation of Taijiquan Yin-Yang Illustrations 太極拳陰陽圖說

What is Taijiquan? It is from the Xin and Yi's Taiji that Yin and Yang were divided. What are Yin and Yang (in Taijiquan)? They are the Two Polarities of Taijiquan and are the Gongfu of internal (i.e., Yin) and external (i.e., Yang). The Xin, Yi, and Qi, which are contained internally, belong to Yin while the external manifestations belong to Yang. Again, from the Xin and Yi's Taiji, the internal (Yin) and external (Yang) are divided and therefore form externally two polarities and internally two polarities; the Four Phases of Taijiquan. Furthermore, from the Xin and Yi's Taiji, both the internal and external Two Polarities can be divided into internal and external Bagua (i.e., Eight Trigrams). Consequently, the Sixteen Trigrams of Taijiquan are derived and emerge.

太極拳者，由心意之太極，而分陰陽。陰陽者，太極拳
之兩儀，內外功夫也。內含之心、意、氣為陰，外象之
顯現為陽。再由心意之太極，內外在行分野，而成外兩
儀與內兩儀太極拳之四象也。進之，由心意之太極，內
外各兩儀再分野成內外四象，因之，太極拳之八卦定形
矣。再進而演化之，由內外之各四象再演變成內外各八
卦之象。太極拳之十六卦現形矣。

From Wang, Zong-Yue's Taijiquan classic, we know that what is Taiji in Taijiquan is actually the mind. According to Chinese custom, we have two minds, one is called Xin (心) (i.e., emotional mind) and the other is called Yi (意) (i.e., wisdom mind). Xin is classified as Yang, and can make your emotions disturbed, while Yi is classified as Yin and makes you calm and thoughtful.

In Taijiquan, the mind (i.e., Taiji, 太極) discriminates the Yin and Yang Two Polarities (Liang Yi, 兩儀), and from the mind's action (i.e., Taiji), these Yin and Yang polarities will again be divided into Yin-Yin and Yin-Yang, Yang-Yin, and Yang-Yang. These are the Four Phases (Si Xiang, 四象). Again, from the action of the mind (i.e., Taiji), these Four Phases are divided into Eight Trigrams (Bagua, 八卦), and so on.

From this you can see that through the mind's action, Taijiquan can be divided into Two Polarities (Liang Yi, 兩儀): external manifestation (i.e., Yang) and internal cultivation (i.e., Yin). The internal cultivation includes regulating the mind—which is to lead the Qi to circulate inside the body, and also the cultivation and the purification of the spirit. The external physical actions are the manifestation of the mind that are carried out with circulating Qi and upraised spirit.

Again, from the mind, both external and internal aspects of Taijiquan can be divided into Yin and Yang (i.e., Two Polarities) and therefore, form the Four Phases (Si Xiang, 四象) of Taijiquan. In the same way, these internal Two Polarities and external Two Polarities can again be divided into Four Phases and this permits the Taijiquan to be represented in Eight Trigrams (Bagua, 八卦). If we advance one more level, then the internal Four Phases and external Four Phases can again be divided into Eight Trigrams and therefore, the Sixteen Trigrams (Shi Liu Gua, 十六卦) of Taijiquan evolved.

Taijiquan actually includes both internal Eight Trigrams and external Eight Trigrams. This shows us the fourth level or depth of Taijiquan analysis. If a Taijiquan practitioner can reach this level and understand the meaning of these Sixteen Trigrams, then he can say he has reached a proficient level of Taijiquan study. Naturally, from Sixteen Trigrams, Taijiquan can again be divided into Thirty-Two (San Shi Er Gua, 三十二卦) and Sixty-Four Trigrams (Liu Shi Si Gua, 六十四卦), and so on. This can lead you to an even deeper Taijiquan understanding. As a Taijiquan practitioner, you should continue pondering and searching for a deeper and more refined understanding of Taijiquan.

From internal Yin, Yin and Yang can be divided. What is Yin-Yang? It means the Xin and Yi remain calm while the Qi is actively moving. What is Yin-Yin? It means to reach the insubstantial ultimate (i.e., Wuji state) and to keep (the mind) in the state of extreme sincere calmness. This will result in the formation of the internal Two Polarities. From Yin-Yang, it can again be divided into Yin-Yang-Yang and Yin-Yang-Yin. What is Yin-Yang-Yang? It means the Muscle/Tendon Changing (Qigong). What is Yin-Yang-Yin? It is the Marrow/Brain Washing (Qigong). Similarly, Yin-Yin can again be divided into Yin-Yin-Yang and Yin-Yin-Yin. What is Yin-Yin-Yang? It implies Girdle Breathing or Body Breathing (i.e., Skin Breathing). What is Yin-Yin-Yin? It means the Wuji Breathing. Therefore, the internal Four Phases are formed. From the internal Four Phases, the internal Eight Trigrams evolved.

由內之陰，陰陽分。陰陽者，心意靜而氣動也。陰陰者，
致虛極，守靜篤。內兩儀因而成形。陰陽者，可再分野
為陰陽陽與陰陽陰。陰陽陽者，為易筋。陰陽陰者，為
洗髓也。同理，陰陰者再分為陰陰陽與陰陰陰。陰陰陽
者，帶脈息、體息也。陰陰陰者，無極息也。如此，內
四象成形也。由此內四象再演變成內八卦。

The internal Yin can again be divided into Yin-Yang and Yin-Yin Two Polarities. Yin-Yang implies that the Xin and Yi are kept in a calm and peaceful state (i.e., Yin) while the Qi is actively circulating (i.e., Yang). Yin-Yin means the mind is kept at the Real Dan Tian (Zhen Dan Tian, 真丹田) (i.e., physical gravity center) and maintains an extremely calm state. In this case, your mind is in a Wuji state and the Qi is kept at its residence. This is the required state for Embryonic Breathing (Tai Xi, 胎息) which will be discussed later.

The Two Polarities again divide into the Four Phases. From Yin-Yang, Yin-Yang-Yang and Yin-Yang-Yin are discriminated and from Yin-Yin, Yin-Yin-Yang and Yin-Yin-Yin are derived. Internal Yin-Yang-Yang means the practice of Muscle/Tendon Changing (Yi Jin, 易筋) Qigong while Yin-Yang-Yin implies the training of Marrow/Brain Washing (Xi Sui, 洗髓) Qigong. Internal Yin-Yin-Yang refers to Girdle Vessel Breathing (Dai Mai Xi, 帶脈息) (Skin Breathing or Body Breathing) (Fu Xi, Ti Xi; 膚息、體息) while Yin-Yin-Yin involves the practice of Wuji Breathing (Wuji Xi, 無極息) (Cavity Breathing) (Xue Wei Xi, 穴位息). From these, you can see how the internal Four Phases have evolved.

Following the same rules, the external manifestation can also be divided into Yin and Yang. Yang-Yang is the action of the external manifestation while the Yang-Yin is the internal plotting and planning of the strategies. This therefore forms the external Two Polarities. Yang-Yang can again be divided into Yang-Yang-Yang and Yang-Yang-Yin. Yang-Yang-Yang is the manifestation of the hard Jin while Yang-Yang-Yin is the execution of the soft Jin. Similarly, Yang-Yin can again be discriminated into Yang-Yin-Yang and Yang-Yin-Yin. Yang-Yin-Yang is for offense while Yang-Yin-Yin is for defense. Thus, the external Four Phases have evolved. From these Four Phases, the external Eight Trigrams are developed and have become the Eight Doors of Taijiquan's thirteen postures.

外象之顯現，亦可依理而分陰陽。陽陽者，外象之執行。
陽陰者，內在之謀略。外兩儀因而成形。陽陽者，可在
分野為陽陽陽與陽陽陰。陽陽陽者，硬勁之顯現。陽陽
陰者，軟勁之執行。同理，陽陰者再分為陽陰陽與陽陰
陰。陽陰陽者，攻勢也。陽陰陰者，守勢也。如此，外
四象成形也。由此內四象再演變成外八卦而構成太極拳
十三勢之八門也。

Similarly, the external Gong (i.e., Yang) can be divided into Yang-Yang and Yang-Yin. Yang-Yang is the execution or the physical manifestation of the internal mind while Yang-Yin includes the strategies or maneuvers of internal plotting and planning. Yang-Yang can then again derive into Yang-Yang-Yang and Yang-Yang-Yin. Yang-Yang-Yang is the manifestation of hard Jins, while Yang-Yang-Yin is the execution of the soft Jins. Naturally, from Yang-Yin, Yang-Yin-Yang and Yang-Yin-Yin can be developed. Yang-Yin-Yang covers the offensive strategies while Yang-Yin-Yin covers the defensive strategies.

From these external Four Phases, the external Eight Trigrams emerge and have become the Eight Jin Patterns of Taijiquan. These Eight Jin Patterns are commonly called the Eight Doors (Ba Men, 八門) since they deal with the eight directions of fighting in Taijiquan. Together with the Five Phases (Wu Xing, 五行) of stepping movements, they explain why Taijiquan is called "Thirteen Postures" (Shi San Shi, 十三勢).

4. Yin-Yang Theory of Taijiquan 太極拳陰陽論

Yin and Yang are opposite (i.e., relative) to each other instead of absolute. That is Yin can become Yang and Yang can change into Yin. Yin and Yang can be exchanged mutually depending on the observer's Xin and Yi. Xin and Yi are the Dao in Taijiquan. Lao Zi, Chapter 36 said: "Wish to close it, must first open it; wish to weaken it, must first strengthen it; wish to abolish it, must first raise it; wish to take it, must first offer it." It is also said in Taijiquan classic: "withdrawing is releasing and releasing is withdrawing." It means: "Yin is Yang and Yang is Yin." Though they are opposite, they are the two faces of the same object which cannot be separated from each other or exist alone. If it can exist alone, then it is a Wuji state and not the natural rule of Yin and Yang.

陰陽者，對立也，而非絕對也。陰者可陽，陽者可陰。
陰陽之互變，以觀者之心意而定。心意者，太極拳之道
也。《老子‧三十六章》：〝將欲歙之，必固張之；將
欲弱之，必固強之；將欲廢之，必固興之；將欲取之，
必固與之。〞 太極拳經亦云：〝收即是放，放即是
收。〞亦即〝陰即是陽，陽即是陰〞也。雖為對立，而
為一物一理之兩面，不可分離而單獨存立矣。如單獨存
在，則為無極之態而非陰陽自然之理也。

Yin and Yang are opposite to each other but not absolute. How Yin or Yang are defined depends on the perspective of the viewer. Often, what is considered Yang by one person can be Yin to another. Moreover, Yin and Yang are exchangeable and this exchange also depends on how you change your viewpoint. You should also remember that the mind is what is called Taiji or Dao in Taijiquan.

When Yin and Yang concepts are applied in Taijiquan, Yin can be Yang and Yang can be Yin. Yin can also be Yin and Yang can also be Yang. All of these alternative concepts all depend on your mind and consequently, different strategies are derived. That means an insubstantial action can be a setup for a substantial action and vice versa. If you do not have the options of Yin and Yang exchange, then your strategy will be stagnant and be easily defeated by your opponent.

Generally speaking, Taijiquan's Yin and Yang can be: closing and opening; defensive and offensive; bending and extending; inhaling and exhaling; retreating and advancing; insubstantial and substantial; small and big; neutralizing and emitting; refined and coarse; leading and attacking; soft and hard; internal and external; Yi and Xin; raising and falling; looking up and looking down; coming and going; enter and exit; withdrawing and releasing; etc. However, (you) should not be fixed in the rules without knowing the mutual exchangeable theory of Yin and Yang. For example, during combat between the opponent and me, bending can be Yang as offensive, and extending can be Yin as defensive. Raising can be Yang as a substantial action and falling can be Yin as an insubstantial movement. Coming can be Yang as emitting and going can be Yin as storing.

一般而言，太極拳之陰陽可為：合、開；守、攻；屈、
伸；吸、呼；退、進；虛、實；小、大；化、打；細、
粗；引、擊；柔、剛；內、外；蓄、發；意、心；起、
落；仰、俯；來、往；入、出；收、放等。但切不可固
執而不懂陰陽互變之理。譬如在敵我對待之時，屈亦可
為陽為攻，伸可為陰為守。起可為陽為實，落可為陰為
虛。來可為陽為發，往可為陰為蓄。

This paragraph lists many examples of the Yin and Yang aspects of Taijiquan actions. However, you should always remember that Yin and Yang are mutually exchangeable. That means substantial can be insubstantial and insubstantial can be substantial.

If (you) are able to understand the theory of Yin and Yang and knows their applications, then (your) comprehension is deep and (Taiji) knowledge is profound. Insubstantial and substantial are exchangeable and are mutually Yin and Yang. This will make the opponent lose track of catching the (Jin's) coming and going. Then this is the beginning of understanding Jin. The theory of Yin and Yang is hard to change; however, the applications of Yin and Yang are exchangeable. Therefore, (Taijiquan) practitioners should be always researching and pondering the theory of Yin and Yang and searching for the applications of Yin and Yang's mutual exchanges. If (you) are able to catch this knack and apply it skillfully, then (you are) surely a proficient Taijiquan talent.

懂得陰陽之理並知其所用，則其悟也深，知其竅亦淵。
虛實互變，互為陰陽，使敵無可捉摸來龍去路，此為懂
勁之始。陰陽為理者，難變。陰陽為用者，可變。如此，
學者當無時無刻不研究太極陰陽之理與探其陰陽互變之
用。能懂其竅，而能致用，此為太極能者之風也。

You should know that Taiji's Yin-Yang theory is the foundation and the root of the entire Taijiquan's creation and development, you should always ponder the theory and its applications. Theory is the scholarship of the art while the actions are the applications of the theory. Only then can you catch the crucial key to Taijiquan's substantial and insubstantial. Once you are able to apply this Yin-Yang theory into the Taijiquan martial art, you will be able to know the opponent but the opponent will not know you. When you have reached this stage, you have surely understood the applications of Understanding Jin.

5. Yin-Yang Theory of Taiji's Xin and Yi 太極心意陰陽論

Xin and Yi are the Dao of Taijiquan. From the Xin and Yi's Yin, the Yang actions can be manifested externally. However, the students should also know that Xin and Yi themselves also have Yin and Yang. Xin is Yang, active, emotional, confused, floating, and uneasy. Yi is Yin, calm, wise, condensed, sunken, and steady. Xin is the motor force while the Yi is the steering wheel. From Xin, the emotion is agitated, the spirit is raised, and from Yi, the discrimination is clear and the spirit is condensed. One Yin and one Yang mutually apply to each other. In this case, the spirit can be high, yet condensed. The Spirit of Vitality can be uprising.

心意者，太極拳之道也。由心意之陰而顯現陽動于外，
然學者須知心意本身卻亦有陰陽也。心者，陽也，動也，
感情也，散亂也，浮也，躁也。意者，陰也，靜也，機
智也，收斂也，沈也，定也。心者，動力也。意者，掌
舵也。由心，情高，神提。由意，辨清，神斂。一陰一
陽互為用。則神高而斂，精神提起也。

According to Chinese concepts, we have two minds. One is the emotional mind which is called Xin (心) while the other is the wisdom or logic mind which is called Yi (意). Xin makes you excited, sad, happy, and is emotional while Yi makes you calm and offers you logical thinking. Because of this, the Xin is classified as Yang while Yi is classified as Yin. Yang offers you the power while Yi controls how the power is manifested. In Chinese Qigong society Xin is compared to a monkey while Yi is compared to a horse. That is why Xin-monkey and Yi-horse (Xin Yuan Yi Ma, 心猿意馬) are often shown in ancient documents.

If there is only Xin without the Yi's presentation, then, though the emotion and the motor force are high and strong, (you) may expose (yourself) and offer an opportunity for (your) opponent. In this case, you are fighting with emotion. However, if there is only Yi without Xin, then though the Yi is concentrated and the decisions are clear, due to the emotion (i.e., fighting spirit) being low, the fighting morale will not be high. (In this case, you) can be subdued by the fear of (your) opponent's killing awe. From the above, (we) know that the (real) Dao is that Yin and Yang mutually apply to, mutually assist, and mutually harmonize with each other. That means the Dao of Taiji is the mutual harmonization of the Xin and Yi.

如僅存心而意不行，雖性情動力高昂，但必為敵所乘。
此為感情之戰也。然而，若僅存意而卻無心，則雖意專、
決明，但情緒低落，戰志不高，易為敵之殺氣所懾。由
上可知陰陽互用、互助、互調乃為道。亦即心意之互相
調合乃太極之道也。

When you are in a conflicting condition with your opponent, you will need your Xin to raise up the fighting morale and also need your Yi to make a clear judgement and logical decision. Without these two minds' mutual coordination and harmonization, you will lose the fight. This theory can also be applied into your life. You will need both your Xin and Yi to make your life vigorous, harmonious, and wise.

6. Yin-Yang Theory of Movement and Stillness in Taijiquan 太極拳動靜陰陽論

Ancient document said: "The ultimate of movement is stillness, the ultimate of stillness is movement. To move is to generate stillness, and to be still is to generate movement. Therefore, (if you) use stillness as movement, (your) movement will be stronger every day. (If you) use movement as movement, (your) movement will weaken daily. (If you) use movement to drive stillness, (it is) calm and long. (If you) use stillness to drive the movement, (it is) vigorous and strong."

古云：〝動極則靜，靜極則動，動以成靜，故以靜為動，
其動日強。以動為動，其動日弱，而以動馭靜，靜而可
久。以靜馭動，動而可大。〞

When the body is calm and still, the mind can be clear and concentrated. When the mind is concentrated, the Qi led can be abundant and consequently, the physical power manifested can be strong. When you are active and moving, the mind is excited and harder to focus. Naturally, the power manifested will be weak. Therefore, it is said that if you use stillness and calmness to drive the movement, the action can be vigorous and strong.

Moreover, if you know how to move slowly and calmly, you are able to keep the mind calm and peaceful. When this happens, the calmness of the mind can last long. However, if you keep moving fast, the mind's concentration will be shallow, the Qi led will be weakened, and naturally, the power manifested will be weak. The aim of Taijiquan is to keep the mind concentrated and calm within the movements. That is why Taijiquan is also called "moving meditation." The more you practice, the more you are able to concentrate. The mind becomes calmer and therefore, the movements can be stronger and stronger.

> *Yin is the beginning of Yang, and Yang is the start of Yin. When Yin reaches its extremity, it becomes Yang and when Yang reaches its extremity, it turns into Yin. This is the rule of heavenly Dao (i.e., natural way). In the theory of Taijiquan, calmness is Yin and movement is Yang. Within calmness, there is a hidden movement and within the movement, there is a calmness. What is the calmness? It is Yin, it is Yi, and it is internal. What is movement? It is Yang, has shape, and is external. When Taijiquan is used for applications (i.e., power manifestation), storage is Yin. When storage reaches its extremity, it becomes Yang. Emitting is Yang. When Yang reaches its extremity, storage begins. To and fro, they mutually apply to each other.*

陰者，陽之始。陽者，陰之初。陰極而陽，陽極必陰，
此為天道之理。太極拳理者，靜為陰，動為陽。靜中寓
動，動中有靜。靜者，陰也，意也，內也。動者，陽也，
形也，外也。太極拳用者，蓄為陰，蓄極而陽。發為陽，
陽極而蓄。一來一往，相互為用。

When Yin has reached its extremity, it turns into Yang and when Yang reaches its limit, it changes into Yin. This is the natural rule or Dao. This theory is also applied in Taijiquan practice. In order to generate Yang, you must first have Yin and when Yang has been manifested, the Yin must begin again. In Taijiquan, Yin is internal which is related to Yi and Qi while Yang is external, and is the manifestation of Yin. When this rule is applied into Taijiquan applications, Yin is storage while Yang is the manifestation of the power and the execution of techniques. Yin and Yang are mutually generating and supporting each other.

But do remember that there is a hidden Yang within Yin and a (concealed) Yin resides within Yang. Yin is not completely Yin and Yang is not completely Yang. (Consequently,) Yin and Yang can then be mutually exchangeable, regulate each other appropriately, and the Jin and skills can be alive. (If) Yin is completely Yin, the Jin will be stagnant and stiff. (If) Yang is completely Yang, then the Jin manifested will be hard to withdraw.

但切記陰中寓陽，陽中帶陰，陰不全陰，陽不全陽。陰陽才能互變、互調得宜，勁技能活。陰而全陰，勁必呆死。陽而全陽，勁必難收。

In order to exchange Yin and Yang smoothly and skillfully, you should not allow your Yin or Yang to reach its maximum or extremity. When this happens, the exchange will become stagnant. If you allow some Yin within Yang and vice versa, the exchange will be smooth, comfortable, and natural. That is why in the Taiji Yin-Yang symbol, there is some Yin hidden in Yang and some Yang hidden in Yin (Figure 14). It is the same for Taijiquan. Insubstantial and substantial should be able to exchange with each other smoothly and naturally so the Jin manifestation will be alive.

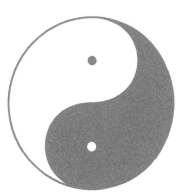

Figure 14. Taiji Yin-Yang Symbol

What is Taiji (in Taijiquan)? It is Yi (i.e., wisdom mind). That means the original natural virtue of Taijiquan is Yin and is calmness. (It) looks for the movement within calmness. From the Yin's containment (i.e., storage) the Yang can be emitted. Calmness is used as a foundation and the movement is used for applications. Use defense as the primary maneuver and use offense for secondary tactics. Search for offense in defense, wait for advantageous opportunity and then emit. Calmness is to store, and movement is to emit. (If you) are able to understand the theory of calmness, then (you) can comprehend the applications of Jin (i.e., martial power). From calmness, the spirit is hidden in Yi, the Qi is stored in the bone marrow, and external Jin is hidden in the postures. From understanding Jin, the advantageous opportunity can be perceived, and from knowing the advantageous opportunity, the Jin can be emitted. When the calmness is deep, the emitted Jin will be strong and when the calmness is shallow, the emitted Jin will be weak. Theoretically, this is not different from bending the bow to store the Jin.

太極者，意也。亦即太極拳之本性，陰也，靜也。由靜中求動，由陰含而陽發。以靜為本，以動為用。以守為主，以攻為輔。守中求攻，待機而發。靜者，蓄也，動者，發也。能懂靜之理，才懂勁之用。由沉靜而神匿於意、蓄氣於髓、隱外勁於勢，由懂勁而知機，由知機而勁發。靜深則勁發強，靜淺則勁弱。此與蓄勁張弓之理無異矣。

We already shown that the Taiji in Taijiquan is the Yi (i.e., the wisdom mind). Yi is internal, which belongs to the Yin aspect of Taijiquan. Therefore, it is calm and peaceful. From this calmness, the Yi can be highly concentrated and its storage can be profound. When this Yi is deep and profound, the feeling will be accurate and refined. You should always remember that feeling is the language of the mind and the body's means of communication. Deep and accurate feeling allows you to manifest the mind's decision precisely and quickly. From this, you can see that the Yin (i.e., the Yi) is the foundation of Taijiquan's Yang manifestation. Taijiquan is a defensive martial art and uses defense as offense. Waiting for opportunity through attaching, connecting, adhering, listening, and following, enables techniques to be executed properly and the power to fully manifest. When this happens, you will know the opponent but the opponent will not know you. This is the stage of Understanding Jin. Taijiquan's Jin storage is the same process as storing power by drawing a bow. If you are calm, firm, and concentrated, the Jin can be stored to its most efficient stage. When this stored Jin is manifested, its execution can be accurate and the power can be strong.

7. Lao Zi's Thesis of Using the Soft to Subdue the Hard 老子以柔克剛論

No one should learn Taijiquan without knowing that the Taijiquan theory of using softness to subdue hardness was originated from Lao Zi's Dao De Jing. Lao Zi; Chapter 78 said: "There is nothing that is softer and weaker than water. However, that which is strong and hard cannot defeat it. This is because there is nothing that can replace it. (The theory) that the weak is able to defeat the strong and the soft is able to triumph over the hard is all well known (by the people) between the heaven and the earth, (however), nobody is able to do it." Again, Lao Zi; Chapter 43 said: "That the softest in the heaven and the earth is able to bore through the hardest. Nothingness is capable of entering the material without any gap. Therefore, I know the benefit of doing nothing." From this, (we) can see that when it is soft, then it is smooth, able to bend, to be gentle, and to vary. When Yi is soft, the Qi is soft and smooth. When Qi is soft and smooth, then there is no place that cannot be reached. Therefore, Lao Zi; Chapter 10 said: "When aiming for the softness of the Qi, can (we) be like a baby?" This emphasizes the softness of Yi and Qi like a baby, so (we) are able to reach the Dao of longevity. When this theory is applied in Taijiquan, then (we) are able to listen (i.e., feel), understand, attach, adhere, follow, connect, and therefore, to be alive. Hence, Lao Zi; Chapter 76 said: "When a human is born, (he/she) is soft and when (he/she) is dead, becomes hard (i.e., stiff). When a plant is just germinating, it is soft and weak and when it is dead, it is dry and emaciated. Therefore, those who are strong and hard belong to the category of death and those who are soft and weak are classified in the category of aliveness. Thus, those who own strong soldiers will die and the wood that is strong will break. Those who are stronger will end in the low place while those soft and weak will be placed in the high position."

習太極者，無不知太極拳以柔克剛之理乃源於老子之道
德經。《老子・七十八章》云：〝天下莫柔弱于水，而
攻堅強者莫之能勝，其無以易之。弱之勝強，柔之勝剛，
天下莫不知，莫能行。〞又《老子・四十三章》云：〝天
下之至柔，馳騁天下之至堅，無有入于無間，吾是以知
無為之有益。〞由此可知，柔則順，能彎、能軟、能變。
意柔，氣柔順。氣柔順，則無所不至也。因而《老子・
十章》曰：〝專氣致柔，能如嬰兒乎？〞強調意氣之柔
如嬰兒然，以達長生之道。此理之應用於太極拳中，則
能聽、能懂、能粘、能黏、能隨、能連、能生。故《老
子・七十六章》曰：〝人之生也柔弱，其死也堅強；草
木之生也柔脆，其死也枯槁。故，堅強者死之徒，柔弱
者生之徒。是以，兵強則滅，木強則折；強大處下，柔
弱處上。〞

The philosophy of using the soft against the hard was originated from Lao Zi (老子). It is from this concept that Taijiquan was created. In this paragraph, a few places of related concepts are excerpted from Lao Zi's *Dao De Jing* (道德經). From development of these concepts, Taijiquan practitioners are able to train and reach the stage of listening, understanding, attaching, adhering, following, and connecting. These are the skills of surviving, and are winning tools in Taijiquan martial applications.

If (you) are able to be soft, then the Xin (i.e., emotional mind) is calm and the Yi (i.e., wisdom mind) is strong. When the Xin is calm, then the body is able to be loose. (If the body) can be loose, then the Qi can be circulating (smoothly). When the Qi is able to circulate smoothly, then live. When the Qi is stagnant, then can become sick and die. The theory of Taijiquan assumes the prior condition that the Xin is calm and the body is soft and loose. (Then) can use the Yi to lead the Qi until it is able to reach everywhere (in the body). The Taijiquan ancestor, Wǔ, Yu-Xiang said: "Transport Qi as though through a pearl with a 'nine-curved hole,' not even the tiniest place won't be reached." This is what he meant. From the abundant Qi circulation, the Jin manifested from the physical body can reach its maximum, and is able to be soft and hard. When it is hard, it is just like steel refined 100 times, no solid (i.e., strong opposition) can resist destruction. When it is soft, it is like a soft whip and the Jin can be directed as wished Able to attack and able to defend. Able to coil and able to neutralize. Use the spirit to govern the Qi and manifest the Jin, and (allow) the hard and soft to mutually support each other. This is the Dao of Taijiquan.

能柔，則心靜意強。心靜，則體能鬆。能鬆，則氣能行。
氣行，則生。氣滯，則病而死。太極拳之理在心靜與身
體鬆柔之前題下，以意引氣，而求氣之無所不至。太極
拳先哲武禹襄曰：〝行氣如九曲珠，無微不到。〞此其
意也。由氣行之沛然順暢，身體之勁道可達高峰，可硬
可軟。其硬如百鍊鋼，無堅不摧。其軟如軟鞭然，馭勁
隨心所欲，能攻能守，能纏能化。以神馭氣運勁，剛柔
相濟。此為太極拳之道也。

Once you are soft, the mind is calm and this will result in the relaxation of the
physical body. When the body is relaxed, the Qi will be able to circulate freely in the
body. In this case, you are healthy and will have a long life. When this softness is
applied to Taijiquan, you are able to use the Yi to lead the Qi smoothly and abundantly. This is the crucial internal key to manifesting strong physical power. Once
you are able to be soft, then you can also be as hard as you wish. Only if you know
how to apply both soft and hard skillfully, can you say you really understand Taijiquan's Jin manifestation.

8. General Theory of Taijiquan Thirteen Postures 太極拳十三勢概論

*From the previous discussion (i.e., refer to article #3), it can be seen that the
external Eight Trigrams in Taijiquan theory refers to the eight postures. Those are
the Jin patterns of the "eight doors." The "eight doors" are four formal directions
(of Jin patterns): Peng (i.e., Wardoff), Lu (i.e., Rollback), Ji (i.e., Press), and An
(i.e., Push) and four corners (of Jin patterns): Cai (i.e., Pluck), Lie (i.e., Split),
Zhou (i.e., Elbow), and Kao (i.e., Bump). These eight patterns, together with
five strategic steppings, become thirteen postures. Then, from these thirteen postures, the thirty-seven postures are developed. Furthermore, from these thirty-
seven postures, hundreds and thousands of applications in kicking, striking,
wrestling, and Qin Na here evolved. Therefore, those who learn Taijiquan must
first be familiar with the theory of Taiji, Yin-Yang, Four Phases, and Eight Doors
and Five Steppings of the thirteen postures, and their derivations. Each posture
and each movement (in Taijiquan), have their foundation and essence that must
not be ignored.*

由前可知，外八卦在太極拳理中為八勢。亦即八門之勁
勢也。八門者，四正：掤、擟、擠、按，四隅：採、挒、
肘、靠。由此八勢，加上五行步伐之配合，而成十三勢。
再由此十三勢而演化而為三十七勢。再由三十七個基本
架勢而變化成上千成百踢、打、摔、拿之應用。因而學
太極拳者，必先熟知太極、陰陽、四象與八門五步十三
勢之理與其衍生之竅。每一勢，每一動中，皆有其根基，
有其精義，不可忽視也。

The Eight Doors of basic Jin or moving patterns include four patterns which deal with four formal directions: Peng (掤) (i.e., Wardoff), Lu (擟) (i.e., Rollback), Ji (擠) (i.e., Press), and An (按) (i.e., Push) and another four patterns which deal with four corners: Cai (採) (i.e., Pluck), Lie (挒) (i.e., Split), Zhou (肘) (i.e., Elbow), and Kao (靠) (i.e., Bump). Together with the five strategic steppings, the Thirteen Postures are established. These thirteen postures or patterns have become the foundation and the root of Taijiquan. Again, from these thirteen postures, countless techniques are derived. Kicking (Ti, 踢), striking (Da, 打), wrestling (Shuai, 摔), and Qin Na (Na, 拿) are the four basic fighting skills which have been developed in all Chinese martial arts styles. Naturally, Taijiquan also includes all of these skills. These skills have therefore become the essence of each movement in Taijiquan. Therefore, as a proficient Taijiquan practitioner, you must continue searching for the applications in these four categories. Only if you know the applications to each movement, then is there a meaning of the movement.

Similarly, the internal Eight Trigrams are eight inner virtues (i.e., energy conduits) in Taijiquan theory. They are the eight main gates of the Qi's exit and entrance. The Eight Gates are four main gates: Baihui, Huiyin, Yinjiao, and Mingmen; and also four minor gates: Tiantu, Jiuwei, Yintang, and Lingtai. From these eight gates, with the coordination of Five Phases' internal correspondences, the internal Thirteen Conduits are established. What are the internal Five Phases? They are: soul, vigor, Spirit of Vitality, supernatural divinity, and ghost. Soul is classified as Yang, belongs to liver, and pertains to wood in Five Phases. Vigor is classified as Yin, belongs to lungs, and pertains to metal in Five Phases. Spirit of vitality is classified as center, belongs to spleen, and pertains to earth. Supernatural divinity is classified as Yang, belongs to heart, and pertains fire in Five Phases. (Finally,) ghost is classified as Yin, belongs to kidneys, and pertains to water. From the adjustment and harmonization of the Spirit of Vitality, Five Phases mutually conquer and support each other. (When this happens,) the stage of cultivating human nature and physical life can reach a peak level.

同理，內八卦在太極拳理中為八德。亦即氣出入之八要門也。八門者，四正：百會、會陰、陰交、命門，四輔：天突、鳩尾、印堂、靈臺。由此八門，加上五行內感之配合，而成十三勢。內五行者，魂、魄、精神、靈、鬼也。魂陽屬肝，五行中為木。魄陰屬肺，五行中為金。精神執中屬脾，五行中為土。陽靈屬心，五行中為火。陰鬼屬腎，五行中為水。由精神之調配，五行相克相輔而成。修性養命可達高峰。

According to Chinese Qigong understanding, a human body has a total of seven major pairs of corresponding Qi gates from which the body's Qi circulatory structure is constructed. These seven corresponding gates are: 1. Huiyin (Co-1) (會陰)-

Baihui (Gv-20) (百會); 2. Yintang (M-HN-3) (印堂)-Qiangjian (Gv-17) (強間)[or Naohu (Gv-18) (腦戶)]; 3. Renzhong (Gv-26) (人中)-Fengfu (Gv-16) (風府); 4. Tiantu (Co-22) (天突)-Dazhui (Gv-14) (大椎); 5. Jiuwei (Co-15) (鳩尾)-Lingtai (Gv-10) (靈臺); 6. Yinjiao (Co-7) (陰交)-Mingmen (Gv-4) (命門); and 7. Long-men (M-CA-24) (龍門)[or Xiayin (下陰)]-Changqiang (Gv-1) (長強)[or Weilu (尾閭)]. Among these seven corresponding gates, two pairs are the most important; Huiyin (Yin)-Baihui (Yang), and also Yinjiao (Yin)-Mingmen (Yang). Huiyin-Baihui is connected through the Thrusting Vessel (Chong Mai, 衝脈) (i.e., spinal cord) which establishes the central balance of the Qi distribution in the body. Yinjiao-Mingmen is also connected through the Thrusting Vessel and joins with Conception Vessel (Ren Mai, 任脈) in the front and Governing Vessel (Du Mai, 督脈) on the back, thus providing a front and rear Qi balance of the body. Therefore, these four gates are the main Qi gates (Figure 15).

Tiantu controls the vocal vibrations and generates the sounds of Hen (哼) (Yin) and Ha (哈) (Yang) for Qi's manifestation. Therefore, it is a gate of expression and its energy is balanced with Yintang, where the spirit resides. When spirit is high in Yintang (i.e., the third eye), the energy manifested will be strong and the alertness and awareness will be high. In addition, Jiuwei and Lingtai connect to the heart. Heart is related to the emotional mind and offers you a strong motor force and helps the spirit to raise up. Therefore, from the Taijiquan sparring point of view, these four minor gates control the Qi's manifestation in the body. Therefore, the Eight Gates are defined. If you are interested in knowing more about Eight Vessels, please refer to the book: *Qigong-The Secret of Youth*, published by YMAA.

The internal Five Phases are: soul (Hun, 魂), vigor (Po, 魄), Spirit of Vitality (Jing-Shen, 精神), supernatural divinity (Ling, 靈), and ghost (Gui, 鬼). Yang spirit is considered as soul (i.e., Hun) while Yin spirit is considered as vigor (i.e., Po). This has been stated in the document: *The Complete Book of Principal Contents of Life and Human Nature, Illustration of Hun and Po*: "Yang spirit is Hun while Yin spirit is Po."[1,5] The explanation of Hun and Po can be found in the document: *The Complete Book of Principal Contents of Life and Human Nature, Illustration of Hun and Po* says: "Hun (i.e., soul) is the spirit of Qi, and can be clean or dirty....Po (i.e., vigor) is the spirit of Jing (i.e., essence), and can be insubstantial or substantial." Qi is the energy. Hun (i.e., soul) is the manifestation of energy (i.e., Qi). When this Qi is manifested uniformly and harmoniously, it is clean. However, if the Qi's manifestation is disordered and chaotic, then it is dirty. Jing (i.e., essence) means hormones. Po (i.e., vigor) originates from the contents of hormones in the body. When the hormone level is high, the vital force is vigorous and substantial. However, when the hormone level is low, then the vital force is weak and insubstantial. It also says: "Liver is related to Hun and Hun is the spirit of the

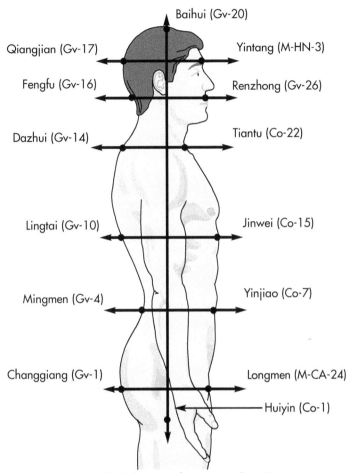

Figure 15. Eight Pairs of Corresponding Qi Gates

liver. Lungs conceal Po, and Po is the spirit of the lungs."[2,5] In the documents, *Praising of the Secret of Dragon-Tiger's Elixir Returning, Gu Shen Zi's Interpretation*: "The earth belongs to Po while the heaven belongs to Hun, these are classified as tiger and dragon. The heaven is Yang, belongs to Hun, and is dragon. The earth is Yin, belongs to Po, and is tiger."[3,6]

Ling (靈) is a word that is very hard to translate from Chinese into English. It is a divine inspiration of the spirit and can make a person sharp in thinking, agile in action, alert in perception, and supernatural in spiritual enlightenment. It is believed that the reason why humans can be so different from animals is because of the high level of Ling which makes our spirit different from animals' spirit. In an ancient document, *All Application Secrets of Real Holy Embryonic Spirit, Chen, Xi-Yi's Secret of Embryonic Breathing* says: "When the spirit is transportable and capable of millions of variations, it is called 'Ling'."[4,5] It also understood that Ling is connected to the heart and therefore, the spiritual mind is called "Xin Ling" (心靈). The root of Ling (Ling Gen, 靈根) implies the root of the tongue (She Gen, 舌根). According to Chinese medicine, the tongue is related to the heart. When the heart is sincere and truthful, the Ling will be high and if we are deceptive and lie, then the Ling will be low. Since Ling is so much related to the spirit (i.e., Shen), when the spirit has reached to a high supernatural level, it is called "Ling Shen" (靈神). This spirit will keep you in a high state of awareness and alertness, which allows you to create and to change.

Gui (鬼) is the ghost and is the remaining energy existing in the space when the physical body is dead. If Hun and Po are strong and the Ling is sharp when a person is alive, his remaining energy (i.e., Gui) will be strong and last for a long time which will allow him to have more time to find a new body for reincarnation. Gui is related to the kidneys. In Chinese Qigong society, ghost path (Gui Dao, Gui Lu; 鬼道、鬼路) means the pathway of the essence (i.e., spirit). This pathway is the penis which is related and connected to kidneys.[5,6]

From the above discussion, you may have already figured out why the Spirit of Vitality (Jing-Shen, 精神) stays in the center of Five Phases and belongs to earth. This is because Spirit of Vitality is the central coordinator of the other four phases. When this central spirit is high, all others will also be high and when this spirit is low, all others will also be low.

9. Practicing Procedures of Taijiquan 太極拳之練習程序

What is Taijiquan? It is a martial Qigong study. Its training procedures are not different from those of other general Qigong (practice) and must follow the (same training) theory. These training procedures are nothing else but: regulating the body, regulating the breathing, regulating the mind, regulating the Qi, and regulating the spirit—five regulatings.

太極拳者，武學氣功也。其練習程序不異於一般氣功，
依理而行。此練習之理與程序不外乎調身、調息、調心、
調氣、調神五調也。

Taijiquan was created in Daoist monasteries and is a Qigong practice for enlightenment cultivation. The only difference is that this Qigong practice can also be applied in martial arts. Since Taijiquan is a Qigong, its training procedures and principles are no different from those of general Qigong practice. These training procedures and principles are: learning to regulate the body (Tiao Shen, 調身), breathing (Tiao Xi, 調息), mind (Tiao Xin, 調心), Qi (Tiao Qi, 調氣), and finally spirit (Tiao Shen, 調神). If you are interested in more of these training procedures, please refer to the book: *The Root of Chinese Qigong*, by YMAA.

What does regulating mean? It means to regulate until harmonized (with others). It (also) means to regulate until it is correct. Therefore, the five regulatings must be mutually harmonized (with each other) and none can exist alone. The five regulatings are unified as one unit, mutually applied to and assisting each other. For example, regulating the body must be harmonized with regulating the breathing. When the body is stiff, the breathing becomes faster, and when the body is soft, the breathing becomes slower. On the other hand, when the breathing is fast, the body is stiff, and when the breathing is loose (i.e., easy), the body is soft. For the same reason, when the mind is restless, the breathing is strong and short, and when the mind is peaceful, then the breathing is slender and long. On the other hand, when the breathing is fast, then the mind is fidgety, and when the breathing is harmonious, then the mind is peaceful.

調者，調之和諧也，調之使正也。因而五調必須互相和
諧，獨一而不存。五調合為一體，互相為用、為助。譬
如調身必與調息和諧，身硬則息急，身綿則息緩。反之，
息速則身僵，息鬆則身軟。同理，心躁則息沛短，心安
則息細長。反之，息快則心煩，息和則心平。

Tiao (調) is a gradually regulating process which proceeds until what is regulated has reached to its harmonious stage with others. All of the regulating processes in Qigong rely on feeling. **Feeling is a language of the mind and the body.** Through feeling, the mind registers problems or errors. It is also from feeling that the mind is able to regulate the body, breathing, Qi, and spirit. From this, you can see that **the mind is the center of five regulating processes and feeling is its tool.**

It is for this reason that deep internal feeling was commonly been known as an important key to Qigong practice. This internal feeling training is known as "Gongfu of internal vision" (Nei Shi Gongfu, 內視功夫). In fact, that phrase means the training of internal feeling. It is called Gongfu because it will take any Qigong practitioner a great deal of time and effort to reach a profound level of this self internal feeling.

If the body is stiff, the breathing is fast, and the mind is fidgety, then the Qi's circulation will not be peaceful. Consequently, it will be hard for the mind to lead the Qi to circulate. If the body is loose (i.e., easy), the breathing is profound, and the mind is calm, then the Qi's circulation is smooth and natural. (In this case), the mind can lead the Qi easily and Qi's circulation can be natural. When the Xin (i.e., emotional mind) and Yi (i.e., wisdom mind) are strong, the spirit can be raised up to a high level, and when the Xin and Yi are weak, the spirit will also stay low.

如身硬、息急、心煩，則氣不安，意難引氣行。如身鬆、
息沉、心靜，則氣順然，以意引氣氣自然。心意強，神
必高提。心意弱，神必低落。

All five regulatings are closely related to and mutually influencing each other. Using the mind as the center, and using the feeling as the communication tool, you can harmonize your body, breathing, mind, Qi, and spirit to a deep meditative stage, which allows you to cultivate your natural being to a profound level and finally reunite with the natural spirit.

From these, (we) can see that five regulatings are the standard means of practicing and learning Taijiquan. However, beginners must start from regulating the body first. From the practice of regulating the body's postures, (you) will be able to understand how to make the (body) soft, gentle, and balanced, maintain central equilibrium, and firm the rooting. This is the first step.

由此觀之，五調乃習太極者練習之準則。然而，初學者，
必先由調身著手。由調身練習拳架，能懂鬆軟、平衡、
中定、與紮根，此為第一步。

In order to allow Qi to circulate freely and naturally, the body must be soft and relaxed. When the body is relaxed, the resistance of Qi's circulation will be low and consequently, Qi can circulate freely and smoothly. Moreover, you must have a physical and mental balance. When they are balanced and coordinated with each other, you will find your center. Only when you have found your center can you have a firm root. All of these are part of the first step in learning Taijiquan movements.

Afterwards, start the practice of regulating the breathing. From regulating the breathing in coordination with the body's regulating, (you) are able to lead the body's regulating to a more profound level. When (you are) regulating the breathing, (you) must aim for a slender, slow, quiet, deep, soft, smooth, and peaceful way which can thus (gradually) lead (you) to the stage of natural regulating without regulating.

之後，即由調息著手。由調息配合調身以使調身更進一
層之境界。調息必求細、緩、靜、深、柔、順、和以達
自然無調而調之效。

After you have regulated your body to a natural state, you can devote more of your mind to your breathing. In regulating breathing, you are aiming for a slender, slow, quiet, deep, soft, smooth, and peaceful manner. When breathing is calm and natural, your mind will reach a deeper state of feeling and the body can be more relaxed. The deepest stage of regulating is **regulating without regulating**. That means you have developed a habit of regulating and your mind does not have to be there to regulate it all the time.

Next, (you should) begin the stage of regulating the Xin (i.e., emotional mind). What is regulating the Xin? It means to regulate the Xin until it is harmonized and peaceful. (Then), from the Yi-horse's control, the Xin-monkey can be stabilized. After that, the Xin and Yi are on the opponent in every posture and movement. (When this happens), the Qi can be led (efficiently) and the Jin can be emitted (effectively). Consequently, the practice of regulating the Qi will happen naturally.

此後，由調心著手。調心者，先調心之和、平。由意馬
之主宰，心猿可定。之後，每勢每動，心意在敵，氣而
能引，勁而能發。由此，調氣成自然矣。

As mentioned earlier, according to Chinese concepts, we have two minds; one is called Xin (心) and means heart and represents the mind of emotions and the other is called Yi (意) which represents the mind of logical thinking and decisions. Xin has commonly been compared to a monkey: which is small and hard to control and calm. Yi has been compared to a horse, powerful yet peaceful and calm. One aspect of Qigong training is learning how to use your logical and wise mind to control the emotional mind. This process is called "regulating the Xin" (Tiao Xin, 調心). When the emotional mind is controlled, the feeling and judgments of your mind can be clear. When the mind is clear, you are able to lead the Qi to circulate in your body smoothly and naturally. Moreover, if your mind is clear, you will be able to use it to harmonize the body, breathing, mind, Qi, and spirit efficiently.

The final goal of practicing Taijiquan is to regulate the spirit. The first target of regulating the spirit is aiming to raise up the spirit of morale against the opponent. When morale is high, the Qi is strong, and the Jin can be withdrawn or released as wished. The final target of regulating the spirit is to reach the stage in which there is no difference of opponent and I, the fight of no fight, and having enemy as no enemy—the state of great peaceful mind. Then, the theory (i.e., meaning) of human life can be comprehended.

最後太極拳練習之境界，乃調神。調神之先的，為提高
禦敵之士氣。士氣高，氣強，勁可收放自如。而極終的
之調神乃至無敵我之中庸境界，無門之門，無敵之敵之
太平心境。則人生之理能貫轍焉。

In combat, the fighting morale is the most important. When morale is high, the sense of enemy will be high, alertness will be sharp, and the techniques executed can be effective and powerful. However, in peaceful time, regulating the spirit means to raise up the Spirit of Vitality and to regulate the spirit until it reaches the neutral state. When your spirit has reached the neutral state, your mind will be peaceful and the meaning of life can be comprehended.

In every regulating procedure, the learners must practice until the stage of regulating without regulating. This is the natural way of following the Dao. If Yi still has to be regulating the body, breathing, mind, Qi, and spirit, then the level of Taijiquan accomplishment will not be profound.

每一層次，學者必調至無調而自調之境界，才順自然而
為道。如意仍須在調身、調息、調心、調氣、與調神，
則太極之境界不為深矣。

The final goal of regulating each aspect is to "regulate without regulating." That means all regulating has become natural and happens by itself. It is like when you are learning how to drive, your mind is in the driving. However, after you have driven for a long time, your driving skills have reached to their natural stage. In this case, you are driving without the mind's whole attention. This is the stage of regulating without regulating. It is the same when you practice Taijiquan, you must practice until no regulating is necessary. Then, your Taijiquan can reach its most proficient level. Naturally, it may take your whole lifetime to reach this goal.

10. Three Heights and Three Postures of Taijiquan 太極拳之三勢與三架

The practice of Taijiquan can be divided into three different heights of stance: high, middle, and low, and three postures: large, middle, and small. Low stances with large postures are practiced by beginners, aiming for comfortable and expanded movements and also emphasizing the establishment of a strong foundation in the lower section of the body. When the lower section is firm and strong, the movements can be loosened and expanded, then should (you) step into the training of the middle stance and middle posture. In the training of middle stance and middle posture, you are searching for the effectiveness of using the Yi to lead the Qi as well as the martial theory and applications of each posture. Therefore, during the practice of middle stance and middle posture, you are constantly looking for the root and the reason of each posture, becoming familiar with the skills and reactions of each movement as if encountering an opponent, and also to aspiring to a higher level of both internal and external cultivation in Taijiquan. When (you) have reached to a level where the manifestation of Listening, Following, Attaching, and Adhering Jins can be carried out naturally as wished, then the stances will become higher and the postures become smaller. Consequently, the body's energy can be conserved and the internal cultivation can reach a more profound state. In this case, creating an advantageous opportunity and establishing a favorable situation are decided by me. The higher levels of Jins such as Controlling, Emitting, Borrowing, and Coiling Jins can be varied without exhaustion and when applying them, there is no end. However, to reach this stage, (you) must have had at least twenty to thirty years of practice and accumulated experience.

太極拳之練習可分高、中、低三勢，大、中、小三架。
低勢大架者為初學者習之，動作求舒展並著重下盤之建
樹。下盤穩固，動作能鬆、能開，即步入中勢中架之練
習。在中勢中架中，求以意引氣之效，求每架每勢武學
上之理解與應用。因之，在中勢中架之練習中去尋求架
勢之根由，熟練每架勢在與人對待時之技術與反應，並
追求更上層次之太極內外之修練。當程度達到聽、隨、
沾、黏之勁隨心所欲而不做作時，架勢漸趨於高勢小架，
以節約體力，以求更深更高之內含境地。此時，造機立
勢在我，拿、發、借、纏等高技之勁技，變化不窮，用
而不竭。然而，欲達此境地，非得二三十年之練習與經
驗。

In Yang style Taijiquan practice, it is well known that there are three different heights of practice: low stance (Di Shi, 低勢), middle high stance (Zhong Shi, 中勢), and also high stance (Gao Shi, 高勢). Normally, a beginner will start with a low stance Di. From the lower stance practice, the lower section of the body will be more tensed so gradually the strength of the legs will build up and the root can reach deeper. Moreover, a beginner will start with a large posture (Da Jia, 大架) from which he will learn to be relaxed and soft. This will make a beginner feel comfortable. However, after you have practiced for some time and wish to reach a higher level of Jin training, you must then practice the middle high stance and middle size posture (Zhong Jia, 中架). From this training, you learn how to step firmly, how to store and manifest your Jins, and how to use your mind to lead the Qi to circulate through the body. However, the most important of all in this middle level training is to search for the meaning or the root of every movement. Therefore, the creation of each movement (i.e., martial applications) must be understood and the sense of opponent (i.e., spirit) must be built up. From understanding this root and essence, you will learn how to train your Jins and manifest them efficiently.

However, the highest level of Taijiquan practice is high stance and small circle (Xiao Jia, 小架). In high stance and small circle, you can conserve your energy to a maximum level. This is very crucial in battle. Endurance has always been the crucial key to survival in a long battle. Moreover, due to high stance and smaller posture, you can reach to the deepest relaxed stage, the mind is highly concentrated, and the sensitivity and alertness can be extremely sharp. However, it is not easy to reach this stage since you must have mastered those Jin skills such as listening, following, attaching, connecting, adhering, coiling, borrowing, etc. to a proficient level. Otherwise, you can be put into a dangerous and disadvantageous situation easily.

11. Yin-Yang Practicing Theory of Taijiquan 太極拳陰陽練法論

As explained earlier, Taijiquan is actually a Taiji Qigong. At the beginning of Taijiquan practice, the movements should be relaxed, soft, and slow, the Xin should be peaceful and the Qi harmonious, and you should use the Yi to transport the Qi. (The training proceeds) from regulating the body, to regulating the breathing, regulating the mind, and regulating the Qi. After (you) have practiced the above four regulatings until the stage of "regulating without regulating," should (you) then start regulating the spirit. Regulating the spirit can be divided into Yin regulating and Yang regulating.

依前所言，太極拳者，太極氣功也。初練太極拳，動作
鬆、柔、緩，心平氣和，以意行氣。由調身、調息、調
心，而至調氣。然以上四調練至不調而自調之境地時，
即步入調神。調神可分為陰調與陽調。

As explained earlier, the entire Taijiquan practicing concept and theory are actually the same as Qigong practice. As a Taijiquan beginner, first you should learn how to be relaxed, soft, and move with a calm mind. In order to reach this goal, you have to move slowly. When you move slowly, your mind can be calm and peaceful, and the feeling can be deep. When the feeling is deep, the mind-body communication will be profound. When this happens, you are able to use your mind to lead the Qi efficiently. From this, you can see that to practice Taijiquan, you must first learn how to regulate your body, breathing, mind, and then Qi.

However, the final stage of Taijiquan practice is not just staying in the stage of using the mind to lead the Qi. In fact, the final stage of Taijiquan practice is no different from that of other Qigong practices; that is, regulating the spirit. The reason for this is very simple. The spirit is the center of the entire being. When the spirit is regulated, the function of the entire body will be healthy and the vitality will be high. However, regulating the spirit can be divided into Yin regulating and Yang regulating.

The Yin regulating of the spirit starts from profound Xin (i.e., extremely calm mind). That is, when (you) practice Taijiquan, the movements gradually get slower, you aim for extreme relaxation of the body, the breathing gradually becomes slower, and the Xin (i.e., emotional mind) moves to extreme calmness. From this, the breath grows longer, the heartbeat slows, the entire body gradually becomes transparent, and the Qi is able to circulate through the (entire body) without any stagnation. When (you) have reached this stage, no place cannot be reached by the Yi and no place Qi cannot be circulated. Inwards, (Yi and Qi) can be condensed into the bone marrow, and upward, (Yi and Qi) can be used to nourish the brain. This is the Dao of reaching the enlightenment and the path of becoming divine.

神之陰調者，由冥心始。亦即練太極拳時，動作漸慢，
身求極鬆，息趨極緩，心向極靜。由此，呼吸漸長，心
跳漸慢，全身漸而透空，氣無所滯。至此意無不到，氣
無不行，內可凝於骨髓，上可補腦洗髓。此為通乎神明
成道成仙之途徑。

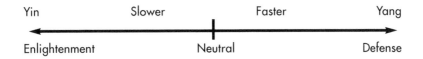

Figure 16. Yin and Yang Sides of Taijiquan Training

After you have learned the entire Taijiquan sequence, you should start to practice the Yin side and Yang side of spiritual cultivation. In the Yin side of spiritual
practice, you must start from regulating your mind (Figure 16). The mind must
reach a deep and profound meditative state. In order to reach this goal, the Taijiquan
movements must gradually become slower and slower; consequently, the body will
be more relaxed, and the breathing will become more slender, slow, and long. When
this happens, the heartbeat gets slower and slower and you will feel the entire body
is becoming transparent. This implies that the Qi circulating in your body is free
without any slight stagnation. When you have reached this stage, you will feel the
disappearance of your physical body, Qi can be led by your mind inward to wash the
bone marrow and also upward to nourish your brain efficiently. In fact, this is the
crucial key to marrow/brain washing Qigong for enlightenment or Buddhahood.

> *In the Yang side of spiritual regulating, the Yang spirit is manifested externally,
> and the Xin (i.e., emotional mind) and Yi (i.e., wisdom mind) are on the oppo-
> nent. From the sense of enemy, the Qi is led outward and manifested in the phys-
> ical body. From this, Jin is formalized for neutralization and emitting, and the
> movements (i.e., actions) become faster and faster, under the conditions of peace-
> ful Xin and harmonious Qi, searching for the Listening and Understanding Jins;
> also under the condition of high morale in the sense of enemy, looking for the
> manifestation of Leading, Neutralizing, and Emitting Jins. This is the Dao of
> Taijiquan's offense and defense.*

神之陽調者，陽神外顯，心意在敵。由敵意而氣外行並
顯化於身。勁由此而化、而發，動作趨快。在心平氣和
中，求聽勁、懂勁。在敵情高昂下，求引、化、發勁之
顯。此為太極拳攻防之道。

As explained in the last paragraph, the Yin side of spiritual cultivation is to find
a peaceful calm mind so the Qi can be led inward to the bone marrow and upward

to the brain. However, in order to use Taijiquan for defense and also for physical strength, you must also practice the Yang side of spiritual cultivation.

When you practice the Yang side of spiritual cultivation, the spirit should be manifested externally. The movements will get faster and faster while keeping the Xin and Yi in the imaginary opponent. When the spirit is highly manifested externally, the alertness and awareness will be sharp, the sense of enemy will be strong, and naturally the fighting morale will be high. In addition, with this external spiritual manifestation, the Jins can be manifested powerfully and precisely. However, you should remember that, though the physical body moves fast and is excited, your mind should remain calm so the Qi circulation will be smoothly led continuously. Only when your mind remains calm, your Listening and Understanding Jins can be executed efficiently. Also, it is only when you have reached a high level of Listening and Understanding Jins that you can execute the skills of Following, Connecting, Leading and Neutralizing. This is the key to Taijiquan self-defense.

> *Yin is the root (of Yang) and Yang is the manifestation (of Yin). Yin belongs to internal, while Yang belongs to external. Yin (in Taijiquan) means to refine (our) human nature (i.e., spirit) and to cultivate the Dao so (we) are able to reach the goal of Buddhahood or enlightenment. Yang (in Taijiquan) means to train (our) physical body and to regulate our mind so they can be used for defense and offense. Ancient people said: "(If we) do not understand the (value of) death, how (do we) know the (meaning) of life?" If a human does not know how ugly killing can be, how can he/she understand the value of life? Yin and Yang must be compared mutually, then we can really know the Dao.*

陰者為根，陽者為顯。陰者為內，陽者為外。陰者，養性培道以成佛、成仙；陽者，練身調意以為防身殺煞。古云：〝不知死，焉知生？〞人不知殺煞之醜惡，焉知生命之可貴？陰陽互比，然後可知道矣。

According to Yin-Yang philosophy, Yin is the root while Yang is the manifestation; Yin belongs to internal while Yang belongs to external. Yin is used to cultivate the mind and spirit so as to understand the meaning of life, while Yang is used to develop a healthy strong physical body and also the capability of self-defense. When the Yin reaches deeply, the Yang's manifestation will be strong. Yin and Yang are relative and balance each other. Those who know the meaning of life will not kill and also, those who know martial arts to a profound level will appreciate life more than others.

> *In conclusion, the theory of practicing Taijiquan is the Dao that, when it is used for defense, it is Yang, and when it is used to comprehend the meaning of life, it is Yin. The deeper the Yin is able to reach, the more the Yang can be manifested. The more the Yang is abundant, the thicker the Yin will be. The great nature of Dao is when Yin has reached its maximum, the Yang is manifested and when the Yang has reached its extremity, the Yin will appear.*

概言之，太極拳練習之理，在防身為陽，在悟人生為陰
之道。陰愈深，陽愈顯。陽愈盛，陰愈厚。陰極陽顯，
陽極陰現之自然大道。

This paragraph summarizes the entire Yin-Yang training concept of Taijiquan.

12. Theory of Taijiquan and Health 太極拳養生篇

*What is Taiji? It is Xin and Yi. Xin and Yi belong to Yin. From Xin and Yi, the
external Yang can be manifested. What is external Yang? It is the body's movements
and reactions. What is Taijiquan? It is the training methods that regulate the body,
regulate the breathing, regulate the Xin, regulate the Qi, and then regulate the spirit. This is also the Daoist method for nourishing life and searching for enlightenment through the processes of: refining the essence and converting it into Qi, refining the Qi and converting it into spirit, refining the spirit and transforming it into
emptiness, and finally crushing the emptiness. From these (trainings), aim to reach
the final goal of double cultivation of human nature and life. The double cultivation of human nature and life means the cultivation of both internal and external.
After the internal regulating of the Xin, Qi, and spirit, then coordinate with regulating of the breathing to harmonize with the external body's regulating.*

太極者，心意也。心意者，陰也。由心意，而外陽顯現
矣。外陽者，身體之動作感應也。太極拳者，由調身、
調息、調心、調氣、而至調神，乃道家練精化氣、練氣
化神、練神返虛、粉碎虛空養生練仙術之法也。由此，
而臻性命雙修之目的。性命雙修乃內外雙修之意也。由
內之調心、調氣、調神再配合調息而外諧和於調身矣。

In Daoist Nei Dan (內丹) (i.e., internal elixir) Qigong training, in order to reach
the final enlightenment, there are four training procedures. These four are: refining the
essence and converting it into Qi (Lian Jing Hua Qi, 練精化氣), refining the Qi and
converting it into spirit (Lian Qi Hua Shen, 練氣化神), refining the spirit and transforming it into emptiness (Lian Shen Fan Xu, 練神返虛), and finally crushing the
emptiness (Fen Sui Xu Kong, 粉碎虛空). To complete these four training procedures,
you must know how to regulate your body, breathing, mind, Qi, and finally spirit.
Moreover, you must also know how to ripen the internal cultivation into external physical health and longevity. This kind of cultivation is called "double cultivation"
(Shuang Xiu, 雙修) and includes the cultivation of human nature as well as physical
life.

*Those who learn Taijiquan must know these theories. Only then can (they) com-
prehend the meaning of life and the natural great Dao through Taijiquan prac-*

tice. Though the martial side of Taijiquan is for strengthening the physical body and also for defense, the scholarly side of Taijiquan is for understanding human nature and comprehending the meaning of life. Only if (you) can cultivate these both internally and externally, can you reach the Dao of balancing physical body and mind, and (also) the double cultivation of human nature and physical body.

太極拳學者，須知此理，才能由習太極拳而悟人生與自
然大道之理。太極拳之武學，固是強身、防身之術。太
極拳之文學，卻是理性悟命之學。能夠內外兼修，才能
達到身心平衡，性命雙修之養生之道矣。

Any Taijiquan practitioner must recognize, understand, and practice this double cultivation. If you are not searching for the deep meaning of the art, then you will always stay in the shallow places of Taijiquan. The final goal of practicing Taijiquan is applying the practice into your life. Your life is Taijiquan and Taijiquan is your life.

13. About Qi Primary Channels, Secondary Channels, Vessels, and Dan Tian
經、絡、脈、丹田考

According to the study of Chinese medicine, the human body has twelve primary Qi channels (i.e., Jing). Among these twelve channels, six of them belong to Yang while the other six belong to Yin. These primary Qi channels are just like the rivers of the Qi('s) flow. What are those Yang primary Qi channels? They are: The Large Intestine Channel of Hand — Yang Brightness; The Small Intestine Channel of Hand — Greater Yang; The Triple Burner Channel of Hand — Lesser Yang; The Stomach Channel of Foot — Yang Brightness; The Urinary Bladder Channel of Foot — Greater Yang; and The Gall Bladder Channel of Foot — Lesser Yang. What are the Yin primary Qi channels? They are: The Lung Channel of Hand — Greater Yin; The Heart Channel of Hand — Lesser Yin; The Pericardium Channel of Hand — Absolute Yin; The Spleen Channel of Foot — Greater Yin; The Kidney Channel of Foot — Lesser Yin; and The Liver Channel of Foot — Absolute Yin. From these, we can see that (the Qi's circulation in) these twelve primary Qi channels follows the limbs up and down. (Among these twelve channels), three Yang primary Qi channels and three Yin primary Qi channels reach to the fingers while another three Yang primary Qi channels and three Yin primary Qi channels reach to the toes. The other ends of these twelve primary Qi channels connect to the six bowels and six internal organs.

依中醫學上之探解，全身計有十二經，中含六陽六陰經，
如氣之河川也。陽經者，手陽明大腸經、手太陽小腸經、
手少陽三焦經、足陽明胃經、足太陽膀胱經、足少陽膽
經也。陰經者，手太陰肺經、手少陰心經、手厥陰心包
絡經、足太陰脾經、足少陰腎經、足厥陰肝經也。由此
可知，此十二經順肢體上下而行，其三陽經、三陰經通
達手指，另三陽經、三陰通至腳趾，而其另一端通達六
腑六臟。

This paragraph describes the twelve primary Qi channels (Shi Er Jing, 十二經) of the human body. If you are interested in learning about the Qi circulatory system in more detail, please refer to the book: ***The Root of Chinese Qigong***, published by YMAA. You can also refer to any Chinese acupuncture or medical book.

> *In addition, there are countless small Qi channels, which are called Luo throughout the body. These small Qi channels branch out sideways from the twelve primary Qi channels. These small channels are like the ditches or streams of Qi. From these (small channels), externally the Qi reaches to the skin as Guardian Qi (Wei Qi) while internally the Qi is transported to the bone marrow as Marrow Qi (Sui Qi). In addition, the body has eight vessels which include four Yin and four Yang vessels. What are vessels? They are lakes or reservoirs which are used to regulate the Qi's flow in the rivers and streams. If the Qi in the vessels is strong and abundant, its regulating capability will be strong. If not, its regulating function will be weak. What are the four Yang vessels? They are: Governing Vessel (Du Mai); Girdle (or Belt) Vessel (Dai Mai); Yang Heel Vessel (Yang Qiao Mai); and Yang Linking Vessel (Yang Wei Mai). What are the four Yin vessels? They are: Conception Vessel (Ren Mai); Thrusting Vessel (Chong Mai); Yin Heel Vessel (Yin Qiao Mai); and Yin Linking Vessel (Yin Wei Mai). Conception, Governing, Thrusting, and Girdle Vessels exists singly while Yang Heel, Yang Linking, Yin Heel, and Yin Linking Vessels exist as a pair.*

再者，全身有無數之小氣道稱之為絡，由十二經分支旁
行而出，如氣之溝渠也，氣由此外達皮膚以為衛氣，內
通骨髓以為髓氣。除此，全身尚有八脈，四陰四陽也。
脈者，湖澤、水壩也。用以調節河川、溝渠之氣流也。
脈中氣強而沛，調節功能強。反之，則調節功能弱。四
陽脈者，督脈、帶脈、陽蹻脈、陽維脈也。四陰脈者，
任脈、衝脈、陰蹻脈、陰維脈也。任、督、衝、帶四脈
存單，而陽蹻、陽維、陰蹻、陰維脈成雙也。

In addition to the twelve primary Qi channels (i.e., rivers), there are countless small secondary Qi channels (i.e., streams) (Luo, 絡) branching out from the primary Qi channels. In order to maintain smooth and abundant Qi circulation in the primary and secondary channels, the body also has eight vessels that are considered to be Qi reservoirs, and are used to regulate the Qi level in the channels.

> *The main function of the Conception Vessel is to regulate the Qi's flow in the six Yin primary Qi channels, while the main function of the Governing Vessel is to manage the Qi's flow in the six Yang primary Qi channels. Therefore, when the Qi storage in the Conception and Governing Vessels is abundant and the Qi circulation in these two vessels is smooth, the Qi('s) circulation in the twelve primary Qi channels is strong. Consequently, the physical body can be conditioned from weak to strong. Those who practice Small Circulation Qigong train to maintain the storage of the Qi in these two vessels at an abundant level, and also to make the Qi circulation in these two vessels smooth. From this, (we) can see*

that Small Circulation Qigong is the most basic and beginning step in training muscle/tendon changing Qigong.

任脈主調六陰經之氣，督脈主營六陽經之氣。因之，任督兩脈存氣強、行順，則十二經之氣流強，物理身體由弱而強健。知小周天氣功者，行功以沛氣壩，以順任督兩脈氣流之行。由此可知，小周天者，易筋之最根本、最初步之基礎功法也。

Of the eight vessels, the Conception and Governing Vessels (Ren, Du Mai; 任、督脈) are the most important. These two vessels regulate the Qi level of the twelve primary Qi channels. Since these twelve primary Qi channels transport the Qi everywhere in the physical body, when the Qi storage is abundant and the circulation is smooth, the physical body will be strong. In Nei Dan Qigong practice, a practitioner will learn how to build up Qi and store it in these two vessels, and will also learn how to mentally lead the Qi to circulate in these two vessels smoothly. From this, you can see that Small Circulation (Xiao Zhou Tian, 小周天) actually is one of the foundations of Muscle/Tendon Changing Qigong.

What is the Girdle Vessel? It is the Qi vessel that circles around the waist area. This is the only vessel which is parallel to the ground (i.e., horizontal). The Qi in this vessel is just like the spread wings of a bird. When the Qi is strong and abundant, the central equilibrium of a posture will be firm, the Guardian Qi will be strong, and the Spirit of Vitality can be raised. (If) the Qi in this vessel is weak, then (you) lose balance and central equilibrium cannot be achieved.

帶脈者，氣脈環繞腰部也。乃身體唯一與地平行之脈。此脈之氣，如鳥翅之開展。氣勢強而沛則中定之勢穩，衛氣強勢，精神上提。此脈氣弱，則失去平衡，中定無著也。

The Girdle Vessel (Dai Mai, 帶脈) is the only vessel situated horizontally, while the other seven are perpendicular to the ground. The Qi in this vessel acts like the wings of a bird, helping you to balance. When the Qi status in this vessel is strong and spread out, the Guardian Qi (Wei Qi, 衛氣) will be strong and you will gain a stronger sense of balance. You will also be able to firm your center and root. This is the key to raising up the Spirit of Vitality.

Theoretically, when the Dan Tian's Qi is abundant, the Qi expanding from the Girdle Vessel will be strong and wide. The Girdle Vessel is considered extremely Yang, while the Thrusting Vessel is considered extremely Yin. When the Qi is abundantly stored in the Real Dan Tian (Zhen Dan Tian, 真丹田), your Guardian Qi is strong and the physical body will be healthy. When the Qi is led upward through the Thrusting Vessel to the brain, the brain can be nourished and the Spirit of Vitality can be raised up to a high level. From this you can see that these two vessels are actually the two facets of the same thing (your life), one is for the quantity of the Qi, while the other is for the quality of the Qi's manifestation (Figure 17). The greater the quantity of the Qi, the higher the quality of manifestation that can be reached.

What are Dan Tians? They are the places where Qi (i.e., bioelectric) can be stored in the body. Dan Tians can be distinguished as Upper Dan Tian, Middle Dan Tian, and Lower Dan Tian. What is the Upper Dan Tian? It is the brain in the head and is also called Mud Pill Palace (Ni Wan Gong) (by Daoists). What is the Middle Dan Tian? It is the cavity of Jiuwei, where the diaphragm is located. The Lower Dan Tian can be discriminated as False Dan Tian and Real Dan Tian. What is the False Dan Tian? It is what is called Qihai cavity by Chinese medicine and Elixir Furnace (Dan Lu) by Daoists. What is the Real Dan Tian? It is called "Yellow Yard" (Huang Ting) or "Jade Ring Cavity" (Yu Huan Xue) by the Daoists and actually is the second human brain (in the guts). Though a human has several Dan Tians, the place which produces Elixir (i.e., Qi) is the Elixir Furnace. The main place of storing elixir is located at the Real Dan Tian. It is what is called Lower Brain or Second Brain.

丹田者，身體蓄氣（生化電）之所也。丹田有上丹田、
中丹田、與下丹田。上丹田者，上腦也，泥丸宮也。中
丹田者，鳩尾穴也，橫膈膜也。下丹田分假丹田與真丹
田。假丹田者，醫家之氣海穴也，道家之丹爐所在之處
也。真丹田者，黃庭也，玉環穴也，下腦也。人雖有數
處丹田，然產丹（氣）之所，在於丹爐也，假丹田也。
主要蓄丹之所，在於真丹田也，亦即人之下腦或第二腦
也。

Dan Tian (丹田) is translated as "elixir field." This means Dan Tians are the places in the body where the Qi can be grown and stored. There are three recognized Dan Tians in the body. One is called the Upper Dan Tian (Shang Dan Tian, 上丹田) and is located at the upper brain. This Dan Tian is the center of the spirit. The second one is called the Middle Dan Tian (Zhong Dan Tian, 中丹田) and is located at the lower part of the sternum, called Jiuwei (Co-15) (鳩尾) (Figure 18), which connects to the diaphragm. The diaphragm is a good electrical conductor that is sandwiched between the fasciae on the top and bottom. Fasciae are poor electrical conductors. When a good conductor is sandwiched by poor conductors, the bioelectricity will be trapped and therefore stored in this area. The Middle Dan Tian has been recognized as the Dan Tian of fire Qi because the Qi there is produced from conversion of post-birth essence, from air and food. In addition, the level of Qi storage there will affect the heartbeat, hormone production of the thyroid gland, and disturb the

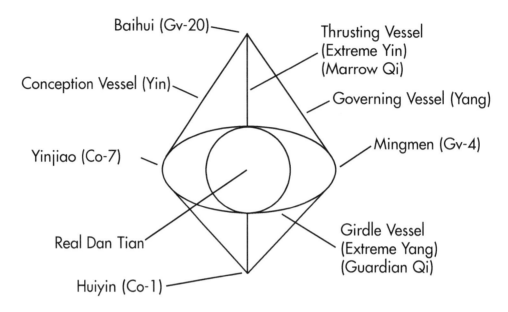

Figure 17. Body's Central Qi Vessel System

emotions. Finally, the Lower Dan Tian (Xia Dan Tian, 下丹田) is located at the lower abdominal area. There are two Lower Dan Tians. One is located on the front where the Qihai (Co-6) (氣海) cavity is on the Conception Vessel (Ren Mai, 任脈). This Dan Tian is also called "False Dan Tian" (Jia Dan Tian, 假丹田) because, though the Qi can be generated there, it cannot be stored there for a long time. Whenever the Qi is built up, it will enter the Conception Vessel and spread to the entire body.

The other Lower Dan Tian, called "Real Dan Tian" (Zhen Dan Tian, 真丹田) is at the center of the abdominal area where the center of gravity (or guts) is located. This place is also recognized as a second brain or lower brain by modern science.[7,8] This Dan Tian has the capability of storing a high level of Qi or bioelectricity. Therefore, this place is where the main human bio-battery is located. It is said that the Qi in the Lower Dan Tian is converted from the Original Essence (Yuan Jing, 元精) which is stored in the kidneys (i.e., both internal and external kidneys). The external kidneys are the testicles or ovaries. Qi produced here comes from the conversion of fat accumulated in the False Dan Tian area (i.e., lower abdomen). The kidneys only produce hormones (i.e., original essence, 元精) in this area. Hormones act as a catalyst in the body's biochemical reactions. Therefore, when the hormone balance in the body is correct, the biochemical reaction will be smooth. The Qi will also be produced naturally and abundantly.

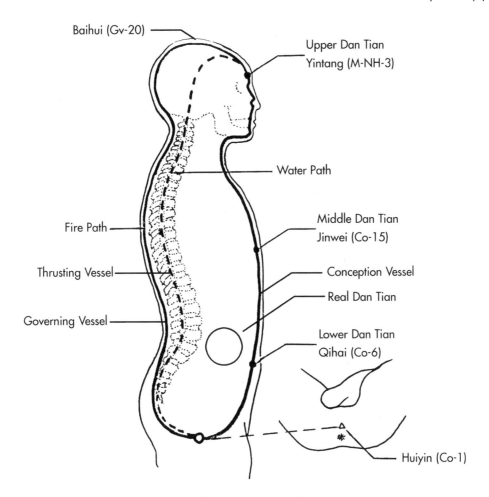

Baihui (Gv-20)

Upper Dan Tian
Yintang (M-NH-3)

Water Path

Fire Path

Middle Dan Tian
Jinwei (Co-15)

Thrusting Vessel

Conception Vessel

Real Dan Tian

Governing Vessel

Lower Dan Tian
Qihai (Co-6)

Huiyin (Co-1)

Figure 18. Three Dan Tians and Real Dan Tian

In the practice of abdominal breathing, due to the abdominal muscles' (i.e., Elixir Furnace's) up and down movements, the fat stored in the abdominal area is gradually converted into bioelectricity (i.e., Qi) through biochemical reaction. Thus, bioelectricity or Qi is produced. But, the reason why this place is called "False Dan Tian" by the Daoists is because, though this place is able to produce bioelectricity, it cannot store it. This is because the False Dan Tian is located on the path of the Conception Vessel. Whenever bioelectricity is produced, it immediately enters the natural path of Small Circulation and then distributes itself to the entire body to be consumed. (Therefore), though it (i.e., abdominal breathing) is able to raise up the quantitative storage of bioelectricity and electric potential (i.e., EMF) and make the physical body strong, it cannot store the bioelectricity to a high energy level. If (you) wish to reach the goals of opening the third eye for enlightenment, becoming a Buddha, or (even) longevity, following the Dao of Small Circulation is insufficient for achieving these goals.

在腹式呼吸中，由於腹部丹爐處肌肉之上下起伏運動，
存在腹部之脂肪漸而由生化化學反應而轉換成生化電。
因之，生化電或氣由之而生。然而，道家稱此處為假丹
田者，乃因其雖能產生電，卻不能蓄電。其因在於假丹
田乃位於任脈上，每每電生，即墮入天然小周天之循環，
而分部到全身肢體上而竭其能。其功用雖能提高身體之
電量與電能而使物理身體強壯，然卻不能蓄電而使達高
電位。如為求達神通、成仙、立佛、與長生，小周天之
道難以成效矣。

The front lower abdominal area (i.e., False Dan Tian) is also called the "elixir furnace" (Dan Lu, 丹爐) because this area can produce the fire (i.e., Qi or elixir). The way Qi is produced is from the up and down abdominal breathing exercises. From the exercises, the fat accumulated in this area will be converted into Qi or bioelectricity through biochemical reaction. Fat is the extra food essence which has already been processed and treated through the body's systems. Fat is a high calorie material that is stored naturally in the body for times when we don't have a food supply for several days. However, as explained earlier, this False Dan Tian cannot store the Qi to a high level since it is located on the Conception Vessel. Once the Qi is built up, it will be distributed to the entire body through natural Small Circulation (fire path). It is because of this that Daoists called this Dan Tian the False Dan Tian.

> In order to open the third eye, reach enlightenment, become a Buddha, and gain longevity, (you) must know how to convert the essence (into Qi) and nourish the brain, refine the Qi and sublimate it upward, refine the Qi and convert it into spirit, and refine the spirit and return it to emptiness. The first step (of reaching these goals) is that (you) must know the Dao of storing the bioelectricity. If the Qi cannot be accumulated to a high energy level, then it cannot be led upward along the Thrusting Vessel to the upper brain effectively. Consequently, the brain cannot reach high resonant frequencies and energy levels. To store the Qi, (you) must know how to use the method of Embryonic Breathing (Tai Xi) to lead the bioelectricity produced in the False Dan Tian (i.e., Elixir Furnace) inward and store it in the Real Dan Tian. What is Embryonic Breathing? It is the breathing method to keep the Yi at the Real Dan Tian. We will discuss this in more detail later.

為求神通、成仙、立佛、與長生，必懂返精補腦、煉氣
昇華，煉氣化神、與煉神返虛之道。其首步在懂得蓄電
之道。氣不蓄至高電量位，不能有效的由衝脈上引至腦，
而腦無法達到高曾次的共振頻率。為能蓄電，必懂得如
何以胎息之法導引由假丹田產生之電入存真丹田。胎息
者，意守丹田之穴位呼吸也。下將專題論之，不在此篇
作專論。

In order to reach immortality, Buddhahood, or enlightenment, you must know how to lead the Qi upward through the Thrusting Vessel (Chong Mai, 衝脈) (i.e., spinal cord) to the brain to nourish the spirit (water path). Each brain cell consumes about 12 times more oxygen than a regular cell. Since oxygen consumption is closely related to Qi (or bioelectricity) consumption, it is reasonable to assume that each brain cell also consumes around 12 times more Qi or electricity than a regular cell. In order to nourish the brain and energize it to a higher state, you will need a great quantity of Qi. Without knowing how to store the Qi in the Real Dan Tian (i.e., second brain) to an abundant level, it is impossible to energize your brain to a higher level and enlighten your spirit. This is why since ancient times, there have been so many Qigong practitioners searching for the way of storing Qi in the Real Dan Tian. These techniques have become known as "Embryonic Breathing" (Tai Xi, 胎息). Since Embryonic Breathing is a huge subject in internal elixir training, we will discuss it in detail later.

14. Thesis of Taijiquan's Muscle/Tendon Changing and Marrow/Brain Washing 太極拳易筋、洗髓論

The meaning of training Muscle/Tendon Changing and Marrow/Brain Washing (Qigong) is to train the Gongfu of refining the essence and converting it into Qi, refining the Qi and converting it into spirit, refining the spirit and returning it to emptiness, and finally crushing the emptiness. Muscle/Tendon Changing (Gongfu) belongs to Yang and is a Gongfu of Small Circulation meditation that converts the essence into Qi to strengthen the muscle/tendon and bones. It also enhances the Qi and blood circulation (in the body). There are two purposes of this (training): 1. to store an abundant level of Qi in the Real Dan Tian and also in the Conception and Governing Vessels; 2. to smoothen the Qi's circulation in these two vessels so that they can regulate Qi levels in the twelve primary Qi channels healthily. Because the Qi in the twelve primary Qi channels reaches the four limbs and hundreds of bones (i.e., entire physical body), its main function is to maintain the strength of the muscle/tendon and bone. When the Qi is abundantly stored in the Real Dan Tian, the Qi's circulation in the Conception and Governing vessels will be strong. When the Qi's circulation is strong in the Conception and Governing vessels, the Qi's circulation in the twelve primary Qi channels will also be strong. When the Qi's circulation in the twelve primary Qi channels is strong, the muscle/tendon and bones will be healthy. From this, (you) can see that Small Circulation meditation is the foundation of muscle/tendon changing.

易筋洗髓之義在於練精化氣、練氣化神、練神返虛、粉碎虛空之返精補腦的功夫。易筋為陽，是練精化氣，以強筋骨，以壯氣血之小周天任督兩脈運行之功夫。其目的有二：在充氣於真丹田與任督兩脈，在於便利氣在兩脈之運行而調十二經氣。十二經通達四肢百骸，乃主筋骨之強健。真丹田氣充，任督兩脈氣旺。任督兩脈氣旺，十二經氣強。十二經氣強，筋骨則健。由此可知小周天乃易筋之本。

There are two major purposes of Qigong training in China. One is to increase the quantity of the Qi. When the Qi reaches abundant levels, the vital force will be strong and clean, and you will be healthy and strong. The second purpose is to increase the efficiency of the Qi's use, by improving the quality of the Qi's manifestation. When the quality of the Qi's manifestation has been improved, the Qi will not be wasted and this will provide you with a root into longevity and spiritual enlightenment. It is believed that Muscle/Tendon Changing Qigong (Yi Jin, 易筋) increases the quantity of Qi and its manifestation in the physical body. When this happens, the physical body can be changed from weak to strong, and health can be maintained. Marrow/Brain Washing Qigong (Xi Sui, 洗髓) improves mental concentration, so the spirit can be raised to a higher level. When this happens, the Qi can be led in the most efficient way to serve different cultivation purposes (to improve the qualitative use of the Qi).

According to Daoist training, there are four stages of cultivation to reach the final goal of enlightenment: 1. Refining the essence and converting it into Qi (Lian Jing Hua Qi, 練精化氣); 2. Refining the Qi and converting it into spirit (Lian Qi Hua Shen, 練氣化神); 3. Refining the spirit and returning it to emptiness (Lian Shen Fan Xu, 練神返虛); and 4. Crushing the emptiness (Fen Sui Xu Kong, 粉碎虛空). The first stage is Muscle/Tendon Changing and the second to fourth are for enlightenment. Once the Qi is converted from essence, then from Small Circulation meditation you learn how to use your mind to lead the Qi to circulate smoothly in the Conceptional and Governing Vessels (Ren and Du Mai, 任、督脈). Since these two vessels regulate the Qi status in the twelve primary Qi channels, Small Circulation serves the purpose of changing the physical body from weak to strong.

> *Marrow/Brain Washing (Qigong) belongs to Yin and is a Gongfu of refining the Qi and converting it into spirit, refining the spirit and returning it to emptiness, and crushing the emptiness, so as to make the bone marrow flourish and to nourish the brain. There are two training purposes: 1. to lead the Qi inward and condense it into the bone marrow to cleanse the marrow; 2. to lead the Qi upward along the Thrusting Vessel to wash the brain and bring the practitioner to the stage of refining the spirit and returning it to emptiness.*

洗髓為陰，是練氣化神、練神返虛、粉碎虛空、以旺骨髓，以補腦髓之功夫。其目的有二：在於引氣內斂骨髓，而達洗髓之效；在於引氣沿衝脈上行，以達洗腦練神返虛之境地。

As explained in the last paragraph, Marrow/Brain Washing has two main purposes. One purpose is to learn how to lead the Qi from the Real Dan Tian along the Thrusting Vessel (Chong Mai, 衝脈) (i.e., spinal cord) upward to nourish the brain, reaching for the goal of spiritual enlightenment. The second purpose is to learn how to lead the Qi to the bone marrow, nourishing the marrow to maintain its healthy functioning.

Bone marrow is the source of blood production. When the Qi in the bone marrow is abundant, then the functional capability of blood production will be high. Blood cells are the carriers of oxygen and nutrition (in the body). When blood cells are healthy and blood circulation is strong and abundant, the body's metabolism will be smooth, and consequently the body will be healthy. In fact, this is the key to health and longevity.

骨髓為造血之源，骨髓氣旺，則造血機能高。血為氧氣
養份運輸之工具。血球健康，血液旺盛，則身體之新陳
代謝順利，身體康健。此實為強身長壽之樞紐。

Bone marrow is the factory of blood cells. When marrow is healthy, the blood cells will be healthy and abundant. Approximately one trillion (10^{12}) cells die every 24 hours in your body. Therefore, you must provide the material, Qi, and also an appropriate environment for the cells' replacement. When this metabolization is healthy and smoothly carried out, the body will be healthy and longevity can be achieved. Therefore, Marrow Washing Qigong is a key to longevity.

The brain is also named Upper Dan Tian, also named Mud-Pill Palace (Ni Wan Gong), or spiritual valley (Shen Gu) (in Daoist society). What is meant by the spirit is the divine spirit. This divine spirit is also named valley spirit (Gu Shen) and is the master of the spiritual valley. When a man is born, the divine spirit resides in the physical body and borrows the feeling of the human body so as to comprehend the Dao of the spirit and the divine. Therefore, when the divine spirit is educated, it can be promoted to a higher level. Repeating, the process becomes the natural rule of reincarnation. The purpose of repeating reincarnation is to reach the great Dao of human-heaven's unification. If (you) wish to reach this stage, (you) must first learn how to refine the Qi and convert it into spirit. From the abundant Qi's nourishment of the brain, the spiritual valley can reach a highly resonant level of vibration. From this resonance, (you) will be able to reach the divine of the heaven and the earth (i.e., nature).

腦一名上丹田，一名泥丸宮，又名神谷。神者，靈神之
謂也。靈神又名谷神，為神谷之主。當人之初生，靈神
寄托於人體，而借人體之感覺，而悟神靈之道。由此，
靈神受教而更上一層。反復如此而為自然迴輪之理。其
反復迴輪之終的，乃臻天人合一之大道。欲達此境地，
必先練氣化神。由旺氣之補腦，神谷可達高程度之共鳴
回響。由此共鳴回響之感應而通天地之靈。

Daoists call the space between the two hemispheres of the brain the "spiritual valley" (Shen Gu, 神谷), while the spirit residing in this valley is called "valley spirit" (Gu Shen, 谷神). This valley acts as an energy resonance chamber that generates vibrations and also receives vibrations from outside. In Daoist society, it is believed that when the brain has been energized to a higher energetic state, the spirit will be raised up, and the frequency band of vibration can be widened. Consequently, the receiving capability will also be more sensitive. This means intuitive spiritual sensitivity, and correspondence with other energy sources will be higher. When this happens, we can comprehend many energy variations around us that cannot be sensed by the untrained. It is from this kind of energy correspondence that we can communicate with natural spiritual energy.

In Buddhist and Daoist societies spiritual education is not from physical contact but from an invisible spiritual energy vibration or resonance. When your vibration frequency reaches a higher level, you will be able to communicate with those people whose vibration frequency is closer to yours. From this mutual resonance, you can understand many things. After a long period of practice, you will be able to re-open the third eye or the heaven eye (Tian Yan, 天眼) and thus be capable of unobstructed communication with the surrounding energy vibrations.

> *From the above, (we can see that) Muscle/Tendon Changing and Marrow/Brain Washing are actually two faces of the same object. One Yang and one Yin, they affect each other and cannot be separated. If (you) only practice Muscle/Tendon Changing, the body will become more Yang and there is a risk of energy dispersion (San Gong). On the contrary, if (you) practice only Marrow/Brain Washing, then the body will turn more Yin and the Guardian Qi (Wei Qi) will be condensed inward, and it is easy to get sick.*

> 由上可知，易筋洗髓兩者實為一體之兩面。一陽一陰互為體用。兩者不能分開。如僅習練易筋，身體為陽，乃有散功之慮。反之，如僅習練洗髓，則身體傾陰，衛氣收斂，容易生病。

Activating more brain cells and raising the brain's energy requires a great amount of Qi or bioelectricity. In addition, bone marrow is a highly electrically conductive material. Both the brain and the marrow will absorb a great quantity of Qi. If you do not have enough Qi to maintain your physical life and lead it inward to the bone marrow and upward to nourish the brain, then your physical body will be weakened and will degenerate quickly. Therefore, the first step in Qigong training is learning how to build up the Qi to an abundant level. Only if you have abundant Qi can you then lead the extra Qi inward to wash the bone marrow and upward to nourish the brain. Muscle/Tendon Changing is used for strengthening the physical body and to increase the quantity of Qi, while Marrow/Brain Washing is used for attuning the spiritual body and improving the quality of the Qi's manifestation.

> *From this, (we can see that) the Yin and Yang of the Muscle/Tendon Changing and Marrow/Brain Washing must be balanced and harmonized with each other; then one can reach the goal of double cultivation of human nature and physical*

life. The Muscle/Tendon Changing and Marrow/Brain Washing of Taijiquan begin from the Yi's Yin and Yang and its knack is regulating the breathing. The most important key to Marrow/Brain Washing is the internal condensation of the Yi. Use the Yi to lead the Qi inward to the bone marrow and also upward to the Upper Dan Tian so as to reach the goal of washing the marrow/brain. This is the practice of Marrow/Brain Breathing (Sui Xi). The most important key to Muscle/Tendon Changing is the Yi's expansion. Use the Yi to lead the Qi and expand it (from the Real Dan Tian) to the skin and beyond; (consequently) the Guardian Qi is enhanced. This is the practice of Skin Breathing (Fu Xi) and is also called Body Breathing (Ti Xi).

由是，易筋洗髓之陰陽必須平衡諧調，才能達到性命雙
修之終的。太極拳之易筋、洗髓始於意之陰陽，其竅在
於調息。洗髓之首要在於意內斂，以意引氣往內至骨髓
並上引至上丹田以達洗髓之目的。此為髓息。易筋之之
首要在於意外張，以意引氣外闊至皮膚之外，衛氣增強。
此為膚息亦稱體息。

There are two meanings for "double cultivation" (Shuang Xiu, 雙修) in Daoist society. One is the cultivation of the physical body and the spiritual body. One is Yang (i.e., physical) and the other is Yin (i.e., spiritual). Both must be cultivated in a balanced way. Only then can you have physical longevity and also have a spiritual center. Another meaning of "double cultivation" is also called mutual cultivation, and means to have a Qi exchange with a partner, to synchronize and harmonize the Qi with the partner. When this is done correctly, the spirit can be raised quickly to a high level.

In Taijiquan training, since Yi is the Taiji, and is the main source of producing EMF (i.e., electromotive force), Yi is then the crucial key to training Muscle/Tendon Changing and Marrow/Brain Washing. With the coordination of the breathing, the Qi can be led outward to the skin surface to strengthen the Guardian Qi (i.e., Wei Qi, 衛氣) and also inward to the marrow to enhance the Qi's storage (i.e., Sui Qi, 髓氣).

Furthermore, (you) must follow the correct breathing method. In Normal Abdominal Breathing, the Qi goes to and fro from the internal organs to the four limbs following the Qi channels. In Reverse Abdominal Breathing, following the secondary Qi channels, the Qi is led outward to the skin (Wei Qi) and also inward to reach the bone marrow (Sui Qi). From this, (you) can see that Muscle/Tendon Changing and Marrow/Brain Washing must adopt the method of reversed breathing in order to reach the expected effectiveness of practice. You can refer to the future discussion of regulating the breathing, and then match this with logical thinking and comprehension. (In this case), you will be able to apprehend the theory of practice suddenly.

再者，必須配合正確之呼吸方法。順腹呼吸者，氣沿經
行由內臟至四肢往返而行。逆腹呼吸者，氣沿絡行外至
皮膚，內斂至骨髓。由此可知，易筋洗髓必須以逆呼吸
為法，才能達到預期之效。學者可參考未來討論之調息
法，再配合理解與邏輯之思考，必能豁然貫通焉。

Breathing is considered to be a strategy in Qigong practice. When breathing is done correctly, the cultivation of Qi can be achieved easily and effectively. In order to lead the Qi to the skin surface and also to the bone marrow, you must use Reverse Abdominal Breathing (Ni Fu Hu Xi, 逆腹呼吸). However, if you are a beginner, you must be careful when you practice Reverse Abdominal Breathing. If you practice incorrectly, tension will be generated at the stomach area. Therefore, you must pay attention to this area and start with a small scale of abdominal movement. Only after you have trained for a while and your mind can control the muscles at the abdominal area effectively, can you then increase the scale of the breathing. Just remember that relaxation is the most important concern—do not hold your breath and do not create uncomfortable tension in the stomach area. Learning Reverse Abdominal Breathing is just like learning how to swim or how to drive. Proceed gradually and cautiously. Once you have grasped the keys to practice, you will enjoy it very much. Knowing this particular method is a crucial key to the practice. If you are interested in learning more about breathing techniques, please refer to the books: *The Essence of Taiji Qigong* and *The Essence of Shaolin White Crane*, by YMAA.

PART II

About Regulating the Body
論調身

1. Importance of Regulating the Body 調身之要

Taijiquan is a martial Qigong. Its first important practicing requirement is regulating the body, next regulating the breathing, then regulating the Xin (i.e., emotional mind), then, regulating the Qi, and finally regulating the spirit. There is an ancient saying: "(When) shape (i.e., body's posture) is not correct, then the Qi('s circulation) will not be smooth. (When) the Qi('s circulation) is not smooth, the Yi (i.e., wisdom mind) will not be at peace. (When) the Yi is not at peace, then the Qi is disordered." From this, (you) can see that from the (correct) regulating of the body, the Qi('s circulation) is smooth and from the smooth Qi circulation, the Xin and Yi are calm and peaceful. It is also said: "The balance of the body and Xin." This means the harmonization of the body and the Xin. When the Xin is clean (i.e., calm without emotional disturbance), the body can be calm. It (also) means: when the body's postures are correct, the Xin is peaceful. In the Daoist book, The Complete Book of Principal Contents of Life and Human Nature, *it is written: "When the body does not move, the Xin will be peaceful by itself. When Xin is not moved (i.e., not being disturbed), then the spirit will stay (in its residence) by itself." This implies that the slower the body moves, the more peaceful the Xin will be. When the Xin is peaceful without being moved, then the spirit will not leave its residence. This is the important key to reaching enlightenment (i.e., Understanding Jin) in Taijiquan. From this, we can see that regulating the body is the first step of learning Taijiquan.*

太極拳，武學氣功也。其練習首要在於調身，次為調息，再為調心，更為調氣，終於調神。古云：〝形不正，則氣不順。氣不順，則意不寧。意不寧，則氣散亂。〞由此可知，由身調而氣順。由氣順而心意寧靜。又云：〝身心平衡。〞此即身心調合，心淨身靜，身正心平之意也。道書《性命圭旨全書‧亨集》云：〝身不動而心自安，心不動而神自守。〞此即意身愈緩，心愈安。心安而不動，則神不外馳也。此即太極拳通乎神明之要徑。由是，可知調身為練太極拳之第一步也。

As explained before, Taijiquan is a martial Qigong which follows the regular, normal training procedures of Qigong practice. These procedures are: regulating the body (Tiao Shen, 調身), breath (Tiao Xi, 調息), mind (Tiao Xin, 調心), Qi (Tiao Qi, 調氣), and then spirit (Tiao Shen, 調神). Regulating the body is the first step in the entire regulating process. However, you must use the mind as the controlling center of your entire being. This is because if the mind is not steady and calm, the thinking cannot be clear and the feeling cannot be accurate. Remember that feeling is the language of mind-body communication. In order to have deep feeling, your body must be calm and the mind must be peaceful. From this, you can see that the process of regulating the body cannot be accomplished in isolation. It must coordinate and harmonize with other criteria. Only if you have provided a relaxed physical body and a calm mind, can your spirit stay in its residence without being disturbed. When this happens, the Spirit of Vitality can be raised.

2. Stationary Postures 定勢 (The Postures of Central Equilibrium) (中定之勢)

Regulate means to regulate until it is regulated to a harmonious stage. Regulating the body means to regulate the entire physical body until it is soft, relaxed, balanced, centered, rooted, and the head is suspended. When the Weilu (i.e., tailbone) is upright, then the body will be balanced without being tilted. When the body is not tilting, the spine will be loose and the body will feel relaxed and seemingly fluid.

調者，調和也。調身者，調和身體之各部位使之鬆軟、
平衡、中正、紮根、頂懸。身體尾閭中正，則身自立而
不傾。不傾，則身不繃緊，脊椎自鬆。

Regulate (Tiao, 調) means to control and refine something until it is harmonized with its surroundings, its peers, and/or its location in spacetime. In Taijiquan, regulating the body means to bring consciousness to it until it can be harmonized with the breathing and the mind. When this happens, the Qi can be circulated smoothly and the spirit can be raised up to a higher potential. In order to reach this goal, the first step of regulating the body is to search for the relaxation, softness, balance, center, and the root of the body. Additionally, in order to raise up the spirit, the head should be upright as if there is a thread suspending it from above, drawing it upward (Xu Ling Ding Jin, 虛領頂勁). Furthermore, in order to keep the Mingmen (Gv-4) (命門) cavity opened, the tailbone (Weilu, 尾閭) must be upright (i.e., tucked in) as well. In this case, the entire body is upright and centered without being tilted. The spine will be loose and the body relaxed. This is the first crucial key to regulating the body.

Relaxation means every section of every joint must be loose. Taijiquan Classic said: "Once in motion, the entire body must be light and agile, (it) especially should (be) threaded together." This means that when the joints are loose, then the body('s movements) can be light. When the body('s movements) are light, then the action can be agile and the entire body's Qi can be united (i.e., act as a single unit). Therefore, it is again said in Taijiquan Classic that: "The root is at the feet, (Jin or movement is) generated from the legs, mastered (i.e., controlled) by the waist and manifested (i.e., expressed) through the fingers. From the feet to the legs to the waist must be integrated, through one unified Qi." From this, (you) can see that in order to reach the goal of the lightness and agility, (you) must first pay attention to regulating the waist (Yao) and the upper thighs (Kua). This is because the waist and upper thighs are the controlling center of the physical body and also the place of the Qi's residence. When this place is loosened, then the body can be soft and the Qi can exit and enter as wished. The waist is just like the steering wheel of a car; it must be able to turn and move. If the waist is stiff and not soft(ened), then the entire body's Jin will lose its control.

鬆意節節關節要鬆。太極拳經云：〝一舉動，週身俱要輕靈，尤須貫穿。〞 此即意關節鬆，則身輕，身輕則動靈，全身可串通一氣也。因而太極拳經再云：〝其根在腳，發於腿，主宰於腰，形於手指。由腳而腿而腰，總須完整一氣。〞 由此可知為求身輕動靈，必先在意於腰與胯。其因概為腰與胯主身之主宰中心，氣結舍之所。此地先鬆然後身能軟，氣能進出自如。腰如開車之駕駛盤，必須轉動自如。如腰死不軟化，則全身之勁必失之主宰。

In order to be loose physically, the mind should first pay attention to the joints of the body. When the joints are loose, you can be relaxed. When you are loose and relaxed, then your action can be light and agile. In addition, when you are loose and relaxed, the Qi can circulate in the body smoothly. When this happens, your entire body can act as a single whipping unit. Taijiquan Jin acts like the whipping of a soft whip. When there is a stiffness in any joint, the whipping power will be reduced.

All of the action or power is generated from the feet (i.e., root), directed and controlled by the waist and finally manifested in the fingers. Therefore, the waist area including the upper thighs, is the controlling center of the whipping power. Kua means the upper thighs where they connect to the waist. Kua (胯) can be discriminated as Wai Kua (外胯) and Nei Kua (內胯) which means external or outer upper thighs and internal upper thighs near the groin area (Figure 19). Waist and Kua act as the steering wheel of a car, to control the entire body's power manifestation. Only when these two places are soft and loose can you use them as you wish. In order to make these two places loose and soft, you must learn how to move the hip joints soft-

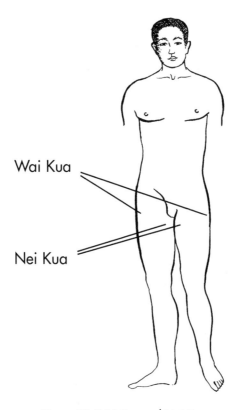

Figure 19. Wai Kua and Nei Kua

ly and skillfully. In fact, it is the softness of the hip joints that allows the waist and Kua to be soft. In *Taijiquan Classic*, it is said: "If you fail to catch the opportunity and gain the superior position, (your) body will be disordered. To solve this problem, (you) must look to the waist and legs."[9] From these two sentences, we can see the importance of the waist and legs.

> *The upper thighs are the connecting place of the upper and lower body. When the upper thighs are firmed, then the root is firm. In order to be firm in the root, the upper thighs must be loose. When (they are) loose, then the upper body and the lower body can be connected and the Yi and the Qi can be sunk to the bottom of the feet. On the contrary, if the upper thighs are tensed, then the lower body will be stiff and stagnant, and the root can be easily pulled. Furthermore, when the upper thighs are tensed, the waist will also be tightened; both are related to each other. In addition, though the waist and the upper thighs are loose and soft, (you) must also pay attention to the groin area. This is because when the groin is not wrapped (i.e., protected) (Guo Dang) then the lower section will not be firm and the root will be shallow. (In this case,) the upper body and the lower body will lose their means of communications.*

胯為上下身連接之所。胯固則根穩。為求根穩，胯必鬆。
鬆則上下相連，意氣能沉於腳底。反之，胯緊，則下身
呆硬，根易被拔。況乎胯繃則腰緊，兩者相互關係也。
不僅如此，雖腰胯鬆軟，仍須注意裹襠以護下陰。況乎，
襠不裹，則下盤不穩，根必淺，上下失去聯絡。

In order to be loose in the waist, the upper thighs where they connect to the waist area must also be loose. This is the place where the hip joints are located and these two joints connect the legs and the waist. When these two joints are tightened, the waist will be tensed. As a result, the connection of the upper body and the lower body will be stagnant and stiff here. Therefore, in order to have a good connection so that you can build up a firm root and the entire body can act as a single unit, you must pay attention to these two joints. They must be loose and relaxed.

Guo Dang (裹襠) means to wrap the groin area. In Chinese martial arts, a common mistake that a person, when loosening up his/her Kua (胯), will also open his/her groin area. This will allow the opponent to attack the groin. Therefore, though you are loose in the hip joints, you must also wrap the groin area to protect this vital area. The way to reach this goal is to keep your knees slightly inward.

After (your) central body has gained its relaxation, (you) should search for the shoulders' sinking and elbows' dropping and aim for the comfort, relaxation, and softness of the arms. When the shoulders are sunk and the elbows are dropped, then the area under the armpits will naturally be protected from the opponent's attack. Furthermore, if the shoulders are not sunk and the elbows are not dropped, then there is no root for the Jin's manifestation. The main Jins are stored in the bows of the spine and the chest; the key to execution is decided in the formation of Peng Jin, in which the chest is drawn in and the back is arced (Han Xiong Ba Bei). If (you) can formalize a Peng Jin, then (you) can store and (also) emit (the Jins). If (you) do not know how to formalize a Peng Jin, then the Jins manifested will be limited to the stagnant muscular force generated from the arms. In this case, the entire body cannot be threaded together as a unified Qi. However, if (you) only know how to store Jin in the two bows of the spine and chest and do not know how to sink (your) shoulders and drop (your) elbows, then the Jin will not be connected (to the body) in the two places of the shoulders and elbows. If (you) can understand the keys of keeping the body upright, loosening (your) waist, loosening (your) upper thighs, wrapping the groin area, sinking (your) shoulders, and dropping (your) elbows, then (you) have comprehended the theory of regulating the body in Taijiquan. If (you) can further understand the theory of how to draw in the chest, arc the back, and control by the waist, then it is not difficult to comprehend the Jin.

身鬆之後，再求沉肩，墜肘，以求臂膀之安舒鬆軟。肩
沉、肘墜則脅下自守而不為敵所乘。況乎，肩不沉，肘
不墜，則發勁無根。主勁蓄於脊於胸兩弓，其竅決於含
胸拔背之掤勁。能掤則能蓄能發，不知掤，則勁僅限於
臂膀之呆力耳，全身不能一氣串連而貫之矣。然者，如
僅知蓄勁於脊胸兩弓，而不知沉肩墜肘，則勁必不串連
而失於臂肩兩處矣。能懂中正、鬆腰、鬆胯、裏襠、沉
肩、墜肘，即已悟太極調身之理。如能再懂含胸、拔背、
主宰于腰之理，則悟勁不難矣。

Once the central body is loosened and you have gained the balance, the center, and the root, your upper body and your lower body will be connected. However, in order to lead the Jin generated from the body to the fingers, you must also know how to sink your shoulders and drop your elbows. If you do not know how to do these things, the joints in the shoulders and elbows will be tensed and consequently, the Jin generated in the body will be stagnant in these two places. When the shoulders are sunk and the elbows are dropped, then there is a root or foundation for the Jin's manifestation. This is because there is a firm connection between your hands and central body.

Furthermore, in order to manifest the Jin to its maximum, you must also know how to store it in the chest and spine. The entire body can manifest six bows (Liu Gong, 六弓), which allow you to store Jin efficiently. The two arms and two legs are four bows. The chest and spine are the other two bows. The storage of Jin in the chest and spine are considered to be basic body movements (Shen Fa, 身法) in any Chinese martial art style. In Taijiquan, this action is called "draw in the chest and arc the back" (Han Xiong Ba Bei, 含胸拔背). This is the crucial key to executing Peng Jin (i.e., Wardoff Jin).

3. Moving Postures 動勢(The Postures of Four Directions) (四面之勢)

The concept of regulating the body in the stepping movements requires, beyond the above theory of regulating the body in the stationary posture, that (you) know the theory of stepping. Stepping (in Taijiquan) means that when (you) step, it is as if you are pushing a car. There is a root in stationary posture, but there is also a root when (you are) in stepping movements. If there is no root, then the Qi will be floating, the body will be uprooting, and the Yi will also drift. In addition, when (you) move, the body should be upright, just as in stationary practice. When stepping, the groin area must be wrapped and the body must be balanced and centered in every step. Advance, retreat, beware of the left, and look to the right, every step is firm and clear without any disorder. (In addition), when stepping, it is as a cat walking: light and agile but not floating. The firm root in stepping is decid-

ed by the ankle('s intelligence), the waist('s looseness), and how it connects to the upper body at the Kua (i.e., upper thighs) area. From the feet to the body, every section is threaded together; must avoid stagnation and stiffness.

調身于動勢者，除上述定步調身之理外，必知行步之理。
行步者，行步穩重如推車然矣。定勢有根，動勢亦要紮
根。無根，則氣浮，身浮，意也浮。不但如此，動時身
體中正如定勢然。行步裏襠，步步上身平衡中定。進退
左顧右盼，邁步不亂，步步分明。邁步如貓行，輕靈而
不浮。行步紮根取決於踝，鬆於腰，由胯接上身。由足
到身，節節貫串，切忌呆死。

To regulate your body when you are moving or stepping is harder than when you are still. However, movement is much more likely to occur in an actual combat situation. Therefore, you must be familiar with the theory and the methods of how to regulate your body while you are stepping. Many of the same principles that govern how to regulate the body in a stationary position also apply when moving. You search for relaxation, balance, and rooting while you are moving. When you need to step, in addition to keeping your body relaxed and balanced, you must step with a firm root. Your root must be firmed, and the body cannot be tilted forward. Only if you can step with a firm root will your mind be settled, will the Qi sink, and can the body consequently be agile. In order to have a firm root while you are moving, you must pay attention to the joints in your hips. When these two joints are loose and actively mobile, the connection between the upper body and the lower body will be natural and firm. This will allow the entire body to unite in an integrated, whiplike way for the manifestation of Jin's. In addition, when the hip joints are loose, the waist will also be loose. This will allow the Qi to exit and enter its residence (i.e., Lower Dan Tian) smoothly and naturally.

However, the hardest part of regulating the body during stepping is that while you are moving, (you) must still be able to exchange (your) steppings with agility and liveliness, so the Jins should be generated from the legs, mastered (i.e., controlled) by the waist and manifested through the fingers (efficiently). (In addition), during stepping, (you) should maintain central equilibrium, be able to change the steps (easily) by following the body('s maneuvers), and emit or neutralize the Jins naturally without any stagnation. Without all of these (criteria), the Jin manifested will not have a firm root and body, Yi, and Qi will be floating.

然者，最難之動步調身者，乃為動步之中，仍能步步轉
換靈活，勁發于腿，主宰于腰，而形于手指。步動之中，
仍有中定之勢，步隨身換，勁之化發，自然無滯。無此，
則勁無根，身、意、氣皆浮矣。

The most important factor in winning, is knowing how to neutralize incoming power and manifest your own power skillfully and effectively. In order to do so, you must have a firm root, central equilibrium, and a unified body. In addition, you must be able to move swiftly and skillfully without stagnation. In Taijiquan, all of these criteria are gained from moving pushing hands drills.

PART III

About Regulating the Breathing 論調息

1. Secret of Regulating the Breathing 調息法訣

Lao Zi, Chapter 5: "Between heaven and earth, isn't it just like a Tuo Yue (i.e., bellows)?" In the human body, the head is the heaven, the Huiyin (i.e., perineum) is the earth or the sea bottom. Between them, isn't it just like the Tuo Yue of the (natural) heaven and the earth? If it is so, then the key to maintaining a human life is just like the millions of lives which must rely on the Tuo Yue between heaven and earth, that is to find the Qi's smooth circulation and rely on it to live. Regulating the breathing is to regulate the exit and entrance of the air in the body's Tuo Yue. From this, the exchange of oxygen and carbon dioxide can be smoothly accomplished. If there is any stagnation in this exchange, then the metabolism of the body's cells will not be carried out efficiently. Consequently, the vital force will be reduced and the cells will age faster.

《老子‧五章》：〝天地之間，其猶橐籥乎？〞人身者，頭為天，會陰為地、為海底。其間猶如天地之橐籥乎？然，則人生命之竅有如天地間之萬生眾命，惟賴天地間之橐籥以求氣之順利運行而賴以生存。調息者，調身體橐籥中空氣之出入也。由此出入，氧氣與二氧化碳可順利之交換。如此交換不順，則身體細胞之新陳代謝無法有效之施行。生命力由之降低，細胞加速之老化。

Tuo Yue (橐籥) (i.e., bellows) is a tube which is used to intensify the fire in a furnace. According to Lao Zi (老子), the space between heaven and earth is just like a Tuo Yue. From circulation of the air, all lives gain continuity. According to Chinese Qigong, a person's head is analogous to heaven (Tian Ling Gai, 天靈蓋) while the perineum (i.e., Huiyin, Co-1) (會陰) is like the earth or sea bottom (Haidi, 海底). Therefore, the body is like a Tuo Yue. Through the nose, oxygen and carbon dioxide are exchanged in the body and consequently, millions of lives of cells can be maintained. Without this exchange, we would die.

According to science, in order to generate a biochemical combustion process, oxygen is required to change the food essence into energy. Without sufficient oxygen, the energy production will be stagnant. In addition, all of the cells in the body requires substantial oxygen. All of the cells have their own life span (e.g., skin cells' life time is about 28 days). Therefore, when the cells die, they must be brought out through exhalation. At the same time, new cells must be generated to replace the dead cells. This smooth process of cell replacement metabolism is the key to health and longevity. The first crucial key is learning how to take in sufficient oxygen and to expel carbon dioxide efficiently. That means breathing correctly. It is because of this that all of the Qigong practices emphasize the training of correct breathing. This process is called "Tiao Xi" (調息) which means regulating the breathing.

> After (you) have regulated (your) body until it has reached a stage of regulating without regulating, then (you) should enter the practice of regulating the breathing. What is regulating the breathing? It means to regulate the breathing until it is calm, slender, deep, continuous, and uniform. When the breathing is regulated appropriately, the Qi's circulation will be smooth and when the breathing is inverse, then the Qi's circulation will be stagnant. If Xin and Yi can be peaceful and calm, then the body's regulating can be regulated to an even deeper stage. Treatise on Comprehending the Real (Wu Zhen Pian) said: "There are three kinds of breathing. From coarse to fine, inhalation and exhalation through the nose is nose breathing. Keeping the center (Lower Dan Tian) ascending and descending, is Qi breathing. (When) extremely calm and return to its root is called Shen breathing (i.e., Spiritual Breathing). Therefore, to number (i.e., to evaluate): the breathing (i.e., nose breathing) is not as high as regulating (abdominal real) breathing, and the regulating breathing is not as high as Shen breathing. When the Shen breathing becomes peaceful, then condense the Shen into the Qi cavity (Huang Ting) (i.e., Real Dan Tian); then the breathing is really deep." (The Daoist) Guang Cheng Zi said: "One exhale, the Earth Qi rises; one inhale, the Heaven Qi descends; real man's (meaning one who has attained the real Dao) repeated breathing at the navel, then my real Qi is naturally connected." (Daoist book) Sing (of the) Dao (with) Real Words (Chang Dao Zhen Yan) says: "One exhale one inhale to communicate Qi's function, one movement one calmness is the same as (is the source of) creation and variation." From the above, (you) can see that when (you) regulate (your) breathing, (you) should regulate it until the regulating is stopped and has reached to the stage of real breathing. What is real breathing? It seems that it is there and as if it is not there, soft without being broken, also named 'internal breathing' (Nei Hu Xi). Though the external ordinary breathing is stopped, it seems that there is an internal scenery of rising and descending in the Dan Tian.

繼調身至調而不調之境地，則步入調息之修練。調息者，
調呼吸之靜、細、深、悠、勻。息調得宜，則氣之行順，
息逆則氣滯。如心意能寧靜，則身體可調至更深之調身
境地。悟真篇曰：〝息有三種：從粗入細，呼吸出入者
鼻息也；規中升降者氣息也；靜極歸根者神息也。故數
息不如調息，調息不如安息。神息既安，則凝神入氣穴，
其息深矣。〞廣成子曰：〝一呼則地氣上升，一吸則天
氣下降，人之反覆呼吸於蒂，則我之真氣自然相接。〞
唱道真言曰：〝一呼一吸通乎氣機，一動一靜同乎造
化。〞由上可知，調息要調無息息，達到真息之境地。
真息者，似有似無，綿綿不斷，一名內呼吸。外面之凡
息雖斷，而丹田之中猶有一上一下之內景。

In order to regulate the breathing well, you must first put the body into the right state. Breathing behavior is closely related to and influenced by the tension or relaxation of the body. Therefore, when you practice Qigong, the first step is to regulate your body. Once you can reach the stage of regulating without regulating, then you can start the process of regulating the breathing.

When you regulate your breathing, you are aiming for breathing that can be: 1. Calm (Jing, 靜), 2. Slender (Xi, 細), 3. Deep (Shen, 深), 4. Continuous (You, 悠), and 5. Uniform (Yun, 勻). First, you learn nose breathing from coarse to fine, until your breathing becomes relaxed, deep, smooth, and natural. Then you enter into abdominal breathing (Fu Hu Xi, 腹呼吸) and eventually enter into Real Breathing (Zhen Xi, 真息).

It is important for a Qigong practitioner to learn the correct ways of regulating his breathing. There are many ways of regulating the breathing. Here, the methods are arranged from the most basic to the deepest and most difficult. To reach the final goal of Embryonic Breathing (Tai Xi, 胎息), you must start with regulating the normal breathing. It is called "Bi Xi" (鼻息), which means "nose breathing." From normal regular breathing, you will enter the abdominal breathing (Fu Xi, 腹息) stage which enables you to build Qi at the False Dan Tian (i.e., Elixir Furnace) (Dan Lu, 丹爐). It is this Qi which will lead you to the door of Real Qigong Breathing practice. This training is called "Qi Xi" (氣息), or "Qi breathing." When you have reached this level, the Dan Tian Qi can move up and down following your breathing. You have then reached the target of "Real Breathing" (Zhen Xi, 真息). Finally, you will lead the Post-birth Qi to the "Huang Ting Cavity" (黃庭穴) (or Yu Huan Xue, 玉環穴) to interact with the Pre-birth Qi and generate the "Holy Embryo" (Sheng Tai, 聖胎). This stage of breathing is called "Tai Xi" (胎息), which means "Embryonic Breathing."

An ancient Daoist Li, Qing-An said: "Regulating breathing means to regulate the breathing until (you) stop."[10] This means that correct regulating means not having to consciously regulate. In other words, although you start by regulating your breath consciously, you must get to the point where the regulating happens naturally by itself and you no longer have to think about it. When you breathe, if you concentrate your mind on breathing, it is not true regulating. When you reach the level of true regulating, no regulating is necessary, and you can use your mind efficiently to lead the Qi. Remember wherever the Yi is, there is Qi. If the Yi stops in one spot, the Qi will be stagnant. It is the Yi which leads the Qi and makes it move. Therefore, when you are in a state of correct breath regulating, your mind is free. There is no sound, stagnation, urgency, or hesitation, and you can be calm and peaceful. When you reach this stage, you have obtained the real key to meditation.

The methods of regulating the abdominal breathing include: Normal Abdominal Breathing, Reverse Abdominal Breathing, Embryonic Breathing, Five Gates Breathing, Girdle Vessel Breathing, Wuji Breathing (also called Real Dan Tian Breathing or Cavity Breathing), Skin-Marrow Breathing, Spiritual Breathing, Hibernation Breathing, and Turtle Breathing, etc. What is Normal Abdominal Breathing? It is breathing by using (the muscles of) the abdominal area in normal breathing. When the nose inhales, the abdomen expands and the Huiyin (i.e., perineum) sinks (gently). When the nose exhales, the abdomen is withdrawn and the Huiyin is lifted up (softly). What is Reverse Abdominal Breathing? It is to use the abdominal area for breathing. However, when the nose is inhaling, the abdomen is withdrawn and the Huiyin is lifted up (gently). When the nose is exhaling, the abdomen is expanding and the Huiyin is sinking (or pushed out gently). What is Embryonic Breathing? It is to store the Qi in the Real Dan Tian. What is Qi? It is bioelectricity. What is the Real Dan Tian? It is the biobattery that stores the bioelectricity. It is the place where the second human brain is located. The entire body's bioelectricity is stored here and supplies the electricity to the whole body. When the electric storage is high, then the vital force is strong and living activities vigorous. We will discuss this subject more later.

調腹息法有正（順）腹息、反（逆）腹息、胎息、五心息、帶脈息、無極息（或稱正丹田息、穴位息）、膚髓息、神息、冬眠息、龜息等等。正腹息者，以下腹部正呼吸也。鼻吸腹張，會陰下沉。鼻呼腹收，會陰上提。反腹息者，亦以下腹部呼吸也。然卻鼻吸腹收，會陰上提。鼻呼腹張，會陰下沉。胎息者，以氣蓄正丹田也。氣者，生化電也。正丹田者，蓄電之生化電池也，人之第二腦也。全身之生化電積於此，由此供給全身生化電之所須。蓄電高，則生命力強，生活活力旺。下將專題論之。

There are many ways of training to regulate the breathing, from simple to deep.

Beginners should first learn to regulate the regular breathing, by starting with Normal Abdominal Breathing (Zheng Fu Hu Xi, 正腹呼吸). This breathing technique is the easiest and most comfortable. Through this breathing, you will learn how to use your mind to control the muscles in the abdominal area efficiently. Only after you have reached a stage where you feel very comfortable and natural should you move into Reverse Abdominal Breathing (Fan Fu Hu Xi, 反腹呼吸) (Ni Fu Hu Xi, 逆腹呼吸). As mentioned earlier, if your mind cannot control the muscles at the abdominal area efficiently and you start Reverse Abdominal Breathing training, the stomach area will be tense, and this can cause pain and stagnation of the Qi in this area.

After you have reached a stage of regulating without regulating Reverse Abdominal Breathing, you should then progress to Embryonic Breathing (Tai Xi, 胎息). Through Embryonic Breathing, you will be able to lead the Qi to the Real Dan Tian (Zhen Dan Tian, 真丹田) (i.e., guts or second brain) and store the Qi there. When the storage of the Qi at the Real Dan Tian is abundant, your vital force will be strong.

Once you have reached the level of Embryonic Breathing, then you can apply the Qi for Five Gates Breathing (Wu Xin Xi, 五心息), Girdle Vessel Breathing (Dai Mai Xi, 帶脈息), Wuji Breathing (Wuji Xi, 無極息), Skin and Marrow Breathing (Fu Sui Xi, 膚髓息), Spiritual Breathing (Shen Xi, 神息), Hibernation Breathing (Dong Mian Xi, 冬眠息), and Turtle Breathing (Gui Xi, 龜息), etc.

> *What is Five Gates Breathing? It is when the Qi exits and enters through the Laogong, Yongquan, and Upper Dan Tian. This is the method of Qi's transportation in Grand Circulation. The (Qi's) exiting and entering through the Laogong is palm breathing, where the Jin (i.e., martial power) is emitted. The (Qi's) exiting and entering through the Yongquan is Yongquan breathing and is also called sole (of the foot) breathing, where the root of Jin is located. The (Qi's) exiting and entering through the Upper Dan Tian is Spiritual Breathing. From the spirit's upraising, the Qi transports upward to the palms and downward to the soles (efficiently); Jin is hence manifested and emitted. This is a state of central equilibrium.*

> 五心息者，由調息氣由勞宮、湧泉、上丹田出入也。此為大周天之運氣法也。由勞宮出入者，掌息也，勁之發也。由湧泉出入者，湧泉息也，踵息也，勁之根也。上丹田出入者，神息也。由神之提，氣上行至掌，下行至踵，勁由之而發，中定也。

The Laogong cavity (P-8) (勞宮), located at the center of the palms, belongs to

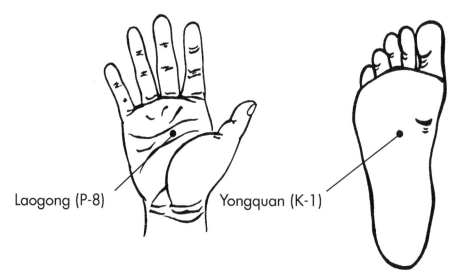

Figure 20. Laogong (P-8) Cavity   Figure 21. Yongquan (K-1) Cavity

the Paricardium Primary Qi Channel (Xin Bao Luo Jing, 心包絡經) (Figure 20) while the Yongquan cavity, (K-1) (湧泉) located at the center of the feet, belongs to the Kidneys Primary Channel (Shen Jing, 腎經) (Figure 21). These four gates are considered as the four major gates which regulate the body's Qi status. Naturally, the Qi led to the palms and soles also provides their sensitive feeling. The fifth gate can be the crown of the head, the Baihui (Gv-20) (百會) (also called Tian Ling Gai, 天靈蓋) or the third eye (Yintang, M-HN-3, 印堂) (Tian Yan, 天眼).

Taijiquan emphasizes central equilibrium (Zhong Ding, 中定). *Taiji Classic* says: "If there is a top, there is a bottom; if there is a front, there is a back; if there is a left, there is a right."[11] This means central equilibrium and means the balance and equilibrium of a point, which is the Real Dan Tian (i.e., center of gravity or physical center). Four gates breathing through the palms and soles provides you with an equilibrium, while the fifth gate raises up the spirit and offers you central balance.

Girdle Vessel Breathing (Dai Mai Xi) is related to Skin (or Body) Breathing (Fu Xi or Ti Xi) and Wuji Breathing (Wuji Xi) is related to Bone Marrow Breathing (Sui Xi). Girdle Vessel Breathing and Wuji Breathing, one is Yang and one is Yin. In Girdle Vessel Breathing, the Qi's circulation is branched out through Luo (i.e., secondary Qi channels) from the primary Qi channels and reaches to the skin, thereby forming the Guardian Qi (Wei Qi). In Wuji Breathing, the Qi is condensed inward from four limbs and hundreds of bones (i.e., entire body) to the Real Dan Tian (Zhen Dan Tian). Hence, the Qi is stored at the Qi residence and condensed to the bone marrow. Since these two ways of breathing are closely related to Embryonic Breathing it will be discussed at the same time with Embryonic Breathing. Other breathing such as Hibernation Breathing (Dong

Mian Xi), Turtle Breathing (Gui Xi), etc., are not related to Taijiquan's regulating of breathing. We will not discuss them here.

帶脈息者有關於膚息（體息）也。無極息有關於骨髓息
也。帶脈息，無極息，一陽一陰。帶脈息，氣由主經脈
外引隨絡外行通達皮膚而成衛氣。無極息，氣由四肢百
骸內收斂至真丹田，氣由之蓄於氣舍，凝於骨髓。此兩
息與胎息有關，將於論胎息時一概論之。其他，如冬眠
息、龜息等者，不在太極拳調息之規範內，不以述之。

When the Qi is led to expand in the Girdle Vessel (Dai Mai, 帶脈), the Guardian Qi (Wei Qi, 衛氣) will also be expanded and strengthened. This will lead the body to a more Yang state since the Qi has been led outward and manifested. However, when the Qi is led to the center of the Real Dan Tian, the Qi can be stored there. In addition, the Qi will also be led to the bone marrow to nourish it. Naturally, the Guardian Qi will be weakened and the body will become more Yin. Since these two breathing techniques are related to Taijiquan, we will discuss them in more detail later.

2. Theory of Normal and Reverse Abdominal Breathing 論順逆腹式呼吸

In regulating the breathing, Reverse Abdominal Breathing is considered Yang while Normal Abdominal Breathing is considered Yin. In Reverse Breathing, inhalation is Yin while exhalation is Yang. When inhaling, the abdomen is withdrawn and the Huiyin (i.e., perineum) is gently held up. When exhaling, the abdomen is expanding while the Huiyin is pushing out softly. (When this happens,) substantial amounts of Qi will circulate sideways along the secondary Qi channels (i.e., Luo) to the skin, leading to what is called Body Breathing (Ti Xi) or Skin Breathing (Fu Xi). When inhaling, the abdomen is withdrawn while the Huiyin is held up gently and softly. The majority of Qi will condense inward along the secondary Qi channels to the bone marrow, leading to what is called Marrow Breathing (Sui Xi). Body Breathing is Yang while Marrow Breathing is Yin. When you exhale, the Yi leads the Qi outward to supply the Qi to the tendons and bones; Jin is emitted. On the contrary, when you inhale, the Yi leads the Qi inward and stores the Qi in the bone marrow. When the Qi is stored deeply, the emitting Jin must be strong. Therefore, if (you) practice Taijiquan for martial arts and wish to emit the Jin from the body, (you) must use Reverse Abdominal Breathing.

調息以反（逆）腹呼吸為陽，正（順）腹呼吸為陰。逆
呼吸，吸為陰，呼為陽。吸，小腹內收，會陰上提。呼，
小腹外張，會陰輕輕下推。主氣沿絡橫行而達皮膚，為
之體息或膚息。吸，小腹內縮，會陰輕輕柔和上提。主
氣沿絡橫行而凝骨髓，為之髓息。體息為陽，髓息為陰。
呼時，意引氣外行而供能于筋骨，勁因之而發。此如推
車然。反之，吸時，意引氣內行而蓄氣于骨髓。氣蓄得
深，勁之發必強。因之，習太極拳，如為武學而欲發勁
于身，必用逆腹呼吸。

Please see Figure 22 for the breathing's Yin and Yang. In Normal Abdominal Breathing, the main Qi flow circulates following the 12 primary Qi channels communicating between the limbs and the 12 internal organs. When this happens, since the Qi is not led sideways to energize the muscles, you are in a relaxed state (Figure 23). However, in Reverse Abdominal Breathing, the main Qi flow circulates sideways to muscles, skin, and bone marrow. Consequently, the body is tensed, and you feel either hot or cold (Figure 24). In Reverse Abdominal Breathing, if exhalation is longer than inhalation, such as laughing with the sound of Ha, then more Qi is led to the skin surface. In this case, you feel hot. Conversely, if inhalation is longer than exhalation, such as when you cry, are cold, or are in fear at the sound of Hen, then more Qi is led inward to the marrow. In this case, you feel cold. From this, you can see that through different ways of breathing, you can change the body's Yin and Yang. That is the reason why breathing is commonly recognized as Kan (坎) (water) and Li (離) (fire) which can adjust the body's Yin-Yang condition.

In addition, when you use Reverse Abdominal Breathing, the majority of Qi will be led sideways to energize the muscles, thus, the Qi is used to manifest the physical power to a higher state. For example, when you push a car or lift a heavy weight, you will change your Normal Breathing into Reverse without even thinking about it. This is the way of Dao (道) (i.e., Nature). Therefore, if you practice Taijiquan just for relaxation, you should use Normal Abdominal Breathing. However, if you have a sense of enemy and an intention to energize the physical body for power manifestation, then you should use Reverse Abdominal Breathing.

Breathing's Yin and Yang in Taijiquan 太極拳呼吸陰陽圖

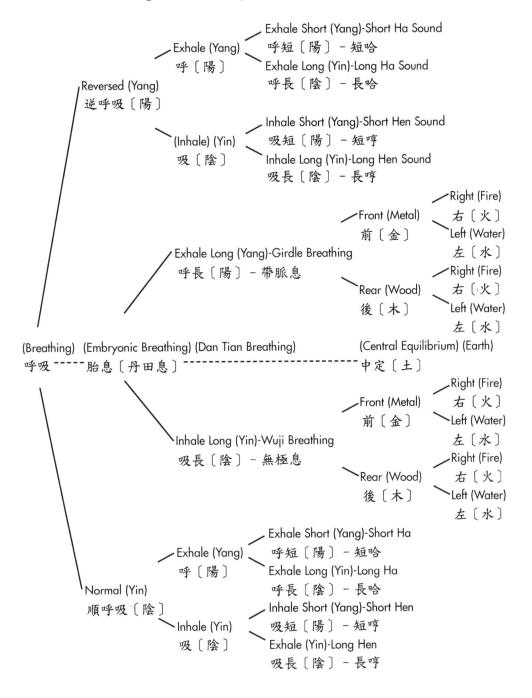

Figure 22. Breathing's Yin and Yang in Taijiquan

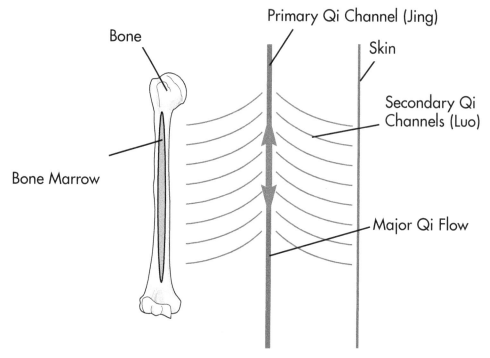

Figure 23. Major Qi Flow in Normal Abdominal Breathing

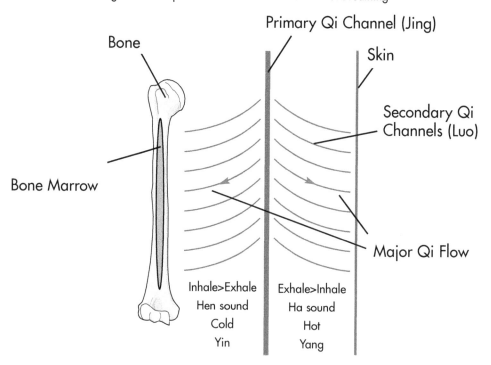

Figure 24. Major Qi Flow in Reversed Abdominal Breathing

In Normal Abdominal Breathing, inhalation is also considered Yin, while exhalation is also considered Yang. When inhaling, the abdomen is expanding and the Huiyin is pushing out gently. When exhaling, the abdomen is withdrawn and the Huiyin is held up gently. In exhalation, the Qi will be circulating along the primary Qi channels and reach to the four limbs; hence it is called Four Gates Breathing. What is Four Gates Breathing? It is Laogong and Yongquan breathing. When inhaling, the majority of Qi will condense inward along the primary Qi channels and reach the internal organs. From this, (we can see that) the majority of Qi will not circulate sideways, the tendons and bones will not be tightened and the Qi is circulating smoothly. Therefore, if (you) practice Taijiquan just for loosening the body and softening the body, Normal Abdominal Breathing is better.

正腹呼吸，吸亦為陰，呼亦為陽。吸，小腹外張，會陰輕輕下推。呼，小腹內收，會陰上提。呼，氣沿經直行而達四肢，曰四心呼吸。四心呼吸者，勞宮、湧泉呼吸也。吸，主氣沿經直行而斂於內臟。因此，主氣不橫行，不繃筋骨，身體鬆爽，氣行無阻。因之，習太極拳，如為鬆身軟身而已，順腹呼吸較佳。

Though Normal Abdominal Breathing is used for Four Gates Breathing (Si Xin Xi, 四心息), it does not mean that Reverse Abdominal Breathing cannot be used for Four Gates Breathing. You should always remember, breathing is only a strategy for leading the Qi. If you have a sense of enemy and have an intention to lead the Qi to the four gates, you commonly also use Reverse Abdominal Breathing. In fact, in order to coordinate with the fifth gate in raising up your spirit, usually, it is more efficient and effective to use Reverse Abdominal Breathing instead of Normal Abdominal Breathing.

Breathing can again be classified as scholar and martial. Scholar breathing is Yin, is calm, slow, slender, uniform, and smooth. Use the peaceful Yi and calm Xin to search for the spiritual condensation. Scholar breathing can be used for both Normal Abdominal or Reverse Abdominal Breathing. Martial breathing is Yang, is fast acting, vigorous, and short. Using the concentrated Yi to direct (i.e., govern) the Xin in searching for the upraising of the spirit, hence reaching the effectiveness of the Jin's emitting. Martial breathing is often used for Jin's emission in the martial arts and therefore, Reverse Abdominal Breathing is commonly used.

呼吸者，再分文武也。文呼吸者，陰也，靜也，緩也，細也，均也，勻也，以意寧心靜追求神凝。文呼吸者，正、反呼吸皆可用。武呼吸者，陽也，動也，快也，猛也，短也，以意專導心追求神提以達勁發之效。武呼吸者，多用於武學以為發勁之用，因而以反呼吸為主。

In Chinese Qigong society, apart from being Normal Abdominal or Reverse Abdominal, breathing can also be classified as scholar (Wen Huo, 文火) or martial (Wu Huo, 武火). In scholar breathing, the length of the breath is relatively longer and thus, the body is more relaxed. In martial breathing, the length of the breath is shorter. Though in martial breathing, the Qi can be built up much more quickly, due to greater physical tension, the body will turn more Yang and the built up Qi will be consumed at a faster rate. In scholar breathing, though the Qi cannot be built up in a short time, due to the relaxation of the physical body, moreover the Qi can be stored easily inside the body. This will make the physical body more calm and Yin.

3. Secret of Embryonic Breathing 胎息法訣 (Wuji Breathing, Girdle Vessel Breathing) (無極呼吸、帶脈呼吸)

What is Embryonic Breathing? It is the Real Dan Tian's breathing, and is also called 'Cavity Breathing.' Embryonic Breathing Classic said: "The embryo is conceived from the hidden or undeveloped Qi. Qi is accepted through the regulated breath of the embryo. When Qi is present, the body may live; when Shen (Spirit) abandons the body and the embryo disperses, death will follow. Cultivation of Shen and Qi makes long life possible. Protect and nourish the spiritual embryo to build up Shen and Qi. When Shen moves, the Qi moves; where Shen stops, the Qi stops. For life to flourish, spirit and energy (Shen and Qi) must interact harmoniously. When the Xin (heart-mind) is not touched (i.e., moved by surrounding environments), not a thought goes or comes. (When thoughts are not going and coming), nature is free. Intelligence in action is the only true path." The Daoist book also said: "When the spirit is conceived in the Qi cavity (i.e., Real Dan Tian) it is called embryo, and when the Qi reaches the Qi cavity it is called breathing. Conceiving the spirit and breathing the Qi, Gongfu gradually advances into Embryonic Breathing. Then there is no exit and no entrance and you will never have ordinary breathing." From this, (you) can see that Embryonic Breathing is the method of storing the Qi and nurturing the (spiritual) embryo. Storing the Qi is the Dao of longevity and nurturing the (spiritual) embryo is the way of reaching the divine and Buddhahood.

胎息者，真丹田呼吸，又稱穴位呼吸也。《胎息經》云：「胎從伏氣中結，氣從有胎中息。氣入身來為之生，神去離形謂之死。知神氣可以長生，固守虛無，以養神氣。神行則氣行，神住則氣住。若欲長生，神氣相住。心不動念，無去無來，不出不入，自然常住。勤而行之，是真道路。」道書亦云：「藏神於氣穴曰胎，氣至氣穴為息，胎其神息其氣，功夫進至胎息，則不出不入，永無凡息矣。」由此可知，胎息乃蓄氣養胎之法也。氣蓄節用乃長生之道，養胎乃成仙立佛之法也。

Embryonic Breathing is a well-known breathing technique that allows you to store the Qi at the Real Dan Tian. The Real Dan Tian is regarded today as the second brain, which can store a bioelectric charge and can be considered a biobattery.[7,8] When the bioelectricity storage has reached a high level, the vital force and energy manifested by the physical body will be strong. Naturally, you will be healthy and have a long life. There are more than 150 Daoist documents about Embryonic Breathing that have been revealed today. This has provided a reliable guideline and informs us of how to practice Embryonic Breathing.

In Qigong practice, generally there are two main purposes. One is to build up the Qi to an abundant level, and the other is to improve the quality of the Qi's manifestation. The purpose of practicing Muscle/Tendon Changing is to build up the Qi and then manifest it to the physical body for strength and health (i.e., long healthy life). This serves the purpose of increasing the quantity of Qi. The practicing of Marrow/Brain Washing is to purify the mind to a higher concentrated state so the usage of the Qi can reach its maximum efficiency. That means to improve the quality of the Qi's manifestation by raising up the Spirit of Vitality. However, in order to raise up the spirit to a higher level, you must know how to store the Qi at the Real Dan Tian to an abundant level by Embryonic Breathing, and how to then lead it up the spinal cord (i.e., Chong Mai, 衝脈) to the brain. This activates the brain cells to a more energized state. From this, you can see that Embryonic Breathing is the key to raising up the spirit and reaching enlightenment.

The secret key of practicing Embryonic Breathing is keeping the Yi (i.e., wisdom mind) at the Real Dan Tian. When the Yi is kept at the Real Dan Tian, the Qi will be stored and the usage (of Qi) will be regulated (i.e., used efficiently). If the Yi is away (from the Qi residence), then Qi will be led out from its residence and be consumed. When Qi is overused, then it will be exhausted, consequently the body will degenerate and the spirit will weaken and wither. Those who are learning the Dao must know this theory. In addition, (they) must also know the Dao of producing the Qi and growing the elixir. If (they) do not know this, then the Qi will also be exhausted. The place where the elixir is produced is what the Daoists called Lower Dan Tian or Elixir Furnace, the Chinese medical family called Qihai cavity, and is known as the abdomen by the general public. From modern science, it is known that this place (i.e., abdomen) is constructed from six layers of muscles and fasciae, mutually sandwiched. The fasciae is also the storage place for fat when too much food is absorbed into the body. Fat is actually post-heaven food essence. From the abdominal up and down exercises, through biochemical reaction, the stored fat will be converted into bioelectricity (i.e., Qi or energy). This kind of abdominal breathing is called "Back to Childhood Breathing," also "Qihai Breathing."

胎息法訣，意守真丹田也。意守真丹田，則氣蓄節用。
意外馳則氣由氣舍外引而為所用。用過之，則竭，身體
老化之，精神衰退之。學道者，必懂此理。不僅如此，
亦必知生氣產丹之道。不知，氣亦竭矣。產丹處，道家
之下丹田或丹爐也，醫家之氣海穴也，亦即大眾所知之
小腹也。由近代科學知此處乃由六層之肌肉與膜互相夾
層而成。然而此膜處亦為多食時身體主要存蓄脂肪之所。
脂肪者乃後天食精也。由小腹上下起伏之反復運動，積
蓄之脂肪由生化化學反應而轉化成生化電（氣）。小腹
呼吸者，返童呼吸也，氣海呼吸也。

All the revealed documents agree that in order to store the Qi at the Real Dan Tian to an abundant level, you must know two main keys. One is learning how to keep your mind at the Real Dan Tian so the Qi will not be led away from its residence. The other one is learning how to produce more Qi in the body.

Whenever your mind generates an idea, EMF (i.e., electromotive force) (Dian Dong Shi, 電動勢) is created. This will lead the Qi either to the brain or to the physical body for manifestation. That means you are consuming the Qi stored in the Real Dan Tian. Once you have learned how to keep your mind at the Real Dan Tian, the Qi will stay at its residence and not be led outward. Consequently, the Qi can be stored.

In addition, you can produce Qi in the body at higher levels. Traditionally, you could use special herbs to increase the quantity of Qi. However, nearly all Daoist Qigong masters believed that the best way to produce the most pure Qi is to convert the essence stored in the body into Qi. As long as you use the abdominal area to control your breathing, the up and down abdominal exercises will convert the stored food essence (i.e., fat) into Qi (Figure 25). Fat is the food essence which has been filtered and purified through your body's system. It has a high calorie content that can be efficiently converted into Qi through biochemical reaction. Breathing with the up and down abdominal exercises is also called "back to the childhood breathing" (Fan Tong Hu Xi, 返童呼吸) since babies move their abdominal areas when they breathe. The abdominal area is called "Elixir Field" (Dan Tian, 丹田) by Daoists and "Qi Ocean" (Qihai, 氣海) by Chinese medicine. In addition, this place is also called "Elixir Furnace" (Dan Lu, 丹爐) because it produces elixir (i.e., Qi).

From this, you can see that abdominal breathing is the key to producing Qi. Normally, there are two kinds of abdominal breathing; Normal Abdominal Breathing (Zheng Hu Xi, 正呼吸) and Reverse Abdominal Breathing (Fan Hu Xi or Ni Hu Xi, 反呼吸・逆呼吸) which have been discussed earlier.

Daoists call the Lower Dan Tian "False Dan Tian." It was named this because, although this place can produce elixir and generate Qi, once the Qi is produced, it immediately enters into the Conception and Governing Vessels' Small Circulation. Consequently, it will be distributed to the twelve primary Qi channels and be used by the physical body. Thus, it is known that, though the Lower Dan Tian is an elixir furnace, it cannot store the elixir (i.e., Qi) efficiently. If the elixir cannot be stored to a higher abundant level, then the Daoist Gongfu (i.e., training) such as "refine the Qi and sublimate it upward," or "returning the essence to nourish the brain" cannot be accomplished effectively. In order to store elixir, (you) must know how to use the method of Embryonic Breathing to lead the elixir produced from the elixir furnace to the Real Dan Tian and store it there. The location of the Real Dan Tian is where, on the top, it is not against the internal kidneys, and, on the bottom, it does not touch the external kidneys. It rests behind the navel and in front of the Mingmen cavity (i.e., behind the Life Door and in front of the Closed Door). This is what the Daoists called the "Jade Ring Cavity," where the embryo is formed. This place is also called the "second brain" by science. (In fact,) this is the place where the large and small intestines are located. When an embryo is forming and growing into a baby, it must rely on abundant Qi and therefore, the embryo is formed in this Qi residence.

道家稱下丹田為假丹田。其因不外乎此處雖能產丹生氣，然一但氣生則馬上進入任、督兩脈之小周天循環，而分部至十二經為身體所用也。因之而知，下丹田雖為丹爐，卻不能有效的蓄丹（電）。丹不能蓄至一高層次，則道家所謂之練氣昇華、返精補腦之功夫必不能有效的施行。為能蓄丹，必懂的如何由胎息之法將丹爐之丹內引至真丹田而蓄之。真丹田之處，上不衝內腎，下不抵外腎，臍後與命門之前（生門之後密戶之前）。此為道家所稱之玉環穴，胎兒成形之所也。此處亦為今科學上所稱人之第二腦也，亦即大小腸內臟之所也。胎兒成形與成長必賴充沛之氣，因之胎於此氣舍也。

If you know how to produce Qi at the abdominal area, but do not know how to lead it inward and store it at the Real Dan Tian, your practice will stay on the Muscle/Tendon Changing level. Though you can increase the quantity of Qi and manifest it into physical health, you will not be able to reach the goal of spiritual enlightenment. In order to do so, you must know how to lead the Qi inward and store it in the Real Dan Tian.

According to Chinese medicine and Qigong practice, the kidneys on the back are considered "internal kidneys" (Nei Shen, 內腎) while the testicles or ovaries are considered "external kidneys" (Wai Shen, 外腎) (Figure 26). In Daoist society, the navel is considered the "Life Door" (Sheng Men, 生門) since it provides life before your birth, and the Mingmen (Gv-4) (命門) is considered the "closed door" (Mi Hu,

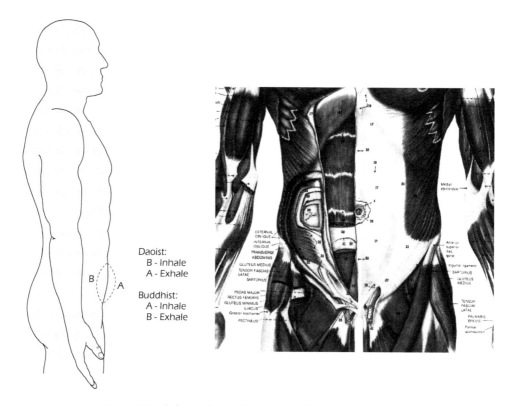

Daoist:
 B - Inhale
 A - Exhale

Buddhist:
 A - Inhale
 B - Exhale

Figure 25. Abdominal Breathing to Start the Fire (Qi Huo)

密戶) which is normally closed. Mingmen is a Chinese medical term meaning "Life Door" since it connects to the life center, biobattery or Real Dan Tian. The Real Dan Tian is also called "Jade Ring Cavity" (Yu Huan Xue, 玉環穴), the place where the embryo is carried by its mother.

The purpose of Embryonic Breathing is to lead the Qi to the Real Dan Tian. The key (to training) is to keep the Yi at the Real Dan Tian and the secret (of practice) is to regulate the breathing. The method of regulating the breathing in Embryonic Breathing is: when (you have) reached the stage of regulating without regulating in (your) Reverse Abdominal Breathing training, then (you) add the Mingmen breathing. That means that when the abdomen is withdrawing and the Huiyin is holding upward, at the same time, the Mingmen is also withdrawing. When the abdomen is expanding and the Huiyin is gently pushing downward, the Mingmen is also expanding. In this case, due to the pressing and releasing massaging at the Mingmen area, the original essence can be smoothly produced from the adrenal glands. Original essence is what (we) call hormones today. Hormones are actually the catalysts which are needed for the body's biochemical reactions. When the content of the body's hormones is normal, then the body's biochemical reaction can be completed smoothly. That means the cells' metabolic process can be carried out efficiently. In this case, the body's Qi will be abundant, the vital force will be strong, and the body's degeneration will be slowed down. This is the crucial key to delaying aging and returning the healthy function (of the body).

胎息之的為引氣內存至真丹田。其竅在於意守真丹田，其訣在於調息。胎息調息之法在調反腹呼吸調至調而不調之境界時，則加以命門之呼吸。亦即當小腹內收會陰上提之時，同時命門之處亦往內收。當小腹外張會陰下推之時，命門亦往外張。如此，由於命門部位之壓放按摩，腎上腺之元精可順利的產生。元精者，今所謂之賀爾蒙也。賀爾蒙者，乃身體中生化反應所須之催化劑。賀爾蒙含量高而正常，則身體中之生化反應順利完成。亦即身體中細胞之新陳代謝可以有效的施行。如此，則體內之氣勢厚，生命力強，身體老化緩慢，此為遲老返機之關鍵。

From the preceding discussion, you know that in order to store the Qi at the Real Dan Tian, you must keep your mind there so the Qi will not be led outward and be wasted. However, when you meditate it is not easy to keep your mind there for a long period of time. To reach this goal, you must first have regulated your body to an extremely relaxed state. Wherever your body is tensed, the Qi will be led there and consumed. Therefore, you must learn how to use your mind to control the muscles in the abdominal area efficiently through abdominal breathing. You must be able to regulate the abdominal breathing until conscious regulating is unnecessary. Then you can begin your Embryonic Breathing.

From my personal experience, the trick to keeping your mind at your center of gravity (i.e., Real Dan Tian) is to begin the breathing training with the abdominal up and down movement in the front, while also keeping the Mingmen area's up and down movement on the back. When this happens, the movement of the front and back will balance each other and this will provide you with a centered feeling. That means the mind can be kept at the center. At the beginning of training, your mind is on the front and the back, however, after you have practiced for a long time and reached a level of regulating without regulating, your mind will move to the center easily. In my experience, using the Reverse Abdominal Breathing techniques with the Mingmen and Huyin's movements is easier than using them with the Normal Abdominal Breathing.

Furthermore, due to the diaphragm's up and down movements in the deep abdominal breathing, the adrenals (i.e., internal kidneys) will be pressed and massaged. Consequently, the original essence (i.e., hormones) will be produced. In addition, due to the Huyin's holding up and pushing down, the Qi will reach

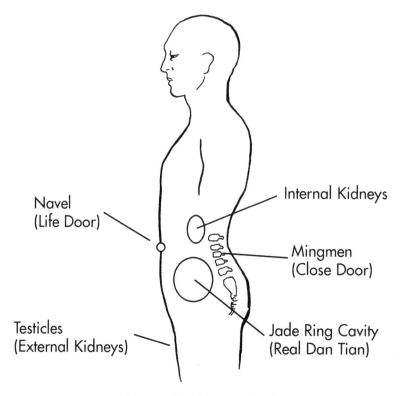

Navel
(Life Door)

Internal Kidneys

Mingmen
(Close Door)

Testicles
(External Kidneys)

Jade Ring Cavity
(Real Dan Tian)

Figure 26. Life Door, Closed Door, and Jade Ring Cavity

the testicles or ovaries (i.e., external kidneys) and consequently, the original essence (i.e., hormones) will also naturally be secreted. This is the process which the Daoists called "to refine the essence and convert it into Qi."

再者，由深腹呼吸橫膈膜之上下運動，腎上腺（內腎）
被壓縮按摩，因而促進元精（賀爾蒙）之產生。不但如
此，由於會陰之上下提推，氣達睪丸或卵巢（外腎）因
而元精（賀爾蒙）亦隨之分泌而出。此乃道家所謂之練
精化氣也。

One of the benefits of this training is produced by the movements of the Mingmen and Huiyin areas. As these areas move, the adrenal glands and testicles are stimulated. Consequently, hormones (i.e., original essence) (Yuan Jing, 元精) can be produced. In addition, due to deep breathing exercises, the diaphragm will also massage the kidneys and stimulate the production of DHEA (Dehydroepiandrosterone) (i.e., hormone produced by the adrenal glands). When the hormone content in our blood stream is high, the body's biochemical reactions will be smooth and metabolization will be carried out efficiently. Naturally, we will be healthier and live longer.

In order to reach the goal of keeping the Yi at the Real Dan Tian in Embryonic Breathing, at the beginning, the Yi is on the Life Door (i.e., navel), Closed Door (i.e., Mingmen), and the Huiyin's up and down exercises. However, when (you) have reached a stage of regulating through no regulating, then the Yi will not be on the movement and will gradually shift to the Real Dan Tian and remain there. After long practice, the Xin is peaceful and the Yi is calm, the spirit is condensed inward, and is not bothered by outside disturbances. This is why Lao Zi said: "Keep physical body and spiritual body in unity, can they not be separated? Specialize in training the Qi to reach its softest, can it be like a baby?" This practice is also "to reach the extreme emptiness and to keep the ultimate calmness sincerely," the great Dao of Embryonic Breathing.

為求達胎息意守丹田之目的，起先意必在生門、密戶之前後與會陰之上下蠕動。然而在調至調而不調之境界時，意即不在動而漸趨至丹田而守之。久而久之，心平意靜，精神內斂，外事不擾。此即老子所謂之：〝載營魄抱一，能無離乎？專氣致柔，能如嬰兒乎？〞亦即〝致虛極，守靜篤。〞之胎息大道也。

In Chapter 10 of *Dao De Jing* (道德經), Lao Zi (老子) emphasizes the unification of the physical body and the spiritual body. When the physical body and the spiritual body are united and in harmony with each other, we will be able to attain the human Dao and live long. In order to reach this goal, we must learn how to breathe naturally and softly like a baby.

In addition, in Chapter 16, Lao Zi states that the way of returning to the origin of our lives involves keeping our minds in the state of extreme emptiness and calmness. That means to keep the mind in the origin of your life, which is the Real Dan Tian.

Embryonic Breathing can again be divided into Yin and Yang. Yang Embryonic Breathing means that the exhalation is longer than the inhalation, the internal Qi is expanding through the Girdle Vessel, and (consequently) the Guardian Qi is strengthened. This is what is called Skin Breathing (Fu Xi) or Body Breathing (Ti Xi) in the Daoist's definition. This kind of breathing is suitable for practice in the fall and winter. The reason is when fall and winter are near, (our) Guardian Qi is getting weaker and our defense against disease is weakened, so it is easy for us to catch a cold. In the seasons of spring and summer, the Guardian Qi is already strong, so if you practice too much Body Breathing, the body will turn too Yang. Furthermore, the Qi stored in the body will be wasted. Yin Embryonic Breathing means that the inhalation is longer than the exhalation. The Yi is aiming for extreme calmness and is kept at the center (i.e., Real Dan Tian). Consequently, the Qi can be condensed inward and stored in the Real Dan Tian and can also reach the bone marrow. This is what is called "Marrow Breathing" or "Wuji Breathing." The practice of this kind of breathing is suitable for the spring and summer. This is because during spring and summer, the external Qi is getting strong, and the need for Guardian Qi is not as high as it is in the fall and winter. This is the time to lead the Qi inward and store it. This can also supply the Qi to the bone marrow, which is required for the production of blood cells.

胎息者，可再分陰陽。陽胎息者，呼長於吸，內氣由帶
脈外張，衛氣加強。此乃道家所謂之膚息或體息也。此
息之習乃適於秋、冬之時。此乃秋、冬之臨，衛氣轉弱，
身體之免疫力低，容易感冒。春、夏之季，衛氣已強，
如多練體息，可使身體趨陽，並徒浪費身中所存之氣。
陰胎息者，吸長於呼，意趨極靜而守中，氣由之內斂而
存於真丹田，而達骨髓。此乃所謂之髓息或無極息也。
此息之習乃適於春、夏兩季。此乃因春、夏之臨，外氣
轉強，衛氣之需不如秋、冬之時。此時正好引氣內存並
供氣給骨髓以生產血球之需。

Once you have practiced Embryonic Breathing to a profound stage and can keep your mind at the Real Dan Tian easily, then you can use it to control the body's Yin and Yang status easily. For example, in Embryonic Breathing practice, if your exhalation is longer than your inhalation, the Qi in the Girdle Vessel (Dai Mai, 帶脈) will be expanded. Consequently, the Guardian Qi (Wei Qi, 衛氣) can be expanded and enhanced. This kind of Embryonic Breathing is called "Girdle Vessel Breathing" (Dai Mai Xi, 帶脈息), "Body Breathing" (Ti Xi, 體息), or "Skin Breathing" (Fu Xi, 膚息). When the Guardian Qi is strong, the immune system is strong. This kind of breathing is more suitably practiced in the winter time.

However, if your inhalation is longer than your exhalation, then you are leading Qi from the surface of the skin to the Real Dan Tian and also to the bone marrow. The Guardian Qi will be weakened and the storage of Qi at the Real Dan Tian can be enhanced and can reach a higher level. This kind of Embryonic Breathing is called "Cavity Breathing" (Xue Wei Hu Xi, 穴位呼吸), or also "Marrow Breathing" (Sui Xi, 髓息). It can also be called "Wuji Breathing" (Wuji Hu Xi, 無極呼吸) since your mind is on the center of gravity, which is the Wuji state. This breathing is most suitably practiced in the summer time when the body has extra energy.

From the above, (you) can see that Embryonic Breathing is the required practice for those who wish to cultivate the Dao and train the Qi. Taijiquan was originated from the Daoist society. Therefore, in order to reach a higher level of achievement, those who practice Taijiquan must know Embryonic Breathing and practice it diligently.

由上可知，胎息乃修道練氣者必知之術。太極拳乃源於
道門，因之，習太極拳者，為達高層次之成果，必知胎
息並勤練之。

Those who would like to obtain health and longevity should learn Embryonic Breathing. For those who wish to reach the final goal of enlightenment, Embryonic Breathing is a necessary practice. Taijiquan originated in Daoist monasteries, therefore, the final goal of cultivation is to reach spiritual enlightenment.

4. Secret Knacks of Regulating the Breathing 調息竅門

The keys to regulating the breathing and transporting Qi are in two places: the Huiyin and the palate (of the mouth). The Huiyin cavity is the connecting point of the four Yin (Qi) vessels and is the controlling and releasing gate for the four Yin Qi reservoirs. When the Huiyin is pushed out, the Qi in the Yin vessels is released and when the Huiyin is lifted upward, the Qi in the Yin vessels is contained and condensed. For example, when (you) laugh out loud, (your) exhalation is longer than (your) inhalation, and when you exhale, the Huiyin is pushed out naturally, the entire body's Yang is manifested and the Guardian Qi is strengthened; consequently, the body gets hot and begins to sweat. Conversely, when (you) are sad and depressed, the inhalation is longer than the exhalation and when you inhale, the Huiyin is lifted upward naturally, the Marrow Qi is increased and the Guardian Qi is condensed inward, hence the body feels chilly. From these (you) can see that when (you) practice Qigong, coordinating the breathing with the Huiyin's lifting and pushing is one pf the key knacks to governing the entire body's Qi status.

調息運氣之竅，在於會陰與上顎兩處。會陰穴者，四陰
脈之交接點也，乃四陰脈氣壩收放之門。會陰下推，陰
脈之氣外放；會陰上提，陰脈之氣收斂持存。譬如在發
大哈笑聲時，呼氣比吸氣長，並在呼氣時，會陰自然下
推。全身陽發，衛氣增強，身體發熱發汗。反之，在悲
哀沮喪之時，吸氣比呼氣為長，並在吸氣時，會陰自然
上提，髓氣增強，衛氣收斂，身體發冷。由此可知，練
氣功時，如何配合呼吸與會陰之上提和下推，乃控制全
身氣勢之關竅也。

In the past, it was common that a master would keep two secret keys of regulating to himself. These secrets would not be revealed to the student until he/she proved trustworthy. One of the secret keys is learning how to control the Huiyin (Co-1) (會陰) (i.e., perineum). This place is the controlling gate of the body's Yin and Yang. Huiyin means "meet Yin" in Chinese and is the meeting place of the four Yin vessels: Conception (Ren Mai, 任脈), Thrusting (Chong Mai, 衝脈), Yin Heel (Yin-qiao Mai, 陰蹺脈), and Yin Linking Vessels (Yinwei Mai, 陰維脈). When this gate is pushed out, the Qi in these four Yin vessels is released, and when this gate is held up, the Qi in the four Yin vessels is kept in and preserved. Because of this, this gate can control the body's Yin-Yang status. In my personal experience, this place acts as a pump or a piston to a Qi chamber that controls the storage and release of Qi.

> *In addition to this practice, there is another key: the palate of the mouth. Daoists believe that the palate is the connecting place of the Conception and Governing Vessels. Normally, the palate is not connected to the tip of the tongue and (there-fore) the Qi is stagnant at the throat area for uttering sound. Therefore, due to the stagnation of the Qi, the mouth is dry. However, if (you) practice Qigong without the necessity of making a sound, then (you) should touch (your) tongue upward to the palate so as to connect the Conception and Governing Vessels. This is what is called "building the magpie bridge," or "releasing the heavenly water." When this happens, the root of the tongue will generate saliva to moisturize the throat and to calm down the Yang fire, and allow the Qi to be transported between Conception and Governing Vessels without stagnation.*

除此一竅，還有一竅在上顎。道家認為上顎乃任督兩脈
交接之所。平時，上顎與舌尖之端，並不隨時相接，氣
滯於喉以供發聲之用。因此，氣滯口乾。然在練氣功時，
口不須發聲，當以舌端上頂上顎以接連順通任督兩脈之
氣。此為搭鵲橋也，放天池水也。此時，舌根生津，以
潤喉口，以降陽火，任督兩脈之氣可以通行無阻。

Another key that a master kept secret is the position of the tongue during Qigong practice. The Conception and Governing Vessels are not well connected in the mouth area. For the Qi to circulate smoothly without stagnation, the tongue should touch the palate of the mouth. This connection is called "building the mag-pie bridge" (Da Que Qiao, 搭鵲橋). According to a Chinese story, long ago a Cowherd (Niu Lang, 牛郎) and a Weaving Maid (Zhi Nu, 織女) would meet once a year on the seventh day of the seventh moon on a bridge across the Milky Way. The bridge was formed by sympathetic magpies. This story has become a symbol of Yin and Yang's interacting or connecting in Qigong practice. When Yin and Yang meet, then the body can be harmonized.

When the tongue touches the palate of the mouth, saliva will be generated. Since the head is considered the heaven while the perineum is considered the sea bottom, the saliva produced is called "heavenly water" (Tian Chi Shui, 天池水) and the area under the tongue is called "heaven pond" (Tian Chi, 天池). When the saliva is generated to a comfortable amount, you should swallow it and use the mind to lead it down to the

Real Dan Tian. This will help you lead the fire Qi downward to cool down the body.

> *If those who are learning Taiji can apply the above two keys into their regular natural (breathing), then the accomplishment of Taiji Qigong can be achieved within days (i.e., expected). These two keys were also the keys that the ancient masters kept as secrets. They were not passed down to those disciples who were not loyal and moral.*

學者如能配合上述二竅於自然之中，則太極氣功之造詣可指日而成。此二竅乃昔時為師者藏訣之所，非有忠有德之徒，不隨便授之也。

At the beginning, it is hard to control your Huiyin's movement smoothly and naturally. In addition, due to the positioning of the tongue, an uncomfortable and tense feeling may be experienced at the root of the tongue. However, after you practice for some time, you will see it will become easier and more comfortable.

PART IV

About Regulating the Emotional Mind 論調心

1. Importance of Regulating the Emotional Mind 調心之要

What is regulating the Xin (i.e., heart, emotional mind)? It calls for using the Yi (i.e., rational thinking, logical mind) to regulate the Xin. Xin belongs to Yang and is active while Yi belongs to Yin and is calm. Dao Treasure, Thesis of Sitting and Oblivion *states: "Xin is the master of the entire body and the commander of a hundred spirits (i.e., all spirits); when it is calm, wisdom is generated and when it is active, then confused. Delusion is generated (i.e., decided) within the action and calmness (of the Xin)." This Xin means Xin and Yi. If the Yi is unable to regulate the Xin, then the Xin easily becomes active, oppressive and impatient, confused and depressed, and it cannot control itself. Thus, the Yi also cannot be calm and peaceful. When the Yi is not calm and peaceful, then the Qi is hard to lead.*

調心者，以意調心也。心者，陽也，動也。意者，陰也，靜也。《道藏・坐忘論》：「夫心者一身之主，百神之帥，靜則生慧，動則生昏，欣迷動靜之中。」此心者即心意之謂也。意不能調心，則心動、悶躁、昏沉、而不知自我。意亦不能寧靜。意不寧，則氣難引。

According to traditional Chinese concepts, we have two minds, one is called "Xin" (心) (i.e., heart or emotional mind) and the other is called "Yi" (意) (i.e., logical, rational, and wise thinking). Regulating the mind means using the Yi to regulate emotional disturbances (i.e., Xin). When the Xin is regulated, you can be calm and the Yi can be strong. Conversely, if the Xin is disturbed and confused, the Yi will also be unsteady. In this case, the Yi will not be able to lead the Qi effectively.

Ancient ancestors said: "When teaching a person the great Dao, first teach him/her how to stop the Nian (i.e., thoughts); if the initiation of Nian cannot be stoped, then the teaching will be in vain." This is the Gongfu of regulating the Xin. Confucius also said: "First must be calm, then there is steadiness. When there is steadiness, then there is peace. When there is peace, then (you are) able to think. When (you are) able to think, then (you will) gain." This means in order to gain, (you) must first be able to keep the Xin and the physical body calm and peaceful. In order to be calm and peaceful, (you) must first have the Gongfu of stabilizing the Xin and getting rid of the Nian. However, in order to gain steadiness, (you) must first begin from the word of calmness. When there is calmness, then the mind is bright. When the mind is bright, then (you are) able to differentiate. When (you) can differentiate, then (the occurrences) will be clear. When it is clear, then (you) will not be confused.

古云：〝大道教人先止念，念頭不住亦徒然。〞此即調
心之功夫也。孔子亦曰：〝先靜爾后有定，定爾后能安，
安爾后能慮，慮爾后能得。〞此即謂要能有所獲，必先
能心身安寧。要能心身安寧，必先能有定心去念之功夫。
然而，要能有定，首先必從靜字著手。靜而明、明而辨，
辨則清，清則不惑也。

Nian (念) is the thought that lingers in your mind and that you cannot dismiss. For example, when you have an idea, it is a thought. However, if this idea continues to disturb your emotion, then it is a Nian. "Nian Tou" (念頭) means the initiation of the Nian, that is the beginning of a new thought.

In order to stop the initiation of a new thought, first you must be calm both physically and mentally. When this happens, a peaceful mind will be generated. Only if you have a peaceful mind can the Yi be clear, concentrated, and strong. Naturally, with this clear Yi, you will not be confused.

After reaching the goal of regulating the Xin, (you) should regulate the concentration of the Yi. When the Yi is concentrated, the Qi can be led and be used efficiently. However, when (you) have reached a stage of regulating without regulating, then the Yi is not in the leading of the Qi but in the spirit. For instance, if (you) wish to lead the Qi to the palm, the spirit is on the opponent. When the Yi is strong, the Qi will be abundant and circulate smoothly and naturally. Taijiquan ancestors said: "Yi is on the spirit and not on the Qi. If on the Qi, then the Qi is stagnant." This is what it means.

在心調之後，即調意之專。意專則氣能引而為我所用。
然而在進入調而不調之境地時，意不再在引氣，而在精
神。比如，欲引氣至掌，精神在敵，意強氣旺，氣行自
如。太極拳先哲云：〝意在精神，不在氣，在氣則
滯。〞此即意也。

In order to increase the concentration of the Yi, you must first regulate the Xin. After the Xin is regulated, you learn how to concentrate your Yi to a higher level.

After you have reached a stage of using your Yi to lead the Qi without any effort, then you should practice raising up the spirit. In Taijiquan, in order to lead the Qi strongly to support the physical manifestation, the spirit of fighting must be high. That means the sense of enemy is high and you are in a highly alert and aware state.

2. Thesis of Monkey Xin and Horse Yi 心猿意馬論

What is Xin? It belongs to Yang, easily active and excited. It is emotional, hard to keep steady, easily impatient and impetuous, and cannot be calm and settled. What is Yi? It belongs to Yin. It is quiet, settled, wise and logical, patient, calm, steady, and not confused. Ancient people said: "The Xin is like a monkey while the Yi is like a horse." This means that, though a monkey is small and weak physically, the level of its impatience and unsteadiness can make a person scared. Conversely, though a horse is big and powerful physically, it can be calm. Both Xin and Yi and used by a person. What does Xin-monkey and Yi-horse mean? It means: to use the Yi-horse to control the Xin-monkey. For example, when (you) are driving (your) car and encounter a big traffic jam. (You) wait and wait. After a while, the Xin gradually becomes unsteady, followed by impatience, and finally you lose your temper. This is caused by the Xin-monkey. At this time, the Yi-horse will take over and ask the Xin: "Will the unsteady and impatient Xin be able to solve the problem of the big traffic jam?" The answer is obvious. It cannot. Then the Yi-horse advises and says: "If this is the case, then why do (you) become unsteady and impatient, which is harmful to your health? Why don't (you) listen to the music from the radio to remove the anxiety of the Xin? Alternatively, (you) could just calm down (your) Xin and regulate (your) breathing for Qigong practice." (If you do so), before you even realize it, the traffic jam will dissipate. This is only an example of using the Yi-horse to subdue the Xin-monkey.

心者，陽也，易動也，易興奮也，感情也，難定也，易浮躁也，不靜也，不沉著也。意者，陰也，靜也，沉著也，理智也，不浮躁也，安寧也，定也，不昏迷也。古云：「心猿也，意馬也。」此意猿雖體小力弱，然其浮躁不寧之能耐卻是大而可畏。反之，馬雖體大力強，卻能心靜意寧的為人所使。心猿意馬者，以意馬克心猿也。比如在開車時遇到大阻塞。等而等之，心漸難寧，接而浮躁，火氣上漲。此心猿之作怪也。此時，意馬接進，反問之，心浮氣躁可去塞車之困擾乎？回答甚為明顯。不能。意馬解之：如是，為何身心煩躁以損身心之健康歟？何不聽聽音樂以解心愁，或靜心調息練練氣功。在不知不覺中，塞車解之。此意馬克心猿之一例也。

In order to use a calm and concentrated mind to lead the Qi, you must first learn how to regulate your emotional mind. However, this is not an easy task. In Qigong practice, the emotional mind remains the main obstacle to progress. When you practice, you must be patient and proceed step by step to deal with the problem. That is why the first stage of meditation is called "self-recognition" (Zi Shi, 自識). In this stage of meditation, the mask on your face drops off and you must face your true self. When this happens, the emotional mind becomes very active.

The second stage of regulating is called "self-awareness" (Zi Jue, 自覺). In this stage, you begin to understand the problem of emotional bondage. The third stage is "self-awakening" (Zi Xing, Zi Wu, 自醒 · 自悟). In this stage, your rational mind has clearly derived an understanding of the emotional problem and is looking for a way of setting you free from the emotional bondage. The last stage is "freedom from emotional bondage" (Zi Tuo, 自脫). These are the four stages of spiritual enlightenment in human life. Progressing through these stages will take a long time. The first step in this practice is through meditation.

> *During sitting meditation or practicing Taijiquan, the greatest challenge is to subdue the Xin-monkey. In order to subdue the Xin-monkey, (you) must offer it a banana. When (you) have a banana, the monkey can be led into the cage and be subdued by the Yi-horse. What is this banana? It is regulating the breathing. From regulating the breathing, the Xin gradually calms down. From the Xin's calmness, the Yi can then be peaceful. From the peaceful Yi, the Qi can be led efficiently. From leading the Qi efficiently, this achievement can be reached. From this, (you) can see the deep relationship between Xin and breathing. We will discuss this topic in the next article.*

> 静坐，練太極拳時，最難是克心猿。為克心猿，必備香
> 蕉。備有香蕉，心猿可引入籠中，遂為意所克。香蕉者，
> 調息也。由調息而心靜，由心靜而意寧，由意寧則氣引，
> 由氣引而功成。由是可知，心息之深切關係。下篇將專
> 題論之。

During meditation, if the emotional mind continues to bother you, then you should pay attention to your breathing. Breathing is the banana. It is a treat for the body, and its way to calm down the emotional monkey mind. We will discuss more of this subject next.

3. Thesis of Mutual Dependence of Emotional Mind and Breathing 心息相依論

> *What is regulating the Xin (i.e., emotional mind)? It means to use the Yi (i.e., rational mind) to regulate the Xin. Xin belongs to Yang and is active while Yi belongs to Yin and is calm. When using the Yi to regulate the Xin, breathing is the key. When the Yi pays attention to the breathing, then Xin can calm. Vegetarian Guest Requests About Listening to the Xin said: "The Xin has been attaching to the objects for a long time. Once it is separated from (these objects),*

it cannot be independent. Therefore, (you) must use the Gongfu of regulating the breathing to leash this Xin; then the Xin and the breathing will mutually depend on each other. When (you) regulate, it does not mean to use (only) Yi. It means only to keep the mind on the inhalation and exhalation. Once the Xin is parted from the object and moves independently, then regulating the breathing is no longer necessary. Only keep the breathing soft as it is there and as if it is not there. After a long time (of practice), it will become natural and you will become skillful." From this (you) can see that the key to regulating the Xin is in regulating the breathing.

調心者，以意調心也。心者，陽也，動也。意者，陰也，靜也。以意調心，其竅在於息。意注於息，則心能靜。《聽心齋客問》：〝心依著事物已久，一旦離境，不能自立。所以用調息功夫，拴系此心，便心息相依。調字亦不是用意，只是一呼一吸系念耳。至心離境，則無人無我，更無息可調，只綿綿若存，久之，自然純熟。〞由此可知，調心之竅在於調息。

The regulation of the emotional mind—bringing it into a calm, peaceful, and harmonious state—depends on the role your Yi (意) (i.e., rational mind) plays in the regulating process. If you can keep your Yi on your breathing, then gradually and slowly, you can calm down the Xin (心) (i.e., emotional mind). This is the reason that breathing is considered to be a strategy in Qigong practice. When breathing appropriately and correctly, you can calm down the Xin and strengthen the Yi and Shen (神) (i.e., spirit). Under this condition, the Qi can be led as smoothly and freely as you wish.

The method of regulating the Xin can be described as "the eyes observe the nose and the nose observes the Xin." "The eyes observe the nose" does not mean literally to use the eyes to look at the tip of the nose, but to keep the spirit of the eyes looking internally (i.e., eyes' sight condensed inward) and the Yi paying attention to the breathing. When the eyes are not looking outward, then the Yi can focus on the internal vision. Consequently, the spirit and the Yi can be condensed. "Using the nose to observe the Xin" means the meeting of the breathing and the Xin (i.e., harmonize and coordinate with each other), which finally leads to a stage of using the Yi to govern the Xin, the stage where Xin and breathing mutually depend on each other. The key to this practice is presented at the beginning of the regulating—pay more attention to the inhalation and allow the exhalation to be natural. This means keeping the Yi on the inhalation, which will allow the Guardian Qi to condense inward, the heartbeat to slow down, and the body temperature to decrease. When (you) have regulated the breathing until regulating is unnecessary, then the breathing will be deep and profound. The Complete Book of Principal Contents of Human Life and Temperament said: "If (one) can reach the stage of deep breathing as a truthful man (i.e., those who have reached the Dao), then the Xin and the breathing will mutually depend on each other. When the breathing is regulated, then the Xin will be calm." In fact, mutual dependence of the Xin and the breathing is the key method of calming the body and human nature. It is the beginning of spiritual cultivation in self-recognition, self-awareness, self-comprehension, self-awakening, and self-freedom (from spiritual bondage).

調心之法在於 "眼觀鼻，鼻觀心"。眼觀鼻者，非眼之
注視鼻端之觀也。而是眼神內視，意觀注鼻息。眼不外
觀，則移意於內視，神意可收斂。鼻觀心者，以息會心，
而達至由意馭心之心息相依之境。其竅在於初調之時，
以吸氣為重，呼氣任其自然。此即意在於吸，使衛氣內
斂，心跳減緩，體溫下降。當調至不調而自調之境地時，
則其息也深矣。《性命圭旨全書‧蟄藏氣穴，眾妙歸
根》："合真人深深之息，則心息相依，息調心靜。"
心息相依是靜身靜性之法，是修行自識、自覺、自悟、
自醒、自脫之初步。

When you bring your mind from outside of your body to inside your body, it is called "Nei Shi" (內視) and means "internal vision." That means paying attention to the internal feeling of the body. The deeper and more sensitive this feeling, the more you can sense the connection between your mind and your body. Feeling is the language between your mind and body. The more you can understand this language, the better your mind can communicate with your body. Naturally, it will take you a lot of practice and experience to reach a profound level of feeling. That is why this internal feeling training is called "Gongfu of Internal Vision" (Nei Shi Gongfu, 內視功夫).

4. Thesis of Comprehending the Human Nature through Taijiquan 太極拳悟性篇

What is a person's original nature (i.e., temperament)? At the beginning, in birth, it is natural, pure, innocent, truthful, and is the Dao. After birth, because of the influence and education of the environment, (your) original human nature is gradually concealed. After a long time, you have forgotten your original human nature. What is Taijiquan? It is a Daoist martial Qigong. Its ultimate goal is to keep apart from laymen society, to awaken the human (original) nature, and finally become divine. If a human wishes to reach this stage, (he/she) must first return (his/her) nature back to its pre-birth state; then (he/she) can return (himself/herself) from the Yin and Yang states to the unified Wuji state of heaven and human. If (one) wishes to return (his/her) human nature to this pre-birth state, (he/she) must see through to the true face of the post-birth human nature, and keep in mind the clean (i.e., pure) idea of standing apart from worldly affairs.

人之本性者，人之初也，自然也，純也，天真也，真實
也，道也。人生之後，受環境之感染教育，本性才漸被
曚蔽，久之忘吾本性矣。太極拳者，道家武學氣功也。
其終的在脫離凡俗而悟性成仙。人欲達此境界，必先返
先天之性，才能由陰陽太極返回無極天人合一之地。欲
返此先天之性，必先看透本事之後天人性，而存出世之
淨念。

We can distinguish the mind into subconscious mind (Qian Yi Shi, 潛意識) and conscious mind (Cun Yi Shi, 存意識). The subconscious mind can be classified as Yin, which you were born with, while the conscious mind can be classified as Yang, which is generated from your education and social conditioning. Normally, when you are awake and your physical body is lively, the mind that governs the thinking and physical action is the conscious mind. However, the subconscious mind, which is originated from the deep feeling inside of your spiritual being, is truthful. Through feeling, the subconscious mind always directs you to a right path of truth. When your physical body is calm and the conscious mind ceases its activities, your subconscious mind awakens. This can happen when you are sleeping or in a deeply profound meditative state. When the subconscious mind is awakened, the mask on your face drops off and you face yourself. This is the first step in meditation, self-recognition (Zi Shi, 自識).

Practicing Taijiquan is the same as other Qigong practices: from regulating the body, breathing, mind, Qi, and spirit, it aims at the goal of eradicating the laymen nature and returning to the original pre-birth nature, from Taijiquan practice to comprehending the meaning and the goal of life. If the goal is not as such, then it is near sighted in Taijiquan practice. From regulating the body, (you) are looking for the comprehension of your body's physical structure and function. From (keeping the body) loose, soft, and calm, (you) are searching for the higher level Gongfu of internal vision (i.e., internal feeling).

太極拳者，同乎其他氣功，亦於調身、調息、調心、調
氣、和調神中去除凡性，而歸本性，由太極之練習去體
會人生之本意與目的。如非此，則習太極之意短視矣。
由調身瞭解本身物理之理與作用，由鬆、軟、與靜而達
至高層之內視功夫。

Since Taijiquan originated in Daoist monasteries, its final goal is to get rid of emotional desires and bondages that are generated from the conscious mind; it aims to search for the truth of human nature. For example, the jealous, selfish love generated from the conscious mind must be eliminated while the natural, giving love originating from true connection should be retained and understood. Only under conditions free from emotional bondage can one approach the truth of human nature. Therefore, the initial goal of practice is to understand the meaning of your life and search for the truth of your being.

> *From regulating the breathing, the Xin can reach its calmness; from the Xin's calmness, the Yi can comprehend; from the Yi's comprehension, the conscious mind is clear; from the clarity of the conscious mind, the awareness is bright (i.e., clear); from the brightness of the conscious awareness, the human nature can be awakened; from the awakening of the human nature, the spirit will be enlightened; from spiritual enlightenment, (you) can reach the divinity of nature; from reaching the natural divinity, (you) can stand aloof from human society; from standing aloof from human society, (you) can reach the goal of unification between heaven and human.*

> 由調息而心靜，由心靜而意會，由意會而識清，由識清而覺明，由覺明而性悟，由性悟而神醒，由神醒而通乎神明，由通乎神明而求超脫，由超脫而臻天人合一之境界。

This paragraph offers a cultivation process for spiritual enlightenment. First, regulate your emotional mind (i.e., Xin) and make it calm down and reach a peaceful state. This will provide you with a clear rational mind (i.e., Yi). From the clear rational thinking, you will see yourself without confusion, and your awareness of your spiritual being can be lucent. This will lead you to a stage of self-awakening. From spiritual self-awakening, you will be able to build up a connection with the natural spirit and finally reach the stage of unification of heaven and human (Tian Ren He Yi, 天人合一).

PART V

About Regulating the Qi
論調氣

1. Theory of Using the Yi to Lead the Qi 以意引氣論

Regulating the breathing means to regulate the breathing until it is smooth, abundant, uniform, and fluid. To regulate it, the Yi is the most important. When the Yi is strong, (the circulation of) the Qi is strong. When the Yi is peaceful, the Qi can be led smoothly. When the Yi is calm, the Qi can be uniform, smooth and fluid. Qi is bioelectricity. Yi is the electromotive force (EMF) (i.e., electric potential difference). From Ohm's law, we know that:

$$V = I \times R$$

V=Electric Potential Difference
I=Current
R=Resistance

From this, we can see that when the electromotive force is strong, the current will be abundant and when the electromotive force is weak, the current will also be feeble. In addition, when the resistance is high, the current will be low, and when the resistance is low, the current will be high. Consequently, when the Yi is strong, the Qi is strong, and when the Yi is weak, the Qi is weak. When the body is relaxed, the resistance is low, and the current is high, and when the body is tense and stiff the resistance is high, and the current is low.

調氣者，調氣之行順、沛、均、與勻。其調之，以意為先。意強，氣沛。意寧，氣順。意平，氣均勻也。由今之科學上之瞭解知，氣者，生化電也。意者，生化電流之電動勢（電位差）也。由歐姆定律知：

$$V = I \times R$$

V: 電位差（電動勢）
I: 電流量
R: 電阻

由是可知，電動勢強，電量則沛；電動勢弱，電量則竭。
不但如此，電阻高，電量小；電阻低，電量大。因之，
意強，氣強；意弱，氣弱。身體鬆軟，電阻低，電流高。
身體繃硬，電阻高，電流低。

The purposes of Qigong training are to increase the flow rate of the Qi's circulation (i.e., abundance of I) and also to improve the quality (i.e., efficiency) of the Qi's manifestation. From the formula, you can see that in order to increase I, you must increase V and also decrease R. In order to increase V, the Yi must be more concentrated. In addition, in order to decrease R, the body must be relaxed and soft. This is the theory of Taijiquan: "relaxed physical movements with a concentrated mind." This is a way of "moving meditation."

> The way of strengthening the Yi is through meditation training. The body relaxes through training the postures. Wǔ, Yu-Xiang said: "Transport Qi as though through a pearl with a 'nine-curved hole,' not even the tiniest place won't be reached." To reach the level of transporting Qi to everywhere as wished, the Gongfu of Yi's internal vision must be high and deep. Only if the Yi can reach everywhere (in the body), can the Qi be led everywhere. This Gongfu must also be gained from training Qi in still meditation. Furthermore, in order to gain the uniformity and fluidity in Qi circulation, the transportation of Qi must be soft and smooth. The key is in the uniformity and fluidity of the breathing, the body's relaxation and softness, the Yi's peace and calmness, and the spirit's condensation and upraising. The Song of the Spiritual Origin of the Great Dao sings: "Concentrate (your) attention to reach the Qi's softness, the spirit will stay for a long time. To and fro of the real breathing will also be natural." This is the Dao of the unification of the spirit (i.e., Shen) and the Qi.

意之強，由靜坐練之。身之鬆軟，由練架得之。武禹襄
云：〝行氣如九曲珠，無微不到。〞為求氣之無所不到，
意之內視功夫必須高深。意之無所不到，才能導致氣之
無所不到。此功夫亦由靜坐練氣中得之。再者，為求氣
之均勻，氣之行必須柔順。其要在於呼吸之均勻，在身
體之鬆柔，在意之寧靜，在神之內聚與上提。《大道靈
源歌》曰：〝專氣致柔神久留，往來真息自悠悠。〞此
是神氣相合之道也。

In order to increase the electric potential difference, you must first know how to increase the concentration of your Yi. The best way to increase concentration is through still meditation training. In addition, in order to reduce the resistance of the body, you must know how to relax and be soft in your movements. When you are soft and relaxed, the Qi can flow smoothly without stagnation. In order to increase the efficiency of leading the Qi with the Yi, you must have a very sensitive inner feeling. The deeper the feeling, the more powerfully your mind can lead the Qi.

In addition, when Qi is flowing in your body, it should flow smoothly and feel natural, which allows you to relax continuously, which in turn makes the body more transparent to the Qi flow. It is known that when your breathing is smooth and correct, the Qi's circulation can be smooth and natural. When you can regulate your mind and Qi until they are harmoniously coordinated with each other, and are coordinated with correct breathing, the Qi can be led effectively and efficiently. This is one of the main goals in Taijiquan training.

2. Secret of Small Circulation 小周天訣

In the Small Heavenly Circulation (or simply called Small Circulation), the Qi circulates in the Conception and Governing Vessels, and when the cycle is completed, re-cycles again repeatedly. (In fact), this Small Circulation occurs naturally in everyone. The Conception Vessel is mainly responsible for regulating the Qi in the six Yin Primary Qi Channels (i.e., Yin Jing) while the Governing Vessel controls the six Yang Primary Qi Channels (i.e., Yang Jing). It is known (from Chinese medicine) that (through) these six Yin and six Yang, a total of twelve primary channels, (the Qi circulates) outward to reach the entire body's extremities and inward to communicate with the twelve internal organs and bowels. When the Qi's storage is abundant in the two Qi reservoirs— Conception and Governing Vessels, then the Qi in the twelve Primary Qi Channels (i.e., Jing) and their branches (i.e., Luo) will also be abundant. If the Qi's circulation in the twelve Primary Qi Channels and their branches is abundant and smooth, then the Guardian Qi (Wei Qi) can expand strongly, the physical body can be strong and healthy, and the immune system can be strong.

小周天氣行者，氣行任、督兩脈，周而復始之謂也。天
然之小周天循環，人皆有之。任脈主調六陰經之氣，督
脈主管六陽經之氣。知六陰六陽十二經外通達全身肢體，
內通達十二臟腑。任、督兩脈氣壜之存氣充沛，則十二
經與其絡支流之氣旺。如氣在十二經與其絡之運行強順，
則衛氣充張，身體強健，抗病力強。

Small Circulation (Xiao Zhou Tian, 小周天) is also commonly called "Microcosmic Meditation." There are two main purposes of Small Circulation meditation training. The first one is to increase the quantity of the Qi flow in the Conception and Governing Vessels. Since these two vessels are the Qi reservoirs that regulate the twelve primary Qi channels, when the Qi's circulation in these two vessels has reached an abundant level, the Qi circulation in the twelve primary Qi channels will also reach a higher level. When this happens, the physical body, including the internal organs, will grow to reflect the new energy situation. Consequently, the physical body becomes stronger and stronger. This means the first purpose is to increase the quantity of Qi.

The second purpose is to improve the smoothness of the Qi's flow, or to improve the efficiency or quality of the Qi's usage. To reach this goal, the mind must be strong and concentrated. In order to improve the quality of this Qi circulation, first you must widen the Qi channels in these two vessels. There are three gates in the path of the Small Circulation that could affect the smooth Qi circulation when you are aged. Therefore, to widen these three gates is crucial to the training. The process of widening these three gates is called "to unobstruct the three gates" (Tong San Guan, 通三關) in Small Circulation meditation practice (Figure 27).

Furthermore, we know that through the twelve primary Qi channels, the Qi can reach the entire body including the extremities. Therefore, when the Qi is abundant and circulating in these two vessels and the twelve primary Qi channels, the level of Qi in the entire body can be raised up to a strong level. When this happens, the physical body can be conditioned from weak to strong and the Guardian Qi (Wei Qi, 衛氣) can be enhanced. Consequently, the function of the body's immune system will be healthy.

> In the natural Qi circulation, the majority of Qi circulates in the twelve Primary Qi Channels during the daytime and reaches the entire physical body. At this time, the exhalation is longer than the inhalation, the internal Qi is led outward through the twelve Primary Qi Channels, the body temperature rises, the heart rate increases. However, during sleep, inhalation is longer than exhalation, the internal Qi is led inward to Thrusting Vessel (Chong Mai) (i.e., spinal cord) from the twelve Primary Qi Channels, the body temperature decreases, and the heart rate slows down. The Qi is led to the Thrusting Vessel, at the top it reaches the Baihui (i.e., crown) and at the bottom it reaches the Huiyin (i.e., perineum). Consequently, the pineal gland, pituitary gland, adrenals, pancreas, testicles, and ovaries receive the nourishment of the abundant Qi and produce hormones. What are hormones? They are related to the Original Essence and are the catalysts of the body's biochemical reactions. When the content of hormones is high, then the body's vital force is strong. When the content of hormones is low, the body's biochemical reactions will be stagnant and the body's metabolism will be weak. From the above, it is known that normally the Qi that is circulating strongly in the twelve Primary Qi Channels during the daytime is classified as Yang. The Yang physical body is active while the Yin spirit is calm. The Qi circulating in the Thrusting Vessel during the nighttime is classified as Yin. The Yang physical body is calm while the Yin spirit is active.

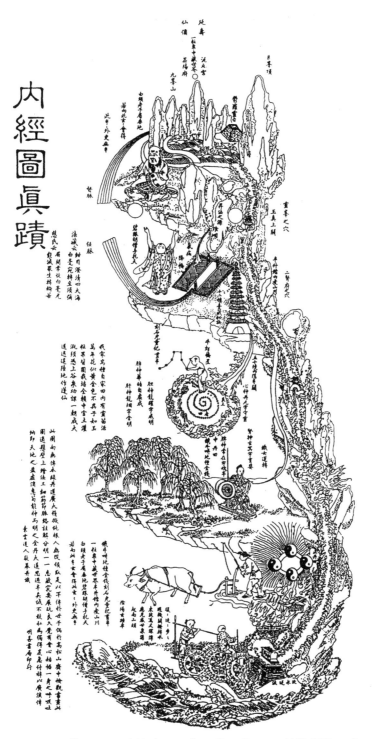

Figure 27. Illustration of Meditation from Tang Dynasty (618-907 A.D.)

天然氣之運行，白天氣注在十二經，而通達全身。此時
之鼻息呼長於吸，內氣由十二經外引，體溫上升，心臟
跳動加強。然晚間睡眠之時，鼻息吸長於呼，內氣由十
二經內引至衝脈，體溫下降，心臟跳動減緩。由於氣之
注於衝脈，上達百會下通會陰，松果腺、腦下腺、腎上
腺、胰腺、卵巢或睪丸受旺氣之滋補而產生賀爾蒙。賀
爾蒙者，關乎元精也，乃身體身化反應之催化劑也。賀
爾蒙之含量高，則生命力強。賀爾蒙弱，則身體之生化
反應慢，新陳代謝之機能弱。由是可知，一般身體之氣
勢乃為白天主任督兩脈與十二經為陽，陽體動而陰神怠。
晚上主衝脈為陰，陽體靜而陰神動。

Normally, when you are awake, your exhalation is longer than your inhalation. When you sleep, your inhalation is longer than your exhalation. Therefore, in the daytime, the Guardian Qi expands outward, the body temperature rises, and the heartbeat is faster. While you sleep, the Guardian Qi is condensed inward and weakened, the body temperature decreases, and the heartbeat is slower. In addition, during the daytime, as a result of physical activities, the Qi circulates strongly in the Conception and Governing Vessels (i.e., fire path) (Huo Lu, 火路) and is therefore distributed to the twelve Primary Qi Channels. In the nighttime, the physical body is relaxed and the major Qi flow is condensed inward, heavily circulating in the Thrusting Vessel (Chong Mai, 衝脈) (i.e., spinal cord) (i.e., water path) (Shui Lu, 水路) (Figure 28). When this happens, all the glands on the path of the Thrusting Vessel produce hormones. Since hormones are considered to be catalysts in the body's biochemical reactions for metabolism, when the hormone levels are high and adequately produced, the aging process can be slowed down.

From this, you can see that during the daytime, your physical body is active and is classified as Yang while during the nighttime, your physical body is resting while your spiritual body is awakened and is classified as Yin. Due to the nourishment of Qi to the brain in the nighttime, brain cells are nourished and activated, and dreams occur.

Small Circulation is again divided into Yin and Yang. The Conception Vessel is Yin while the Governing Vessel is Yang. During the daytime, the Qi is focusing on the circulation in the Conception Vessel, which therefore harmonizes the external Qi's Yang. During nighttime, the Qi is focusing on the circulation in the Governing Vessel, which is therefore balanced with the external Qi's Yin. From this, it is understood that the natural Qi circulation in Small Circulation is as follows: Zi (i.e., midnight) the major Qi flow is on the Baihui and reaches the Huiyin through the Thrusting Vessel. Chen (i.e., dawn) is on the palate (of the mouth) where it is to match the exchange of the external Yin and Yang. Wu (i.e., noon) is on Jiuwei (i.e., lower section of sternum). Jiuwei is known as Xinkan cavity in martial society and is called Middle Dan Tian, the Qi storage place of

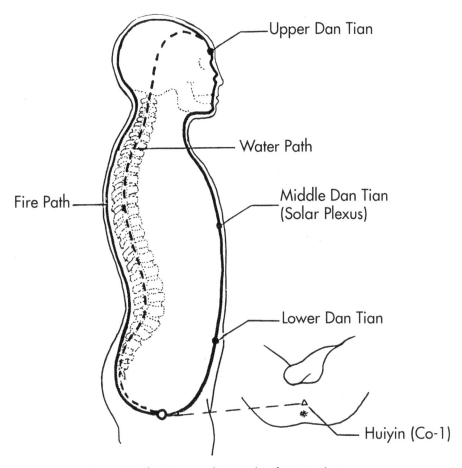

Figure 28. The Water and Fire Paths of Qi Circulation

the post-heaven Qi. At noon time, the major Qi flow is here and the Yang body (i.e., physical body) is at its extreme Yang. Normally, an afternoon nap can calm this down. Qiu (i.e., dusk) is on the Huiyin which is again to match the external Qi's Yin and Yang exchange. During the night, the Qi ascends upward from the Huiyin and reaches the Baihui again during midnight and therefore completes a cycle of circulation.

在小周天之運行中，陰陽再分。任脈為陰，督脈為陽。
白天氣主行於任脈以調合外氣之陽。晚上氣主行於督脈
以平衡外氣之陰。如是可知，天然小周天之運行為，子
時在百會，由衝脈通達會陰。辰時在上顎以配合外氣之
陰陽對調。午時在鳩尾。鳩尾乃武學上之心坎穴也，是
中丹田後天氣聚氣之所。午時，氣注於此，陽體發熱趨
太陽。午睡可平此陽。酉時在會陰以配合外氣之陽陰對
調。晚間氣由會陰上行，子時再由百會始而完成一周天
之行。

Usually, there are four timings that provide you with the information on how the natural Qi Small Circulation is occurring. These four timings are: midnight (Zi Shi, 子時) on the Baihui (Gv-20, 百會), sun rise (Chen Shi, 辰時) on the mouth area (i.e., palate) (Shang E, 上顎), noon (Wu Shi, 午時) on the Jiuwei (Co-15, 鳩尾), and sun set (Qiu Shi, 酉時) on the Huiyin (Co-1, 會陰) (Figure 29). You may notice that all three gates are located on the Governing Vessel. In addition, it takes only about six hours from Huiyin to the Baihui, six hours from the Baihui to the mouth, six hours from the mouth to Jiuwei, and six hours from Jiuwei to Huiyin.

> *However, in order to have abundant Qi storage and smooth circulation (in the Conception and Governing Vessels), those who practice Nei Dan (i.e., internal elixir) Qigong must practice the Gongfu of Small Circulation meditation. From the abdomen—elixir furnace (i.e., Dan Lu) starting fire (i.e., producing Qi or elixir) to reach the abundant level of Qi. From the Yi's leading to lead the Qi's smooth circulation. From this to accomplish the efficacy of Small Circulation practice. However, those who practice (Small Circulation) must know that it was often heard in ancient times that many who practiced Small Circulation encountered problems from going into the fire (i.e., Zou Huo) and encountering the devil (i.e., Ru Mo). They became disabled or even lost their lives. The reason is the difficulty of passing the Qi through the Three Gates (i.e., San Guan). What are the Three Gates? They are Weilu (or Changqiang cavity), Jiaji (or Lingtai cavity), and Yuzhen (or Naohu cavity). Therefore, those who practice Small Circulation meditation must learn it from a good and experienced teacher. Make sure not to practice by yourself, it could result in sickness. Be cautious! Be cautious! In order to be safe, (I) will discuss this practice in detail in a future book.*

然練內丹氣功者，為求氣脈之氣沛與行順，而習小周天靜坐之功。由小腹丹爐之火起以求氣脈之沛然，由意之導以引氣之行。由此，可達小周天之效。然習者須知，古時習小周天者，數聞走火入魔之病，而生殘疾甚而喪命。其因在於三關之困，難以通之。三關者，尾閭（長強穴）、夾脊（靈臺穴），與玉枕（腦戶穴）也。因之，習小周天者，必從有經驗之良師學之。切不可妄自為之以為病害。慎之！慎之！為求安全，以後將專書討論之。

In order to increase the quantity of the Qi and bring it to an abundant level, you must know where to produce the extra Qi. The lower abdominal area, the location of the Lower Dan Tian (Xia Dan Tian, 下丹田) (i.e., lower elixir field), known as Qihai (Co-6, 氣海) by Chinese medical society, and also known as Dan Lu (丹爐) (i.e., elixir furnace) is actually the place where the Qi can be produced. Through the abdomen's up and down exercises in abdominal breathing, the food essence stored as fat can be converted into Qi through biochemical reactions. In addition, the glands such as the adrenals, pancreas, and testicles (or ovaries) will produce hormones (i.e.,

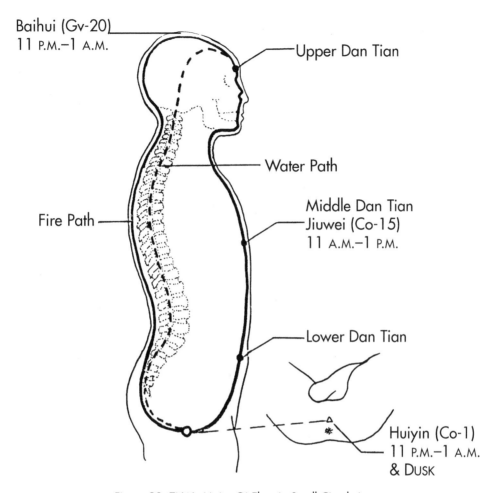

Baihui (Gv-20)
11 P.M.–1 A.M.

Upper Dan Tian

Water Path

Fire Path

Middle Dan Tian
Jiuwei (Co-15)
11 A.M.–1 P.M.

Lower Dan Tian

Huiyin (Co-1)
11 P.M.–1 A.M.
& Dusk

Figure 29. Zi-Wu Major Qi Flow in Small Circulation

original essence) (Yuan Jing, 元精) that expedite the biochemical reactions in the body.

When the Qi's storage has reached an adequate level, then you concentrate to lead the Qi to circulate, and this will provide you with higher quality Qi circulation and manifestation of it into physical strength. However, you must understand one important thing. When you learn Small Circulation meditation, in order to avoid dangers, in addition to knowing the theory thoroughly, you also need an experienced teacher. There are three gates which can cause serious problems if you don't know how to handle them. These problems are called "walk into the fire and enter the demon" (Zou Huo Ru Mo, 走火入魔). "Walk into the fire" means the Qi has entered into the wrong place and is causing problems, and "enter the demon" implies false, fantastical thought generated during the meditation that could lead to a serious imagination problem.

The Three Gates (i.e., San Guan, 三關) have different names originating from different Qigong societies from ancient times. The names Weilu (尾閭) (i.e., tail-bone), Jiaji (夾脊) (i.e., squeeze the spine), and Yuzhen (玉枕) (i.e., jade pillow) were given by Daoist society. The same cavities were named Changqiang (Gv-1) (長強) (i.e., long strength), Lingtai (Gv-10) (靈臺) (i.e., spirit's platform), and Naohu (Gv-17) (腦戶) (i.e., brain's household) in acupuncture. For the same cavities or locations, there are many other names given by martial artists, Buddhists, and scholarly societies. For example, the gate is called Jiaji by Daoists, is called Mingmen (命門) (i.e., life door) by martial artists, and Lingtai in Chinese medicine. The same name Mingmen (Gv-4) (命門) is used by medical society for the cavity that is located between L2 and L3 of the spine.

3. Secret of Grand Circulation 大周天訣

Grand Circulation is the practice that can be started right after a person has passed through the "three gates" in Small Circulation meditation practice. Grand Circulation can be classified into: within self-body's Grand Circulation; Grand Circulation of Qi's exchange with the external world or with a partner (i.e., double cultivation) (Shuang Xiu); and Grand Circulation of the unification of Heaven and human. Here, I will only discuss the self-body's Grand Circulation that is related to the martial arts, such as Yongquan Breathing, Four Gates Breathing, and Five Gates Breathing. Other Grand Circulation practices, such as Qi's exchange with the environment or heaven-human unification, will be specially discussed in a future book.

大周天者，在小周天之練習通了三關之後，即可著手練習大周天。大周天者可分為己身之大周天，與外界換氣或與他人雙修之大周天，和與天人合一之大周天練習。在此，吾僅為與武學上有關之湧泉息，四心息，與五心息作個討論。其他與外界換氣和天人合一之大周天練習，將專書論之。

There are many practices that can be defined as "Grand Circulation" (i.e., Macrocosmic Meditation) (Da Zhou Tian, 大周天), including the grand Qi circulation in your own body, the Qi mutual exchange between you and your partners (Shuang Xiu, 雙修) (i.e., double cultivations), and the mutual Qi exchange between you and nature. The final goal of Qigong practice is to reunify human and nature.

A. Yongquan Breathing 湧泉息

In Yongquan breathing, in coordination with Real Dan Tian breathing, (you) use the Yi to lead the Qi from the Real Dan Tian to the Yongquan cavity. There it communicates with external Qi. External Qi enters through the Yongquan cavity and the Yi leads it back to the Real Dan Tian. This is what Zhuang Zi called: "sole breathing." Zhuang Zi said: "Normal people's breathing uses the throat while truthful persons' breathing uses the sole." Truthful persons imply those Dao searchers who have trained the Qi and have reached a profound stage of (spiritual) purity and truth. In order to practice Yongquan breathing, (you) must first understand the keys of Embryonic Breathing. Under the condition of soft and slender breathing, use the Yi to lead the Qi to the soles and then return it back (to the Real Dan Tian). Han Xu Zu said: "What is sole breathing? It means continuous without broken, soft and slender as it is existing." From this, (you) can see that, with the prior condition of a profound level of regulating the breathing, Yi is the foundation of success in Yongquan breathing. When Yi is strong, the Qi is sufficient and when Yi is weak, the Qi is deficient.

湧泉息者，即是在配合真丹田呼吸下，以意引氣由真丹田至湧泉穴與外氣相通，再由湧泉穴由外納氣意引歸返真丹田之謂也。此亦即莊子所謂之踵息矣。莊子曰：〝常人之息以喉，真人之息以踵。〞真人者，尋道撲實練氣至深之人。為求湧泉之息，必先懂胎息之竅，在綿綿呼吸中，以意引氣來回足踵也者。涵虛祖曰：〝踵也者，相接不斷，綿綿若存也。〞由此可知，在深度的調息前題下，意為湧泉息之本。意強，氣厚，意弱，氣薄。

The Yongquan (K-1) (湧泉) (i.e., gushing spring) cavity belongs to the Kidney Primary Channel (Figure 30). Like the Laogong (P-8) (勞宮) (i.e., labor's palace) cavity at the center of the palm, the two Yongquan cavities on the bottom of the two soles are two major Qi gates that regulate the body's Qi condition. In addition, these two gates also build up a firm foundation for rooting. In Taijiquan, in order to build up a firm root, not only must you have high sensitivity in the connection of your soles to the ground, you must also be able to use your mind to lead the Qi downward beyond the soles and into the ground. It is like a tree growing its root. In order to make this happen, you must practice Yongquan breathing for a long time. This will allow your root to grow deeper and gradually, the Qi can also reach deeper as well. Yongquan breathing is not only good in establishing a firm root for martial arts, but it is also beneficial in maintaining health.

Success depends on how strong and concentrated your Yi is. The stronger you can establish your imaginary target, the stronger the Qi will flow. However, even when the Yi is strong, the breathing must be soft and slender so the Qi's flow can be smooth and continuous.

The practice of Yongquan breathing can be done either lying down or standing. However, (you) must not cross (your) legs. If the legs are crossed, the Qi will be

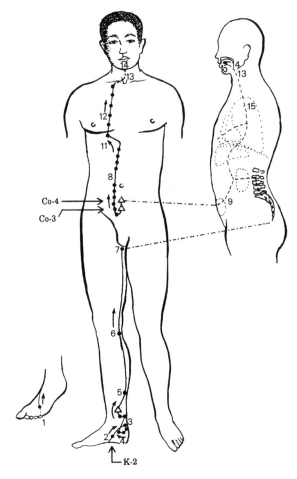

Figure 30. The Kidney Channel of Foot-Lesser Yin

stagnant at the Kua area (i.e., area around hip joints). When (you) practice while lying down, first, inhale deeply and lead the Qi into the Real Dan Tian, and then softly and slowly exhale while at the same time using (your) Yi to lead the Qi along the legs to reach the Yongquan cavities and then out. The mind is used in the same way as (your) feet to push outward. When the exhalation is near the end, inhale and at the same time use (your) Yi to lead the external Qi from outside inward through the Yongquan cavity and along the legs returning to the Real Dan Tian. The phenomenon of successful (Yongquan breathing) is that (you) feel like the Yongquan cavities are also breathing. Repeat the practice. The more (you) practice, the stronger the Qi's flow will be.

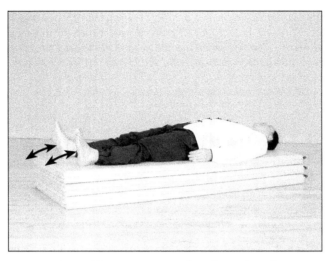

Figure 31. Yongquan Breathing (Lying Down)

湧泉息之練習，可平躺或站立，然卻不可盤腿。盤腿，
則氣滯於胯部也。平躺練習時，先吸氣納入真丹田，再
綿綿緩緩的呼氣，同時以意引氣沿腿至湧泉而出。其意
如以足推出然。待呼至將盡之時，即吸氣並同時以意由
湧泉納入外氣，沿腿回歸入真丹田。其功成之象如湧泉
亦在呼吸然。反覆而行，愈練，氣行愈強也。

When you practice Yongquan breathing, you may either lie down or stand up. When you practice while lying down, the soles are more relaxed and the Qi can exit and enter more easily. The trick to leading the Qi to the soles and beyond is to imagine the feet pushing out without actual physical action (Figure 31). This should be done with the exhalation. When you intend to lead the external Qi in through the Yongquan, you again use your mind to lead the Qi, along the legs, to the Real Dan Tian. After you have practiced for a period of time, you will feel that the Qi's entering and exiting through the Yongquan is just like the breathing of the nose. The more you practice, the more natural and the stronger the Qi's flow will be.

Standing Yongquan breathing practice is commonly used as a rooting training method in martial arts. The method of this practice is a little different from that used in the lying down practice. The difference is that the exhalation is longer than the inhalation. Each time (you) exhale, you squat down slightly and at the same time you use the Yi to lead the Qi to the bottom of the feet and underneath. Each time (you) exhale, the depth is deeper one more inch. When (you) inhale, let it be natural and don't let the Yi lead the Qi back to the Real Dan Tian. If (you) do so, the root will be returning to its shallow place. At the beginning of practice, (you) should stand on the ground. After a long time, stand on horizontally positioned bricks and use the Yi to lead the Qi down to the bottom of the bricks. If (your) Yi and Qi can reach the bottom of the bricks, then stand on vertical bricks. Practice following the same method. If (you) can stand on two or three bricks stacked vertically and the Yi and the Qi are still able to reach the bottom of the bricks, then your root is deep. After the bricks are removed, the Yi and the Qi can reach three feet under (your) feet. It is like the firm root of a big tree.

站立之湧泉息，一般為武學上練紮根之法。其練習方法、
原理與平躺者無異。其不同處在於呼長於吸，並於每呼
時，身體向下微蹲同時以意引氣至足底下深處，每呼一
次，根深一寸。吸時任其自然，意卻不引氣返歸真丹田。
如是，則根返回淺地矣。初習時，站立地上。久之，站
立平磚上，並以意引氣至磚底。在意氣能達磚底後，即
站立在立磚上，依法練習。如能站立在二、三立磚上，
意氣仍能通達磚底，則根深矣。在去磚時，意氣可達腳
底三尺，如大樹之紮根然。

Standing Yongquan breathing is commonly used to establish a firm root in martial arts training. The main difference in this training is that the exhalation is longer than the inhalation. This means that first you inhale deeply and then you exhale slowly and finely while using your mind to lead the Qi to the Yongquan cavity and beyond. The key to establishing a strong Yi is squatting down while imagining you are pushing your feet downward into the ground. When your exhalation is longer than your inhalation, it does not mean you release more carbon dioxide out and take in less oxygen. The difference is that the flow rates are different. When you exhale slower and longer, your mind is more calm and your concentration is stronger. Naturally, the flow rate of the exhalation is less than that of the inhalation.

You should first practice on the ground. After you can feel the Qi deeper than your feet, you should stand on bricks and train with the same methods (Figure 32). If you can stand on two or three vertically stacked up bricks and can lead the Qi to the bottom of the lowest bricks, then your Yi is strong and the Qi can reach deep underneath your feet. If you can reach this level, once you remove all of the bricks and stand on the ground, your root will be at least three feet under your soles.

B. Four Gates Breathing 四心息

Four Gates Breathing is the practice in which Yongquan Breathing and Laogong Breathing are carried out at the same time. The Yongquan cavities are the main gates of the soles' communicating with the external Qi while the Laogong cavities are the key gateways of the palms' communication with external Qi. From the Real Dan Tian the Qi is led upward to the Laogong cavities and downward

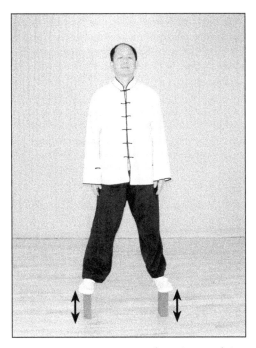

Figure 32. Yongquan Breathing (On Bricks)

to the Yongquan cavities. One upward and one downward, the center is main-tained, and consequently the Jin's manifestation has its root. From this, it is understood that Four Gates Breathing is the secret of the Jin's manifestation.

四心息者，湧泉息與勞宮息並行也。湧泉乃足底通外氣
之中心門戶，勞宮卻是手掌之通外氣之關竅。由真丹田
氣引上行至勞宮，下行至湧泉，一上一下，持中也，勁
有根矣。由此可知，四心息乃勁發之訣矣。

In order to manifest Jin with a firm root and balanced body, you must learn how to keep your center firm. This is called "central equilibrium" (Zhong Ding, 中定). That means to keep your center at one point, and this point is your Real Dan Tian or your physical center of gravity. *Taijiquan Classic* said: "If there is a top, there is a bottom; if there is a front, there is a back; if there is a left, there is a right."[11] This sentence clearly explains the condition of central equilibrium. In order to reach this central equilibrium, you must know Four Gates Breathing. From Four Gates Breathing, you can find your center. Only then can you use this center to direct your Jin with a firm root.

Its practicing method is just like the practice of Yongquan breathing, which can be done both lying down or standing up. However, (you) must not practice with the legs crossed. If the legs are crossed, then the Qi will be stagnant at the Kua area. In lying down practice, first inhale and bring the Qi to the Real Dan Tian, then slowly and softly exhale while at the same time using (your) Yi to lead the Qi (downward) along the legs to the Yongquan cavities and out while also along the arms to the Laogong cavities and out. The Yi acts as if (you are) pushing the palms and soles out at the same time. When the exhalation is near the end, then inhale and at the same time use the Yi to lead the external Qi in through the Yongquan and Laogong cavities, along the original path and return to the Real Dan Tian. The feeling of success is as if the Yongquan and Laogong cavities are also breathing. Practice repeatedly. The more (you) practice, the stronger the Qi's flow will be.

其練習之法如湧泉息然，可平躺或站立，然卻不可盤腿。
盤腿，則氣滯於胯部也。平躺練習時，先吸氣納入真丹
田，再綿綿緩緩的呼氣，同時以意引氣沿腿至湧泉而出，
並沿手臂至勞宮而出。其意如以掌、足同時推出然。待
呼至將盡之時，即吸氣並同時以意由湧泉、勞宮納入外
氣，沿原路回歸入真丹田。其功成之象如湧泉、勞宮亦
在呼吸然。反覆而行，愈練，氣行愈強也。

In lying down Four Gates Breathing practice, simply inhale deeply and then exhale slowly, finely, and softly while imagining you are pushing your palms and soles out without actual physical action (Figure 33). In this case, the Qi will be led naturally to the four gates. Success depends on your Yi and breathing. If you are doing this correctly, you will feel as if these four gates are also breathing with you.

Standing Four Gates Breathing is the method of training internal Jin in martial arts. Its training method is slightly different from that of lying down. The difference is that when (you) inhale, (you) are also leading the Qi upward along the spine. In addition to the natural Qi flow which begins from the Yinjiao cavity and passes through the Huiyin cavity (i.e., Haidi, Sea Bottom) and then upward, (you) are also using (your) Yi to lead the Qi from the Real Dan Tian. Qi exits through the Mingmen cavity and then moves upward along the spine, thus combining with the natural Qi flow. This is the breathing secret of self-grand circulation. In order to lead the Qi to exit the Mingmen cavity and moves upward (along the spine), (you) must first open the Mingmen cavity. This method uses the immortal bone (i.e., sacrum). When the immortal bone is pushed backward slightly, the Mingmen cavity is opened. This body movement is the same as the body movement of natural sighing.

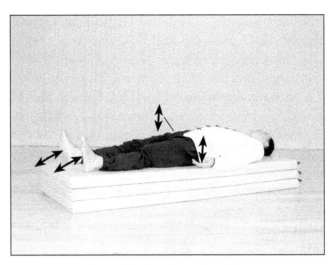

Figure 33. Four-Gates Breathing

站立之四心息，即武學上練內勁之法。其練習方法、原
理與平躺者稍微不同。不同之處，在吸氣時引氣沿脊上
行。如此，除了自然之氣由陰交沿會陰（海底）上行外，
並以意引丹田氣由命門穴出而上行與自然氣合。此是己
身大周天之竅訣也。為引氣出命門而上行，必先開命門
穴。其法在於仙骨（尾椎骨）。仙骨微微後推，命門即
開矣。其身動猶如嘆息然。

When you are doing standing Four Gates Breathing, as in lying down Four Gates Breathing, you may simply imagine that you are pushing your feet and palms downward. In this case, the Yi of pushing will lead the Qi following the natural Small Circulation path from the Real Dan Tian, through Yinjiao (Co-7) (陰交), Huiyin (Co-1) (會陰) (called Haidi, 海底, by Daoists), upward along the spine, Dazhui (Gv-14) (大椎) (or Shenzhu, Gv-12, 身柱) and then dividing into two flows into the arms (Figures 34-36).

However, for martial artists, in order to enhance the Qi's circulation to the arms so that martial power (i.e., Jin, 勁) can be manifested at a higher level, there is another flow of Qi led into the spine through the Mingmen (命門) (Gv-4) cavity (Figure 36). This is one of the paths in self-internal Grand Circulation, and is used by Chinese martial artists. Taijiquan ancestor Wǔ, Yu-Xiang (武禹襄) said: "Power is emitted from the spine" (力由脊發) also, "(The mind) leads the Qi flowing back and forth, adhering to the back, then condensing into the spine."[12] All of this implies that leading the Qi upward through the spine is a way of storing the Jin. The key to Jin manifestation is Four Gates Breathing.

Therefore, when you practice self-internal Grand Four Gates Circulation, first inhale deeply and lead the Qi from the Real Dan Tian to exit out through the Yin-jiao (Co-7) (陰交), downward passing the Huiyin (Co-1) (會陰) to complete the first half of the inhalation process. Then, open the Mingmen (Gv-4) (命門) cavity and lead extra Qi backward from Real Dan Tian through the Mingmen (Gv-4) (命門) to join the Qi led upward from the Huiyin (Co-1) (會陰). In the second half of the inhalation, lead the Qi from the Mingmen (Gv-4) (命門) upward to the Dazhui (Gv-14) (大椎) and Shenzhu (Gv-12) (身柱) cavity. Finally, exhale and lead the Qi out to the palms while also leading the Qi downward to the soles to complete the Four Gates Breathing.

C. Five Gates Breathing 五心息

Five Gates Breathing means that, after (you have) regulated the Four Gates Breathing to the point that regulating is unnecessary, then (you) add the fifth gate's breathing. The first possible fifth gate is the Baihui. The Baihui cavity connects to the Huiyin through the Chong Mai (i.e., Thrusting Vessel). The Chong Mai is what is called the spinal cord and is a highly electrically conductive material. Therefore, though the Baihui and the Huiyin are located in two different places, their functions are connected and act as one. The Huiyin is the most Yin place in the entire body, while the Baihui is the residence of the Yang-Shen (i.e., Yang spirit) and is the most Yang place in the entire body. The Huiyin is the Yin meeting place of the four Yin vessels—Conception, Thrusting, Yin Heel, and Yin Linking Vessels and is the key controlling gate of the entire body's Yin and Yang. To Qi practitioners, it is the secret gate for leading Qi. When the Huiyin is held upward, the Huiyin gate is closed and the body's Qi is condensed inward into the bone marrow, the spirit is converged and the Qi is gathered, the entire body turns Yin, and consequently, the Jin is stored. Conversely, when the Huiyin is pushed out, the Huiyin gate is opened, Qi is released from the four Yin vessels, the Yang spirit is raised up, the entire body turns Yang, and consequently, the Jin is emitted. One store and one emit, this is the key cycle of the internal Jin's storing and emitting.

五心息者，在四心息調至不調而自調之境地時，即加添第五心之息。第五心者，百會也。百會由衝脈相通於會陰。衝脈者，脊髓神經也，特高之電導體也。因而百會與會陰雖於上下兩處，其作用唯一己矣。會陰為陰為全身最陰之所，百會為陽為陽神顯陽之地，亦是全身最陽之處。會陰者，四陰脈，任、衝、陰蹻、陰維脈交會之所，是全身陰陽控制之關，是練氣者引氣之竅門。會陰上提，會陰鎖，氣內斂入骨髓，神凝氣聚，全身趨陰，勁由之而蓄。反之，會陰下推，會陰開，氣由四陰脈外放，陽神上提，全身趨陽，勁由之而發。一蓄一發，此為內勁蓄發關要之鑰。

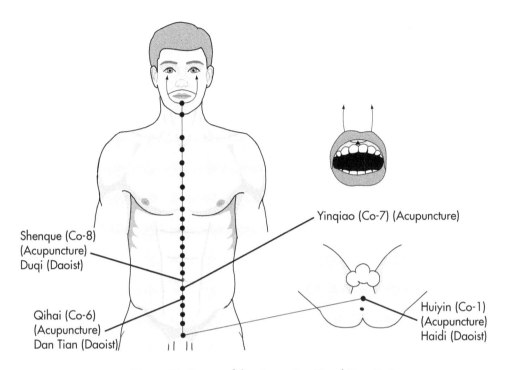

Shenque (Co-8)
(Acupuncture)
Duqi (Daoist)

Yinqiao (Co-7) (Acupuncture)

Qihai (Co-6)
(Acupuncture)
Dan Tian (Daoist)

Huiyin (Co-1)
(Acupuncture)
Haidi (Daoist)

Figure 34. Course of the Conception Vessel (Ren Mai)

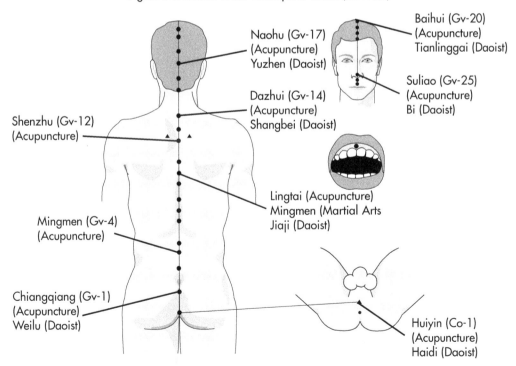

Naohu (Gv-17)
(Acupuncture)
Yuzhen (Daoist)

Baihui (Gv-20)
(Acupuncture)
Tianlinggai (Daoist)

Dazhui (Gv-14)
(Acupuncture)
Shangbei (Daoist)

Suliao (Gv-25)
(Acupuncture)
Bi (Daoist)

Shenzhu (Gv-12)
(Acupuncture)

Lingtai (Acupuncture)
Mingmen (Martial Arts
Jiaji (Daoist)

Mingmen (Gv-4)
(Acupuncture)

Chiangqiang (Gv-1)
(Acupuncture)
Weilu (Daoist)

Huiyin (Co-1)
(Acupuncture)
Haidi (Daoist)

Figure 35. Course of the Governing Vessel (Du Mai)

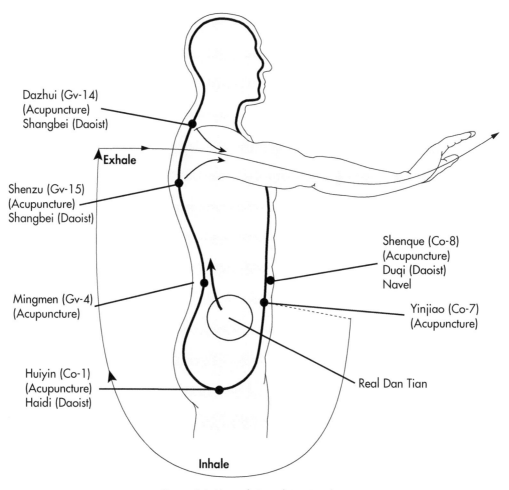

Figure 36. Martial Grand Qi Circulation

The Fifth Gate Breathing is the most important key to the Jin's manifestation. The Yi and the Qi of this gate are balanced with the other four gates, and when the Yi and Qi are strong in this gate, the Yi and Qi of the other four gates will also be strong. Naturally, the Jin's manifestation will be powerful.

The Baihui (Gv-20) (百會) is the residence of the Shen, and the Huiyin (Co-1) (會陰) is the storage place of water. The Shen is Yang while water is Yin. That is why the Shen is commonly called Yang Shen (陽神) while the Huiyin (Co-1) (會陰) is called Sea Bottom (Haidi, 海底) (Figure 35). The Huiyin is the place that connects the Real Dan Tian and the four Yin vessels and thus stores the Qi, while the Shen is the place that governs the effectiveness of the Qi's manifestation. In fact these two cavities are the two poles of the body's central energy through the spinal cord. When this central energy is strong, the body's vital force is strong. Naturally, the Jin manifested will be powerful and precise.

According to Chinese medicine, Huiyin means "Yin Meeting" and is the gate that controls the Qi's storage or release from the four Yin vessels. When the Huiyin is pushing out, the Qi in the four Yin vessels is released, and when this cavity is held upward, the Qi is preserved. This implies that when you store your Jin, you are holding this cavity upward while inhaling and when you emit your Jin, you are pushing this cavity outward while exhaling.

> *Wu, Yu-Xiang said: "(Throughout your) entire body, your mind is on the Spirit of Vitality (Jing Shen), not on the Qi. (If concentrated) on the Qi, then stagnant." This is the fifth gate breathing. Spirit (i.e., Shen) is the master of the Qi's circulation. When the spirit is high, the Qi's circulation is natural, strong, and smooth. When the spirit is low, then the Qi is stagnant, weak, and hard to circulate. This is the secret key to Jin manifestation.*

武禹襄云；〝全身意在精神，不在氣，在氣則滯。〞此
即意第五心之呼吸也。神為氣行之主宰，神高，氣行自
然沛而順，神低，氣滯弱而難行。此為勁發之訣竅也。

When the entire body's concentration is on the spirit, the spirit can be high and the Qi can be led effectively. However, if the Yi is on the Qi, then your mind is not ahead of the Qi and leading the Qi, and the Qi will be stagnant. This will cause the power to stagnate during expression. The key to leading the Qi efficiently is to develop a sense of enemy. This means that you have an imaginary opponent. When your mind is on your opponent, your Yi will lead the Qi there for Jin manifestation. The strength of your Qi depends on the strength of your Yi. However, the strength of your Yi depends on your fighting spirit and morale. When this spirit is high, your alertness and awareness will also be high. Naturally, the Qi can be directed efficiently.

4. Yin-Yang Taiji Ball Qigong 陰陽太極球氣功

> *Taiji Ball Qigong is a martial Qigong training. It has commonly been practiced by both external and internal martial styles. Its purposes are for muscle/tendon changing and also for marrow/brain washing. Muscle/Tendon changing (Qigong) belongs to Yang while marrow/brain washing (Qigong) belongs to Yin. The purpose of muscle/tendon changing training is, through Taiji Ball Qigong's twelve basic movements, to condition those muscles, tendons, ligaments, and bones which are required for different Jin manifestation. Therefore, the training focuses on changing the quality of the muscles, tendons, ligaments, and bones. Change them from weak to strong so the effectiveness of the Jin's manifestation can be achieved. Furthermore, this training can also be used to prevent injuries of the joints and muscles/tendons. Marrow/Brain washing is to train the practitioners in how to use the Yi to lead the Qi efficiently, and also how to lead the Qi to the bone marrow through the joints to achieve the goal of marrow washing.*

太極球氣功武學氣功也。內外家都有習之。其目的在於
易筋，在於洗髓。易筋為陽，洗髓為陰。易筋者，由太
極球十二基本動作架式中，求不同發勁所須筋骨之健。
其著重在肌、筋、骨腱、與骨頭之變質，由弱轉強，以
求勁力之效，並防止骨節與肌肉之受傷。洗髓者，在練
習以意引氣之竅，並由骨節引氣入髓以達洗髓之功。

Taiji Ball Qigong was derived from Da Mo's muscle/tendon changing and marrow/brain washing Qigong. This Qigong was commonly practiced in ancient times when martial arts played an important role in society. Therefore, it was widely practiced by both external and internal styles. The goals of Taiji ball Qigong training are twofold. One is for muscle/tendon changing and the other for marrow/brain washing. Muscle/tendon changing is used to condition the physical body from weak to strong so the Jin manifested can be powerful and effective. Marrow/brain washing trains a practitioner in how to use the mind to lead the Qi to circulate through the entire body more efficiently. In addition, this training also focuses on how to store the Qi in the bone marrow and to lead the Qi upward through the Thrusting Vessel (i.e., Chong Mai, 衝脈) to the brain to raise up the Spirit of Vitality. When the spirit is raised, the fighting morale will be high and the entire body can be a powerful and effective fighting unit.

> The training of this Gong (i.e., Gongfu) can be divided into three levels. The first level is Taiji ball practice without a ball. The training of this level aims for the smoothness of the basic movements, using the Yi to lead the Qi, and also the harmonization and coordination of the internal ball and external ball. The internal ball is hidden internally at the Real Dan Tian which belongs to Yin, while the external ball is manifested externally between the palms and belongs to Yang. From the internal ball's rotating and circular movements, the patterns are delivered to the external ball through the spine. At the beginning, the movements are slow so the effect of using the Yi to lead the Qi can be achieved. When the movements are slow, the feeling can be deep. This means the Gongfu of internal vision (i.e., feeling) can also be deep. When the feeling is deep, the Yi can also reach deeply. In this case, the state of leading the Qi to "no place cannot be reached" can be achieved.

此功之練法可分三段。其初段為無球之太極球練習。此
段之練習在求基本動作之順利，以意引氣，內球與外球
輾轉之調合諧和。內球在真丹田藏於內為陰，外球在手
掌間顯於外為陽。由內球氣之動與動作之輾轉，由脊椎
遞送而至外球。初行時，動作緩慢以求以意引氣之效。
動作慢，感覺深，亦即內視功夫深也。當然，感覺深，
意亦可深，而氣可引至無所不到之境界。

In Taiji Ball Qigong training, there are two balls that you are training. One is located at the Real Dan Tian and the other is between the palms. The motion originates from the internal ball and, through the spine, the action is manifested externally at the ball between the palms. While you are doing this, not only can the movements be directed by the waist, but the Qi can also be led though grand circulation from the Real Dan Tian smoothly to the palms.

At the first level of training, the external ball is formed from the Qi between the palms (Figure 37). Therefore, it is invisible. However, through feeling, you can sense the existence of this ball. At the beginning of the training, the movements must be slow, which allows your Yi to reach a deeper level of activating body movement. In addition, this will help you use your mind to lead the Qi through grand circulation. If your Yi can reach to the skin and beyond (i.e., Guardian Qi) (Wei Qi, 衛氣) as well as to the marrow (i.e., Marrow Qi) (Sui Qi, 髓氣), then you will be able to store the Qi using the bone marrow and also manifest it externally to the skin surface for power manifestation.

After practicing to proficiency in the first level, so that the twelve basic movements can be as smooth as you wish, you can then hold a Taiji ball and again train the twelve basic movements. Generally, a Taiji ball can be made from wood or stone. Those who emphasize training Li (i.e., muscular power) usually use a stone ball while those who emphasize training Qi usually use a wooden ball. Those who practice Taijiquan like to use a wooden ball simply because it can be used to train Qi. At the beginning, use a ball which is smaller, lighter, and less dense. After the muscles/tendons and bones have become stronger, then use a ball which is heavier, larger, and more dense. Also at the beginning, due to the weight of the ball, the muscles are more tensed and consequently the Qi is hard to circulate. However, after practicing for a period of time, the body becomes stronger and this will allow (you) to be more relaxed. Only then (you) advance further and use (your) mind to lead the Qi following the fibers of the wooden ball to communicate between the palms. This can gradually change to go against the fibers and again use the Qi to lead the Qi to communicate between the palms.

在初段功練到一個程度之後，十二基本動作得心應手後，
則手握太極球再依十二基本式練習。普通之太極球可木
製或石製。練力者，多用石製，練氣者，多用木製。練
太極拳者，喜用木製球練氣。初用質鬆、較輕、較小之
球。在筋骨較強後，可用質硬、較重、較大之球。初練
時，因球沉重，肌肉繃緊，氣因而難行。練到一段時間
後，身強體壯，身體輕鬆。此時進一步用意先依質紋而
引氣過球，漸而用意逆紋而引氣過球，以達高層次。

After you have mastered the skills of the body's twelve basic movements and of leading the Qi with the mind efficiently, then you should train using a wooden ball (Figure 38). External styles, which focus on the strength of the muscles and tendons at the beginning, usually use a stone ball for this training. However, internal stylists favor a ball made from wood, which allows them to lead the Qi through the ball more easily and smoothly.

At the beginning of this second level training, due to the weight of the ball, the physical body will be tensed and this will hinder the Qi's smooth circulation. Only after you have conditioned your physical body to a stronger level will you be able to relax your body and allow the Qi to circulate smoothly. At this time, you should use your mind to lead the Qi to pass through the fibers of the wood to communicate with both palms. At the beginning, it is easier to follow the fibers of the wood. After you have reached a profound level, then you lead the Qi against the grain of the fibers. If you are still able to communicate the Qi between both palms, you have reached a profound level of Taiji Ball Qigong.

The last level of practice is returning to the stage of practice without a ball. At this time, because there is no wood, the body can reach to its extreme state of relaxation and softness, the Yi can reach its peak, and the Qi can be lead as you wish without stagnation. In this case, the achievement for both internal and external goals have been accomplished. When using (these skills) to push hands or encounter an opponent, there is more than enough capability to handle the job.

最後段之練習，回到無球之練習。此時，因無木球，身
體可鬆軟至極點。意可達高峰，氣之行隨心所欲。如此
內外兼修，用之於推手應敵，綽綽有餘。

The final stage of Taiji ball training is repeating the twelve patterns without a ball. In this case, your body will be able to reach its maximum relaxation and softness, the mind is strong, and the Qi can be led strongly and effectively.

After you have completed these twelve basic patterns of Taiji ball training, you should mix them any way you like and turn these twelve dead patterns into a living

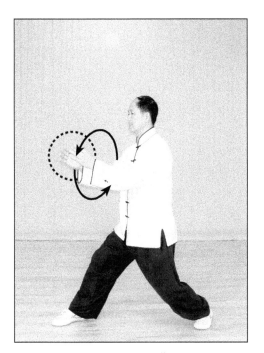
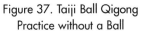

Figure 37. Taiji Ball Qigong
Practice without a Ball

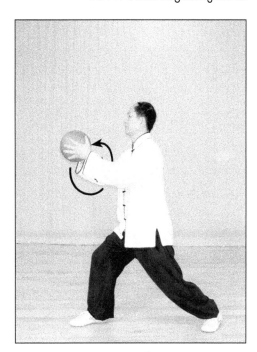

Figure 38. Taiji Ball Qigong
Practice with a Ball

one. Imagine you are pushing hands with someone and apply all of the Taiji ball movements in the actions. In this case, you have made Taiji ball training creative and alive.

PART VI

About Regulating the Spirit
論調神

1. Returning the Essence to the Brain for Nourishing Through Marrow/Brain Washing 洗髓返精補腦篇

In order to raise up the energy resonant vibration level of the brain spirit (i.e., increase vibration frequency band) with the great nature, and also to open the Upper Dan Tian (i.e., Third Eye), you must first know how to convert the essence into Qi, then from the method of "Embryonic Breathing" (Tai Xi) to store the Qi in the Real Dan Tian. When the Qi has accumulated to an abundant level, it can then be led upward along the Thrusting Vessel (Chong Mai) (i.e., spinal cord) to the brain (for nourishing). This is the Gongfu of the Daoist society's training for "returning the essence to the brain for nourishing," "to train the Qi and nourish it to the Shen," and "to train the Qi and sublimate (it to the brain)."

為求腦神與大自然共振能量之提高，與上丹田（第三眼）
之開竅，我必先懂得如何練精化氣，再由胎息之法將氣
蓄於真丹田。當氣蓄至高量時，即可引氣由衝脈上行而
至腦部。此為道家所謂之返精補腦、練氣化神、與練氣
昇華之功夫。

In order to unify your spirit with the natural spirit, you must train in two important parts. The first is to activate more brain cells and raise the energy up to a more highly energized state. When this happens, the resonant vibration energy in the space (i.e., Spiritual Valley) (Shen Gu, 神谷) between the two hemispheres of the brain will be enhanced. Consequently, the vibration frequency band will also be widened. This will increase the sensitivity of the spiritual correspondence with your surroundings and with the great nature.

In order to build up a smooth connection without obstruction, you must also re-open your third eye (Yintang, 印堂; or Tian Yan, 天眼) (i.e., Upper Dan Tian). When the third eye is opened, you will be able to sense and therefore understand the natural energy and spirit. You will also regain the capability of telepathy. This is the Daoist definition of spiritual enlightenment.

To reach this goal, you must first learn how to convert the essence into Qi (Lian Jing Hua Qi, 練精化氣), and nourish the Shen (i.e., spirit) with Qi (Lian Qi Hua Shen, 練氣化神). Essence refers to the post-birth essence stored in the body and also to the hormones. In order to convert these essences into Qi, you must practice abdominal breathing. As discussed before, the abdominal area is considered the "Lower Dan Tian" (Xia Dan Tian, 下丹田) by Daoists or "Qi Ocean" (Qihai, 氣海) by Chinese medical society. This area is also called "Elixir Furnace" (Dan Lu, 丹爐), since through the abdominal up and down exercises, the stored food essence (i.e., fat) can be converted into Qi through biochemical reaction.

However, in order to activate more brain cells, you must first store the Qi in the Real Dan Tian (Zhen Dan Tian, 真丹田) (i.e., biobattery) to an abundant level. Every brain cell consumes at least 12 times as much oxygen as regular cells. Since oxygen is required for biochemical combustion processes in the body, to produce energy (i.e., Qi), it is reasonable to assume that each brain cell also consumes approximately 12 times the Qi of a regular cell. This means that to activate more brain cells and to raise them up to a higher energetic state, it will require a great amount of Qi. The Daoists believed that Embryonic Breathing (Tai Xi, 胎息) was the method of storing the Qi in the Real Dan Tian (i.e., second brain). In Embryonic Breathing, you also stimulate the pancreas, adrenals and testicles for hormone production. It is now known that hormones function as catalysts to the biochemical reactions in the body. Therefore, the function of the body's metabolism can be carried out effectively. When the hormone level is enhanced, the Qi can be produced and stored more efficiently.

What is the brain? It is the master and the center of the human physical body and spiritual body. The brain is constructed from two hemispheres, left and right. The space at the center is called Upper Dan Tian, Spiritual Valley (Shen Gu), or Mud Pill Palace (Ni Wan Gong) by the Daoists. It is the residence of the spirit and therefore called Spiritual Residence (Shen Shi) and is the residence of the Valley Spirit (Gu Shen). Mud Pill Palace refers to what the scientists call brain center, where the pituitary and pineal glands are located. From these two glands, growth hormone and melatonin are produced. Hormones are the catalyst of the body's biochemical reactions. Therefore, if the hormone levels (in the body) can be maintained at the same level as that of youth, then the (body's) metabolism will be carried out smoothly, the function of the body can be healthy, and longevity can be achieved.

腦者，人身體與精神之主宰中心也。腦部之構造由左右
兩腦構成。中心無腦處，道家稱之為上丹田，神谷，泥
丸宮，為人神之室，因而亦稱之為神室。此神室乃谷神
所宅之所。泥丸宮乃今科學上所謂之腦中心腦下腺與松
果腺之所在地也。由此兩腺，生長激素與梅那他林賀爾
蒙產生矣。從今之科學上知，賀爾蒙乃身體中生化反應
中之催化劑也。因而如賀爾蒙之生產量保持年青時之產
量，則新陳代謝順利，身體機能高昂，可保青春。

Daoists consider the entire brain as the location of the Upper Dan Tian (Shang Dan Tian, 上丹田). The space between the two hemispheres of the brain is called the "Spiritual Valley" (Shen Gu, 神谷) and is the place where the spirit resides. Therefore, it is also called "Spirit Residence" (Shen Shi, 神室). The spirit is called "Valley Spirit" (Gu Shen, 谷神). The center of the brain where the pituitary and pineal glands are located is called "mud pill palace" (Ni Wan Gong, 泥丸宮) and can produce essence (i.e., hormones) (Figures 39 and 40).

When the brain energy is raised up to a higher level, the resonance level can also be raised up and the resonance frequency band can be widened. When this happens, the brain's spiritual sensitivity can be raised up to a higher level. When the hormone levels of the body are high, the body's metabolic processes can be carried out efficiently and smoothly.

The Spirit Valley is also known as the resonance center of the brain. When the brain has been charged to a higher energy level, the band of the resonance frequency will be widened and the radiating energy will also be stronger. Consequently, the feeling (i.e., correspondence) of the external environmental echo is strong and the sensitivity is high. The processing capability of the brain can also been raised up to a higher level. The Daoist Gongfu of "returning the essence to nourish the brain" means to increase the charging capability of the brain and to increase the brain's electromotive force (i.e., electric potential difference). When this electric potential difference has reached a high level, the third eye can be re-opened and consequently, the resonant vibration with the external world can occur without obstruction. This is what the Daoist society called "opening the heaven eye" (Kai Tian Yan). When the heaven eye is opened, the aperture to heaven is opened. This is the first step of heaven-human unification.

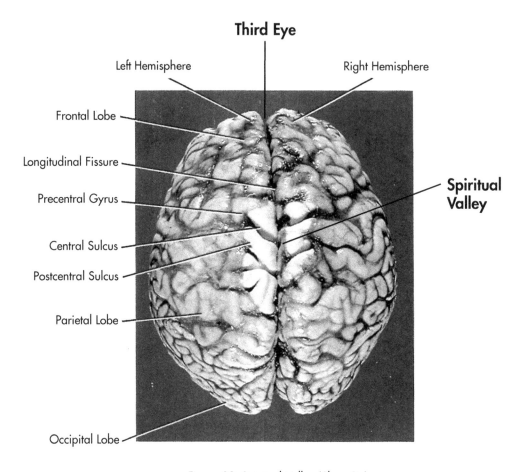

Figure 39. Spiritual Valley (Shen Gu)

神谷亦為科學上所知之腦部振盪中心，腦部的充電量愈
高，則振盪之頻率幅度大，外射線能量大，因而腦部之
外感力強，敏感度高。不但如此，腦部之思考力亦為增
高。道家之返精補腦之功夫，即在加強腦部之充電量，
以增高腦部之電動勢。在電位差達到高電動勢時，能將
第三眼從新開啟，並與外界能量共振交接無阻。此為道
家與佛家所謂之開天眼矣。天眼之開，可開宇宙之竅，
為天人合一之首步。

The Western term "third eye" is called "heaven eye" (Tian Yan, 天眼) in Chinese Qigong. Through re-opening this aperture, the energy vibration of your brain can correspond with the energy around you and with nature. When this happens, you

Pineal Gland   Pituitary Gland

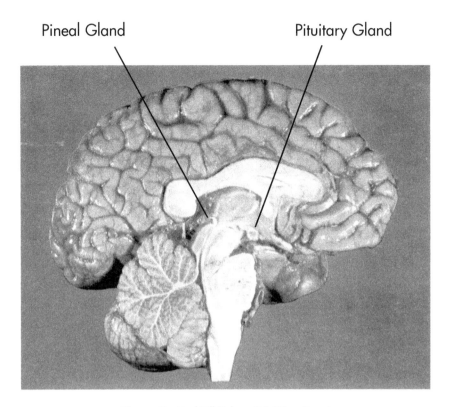

Figure 40. Mud Pill Palace (Ni Wan Gong)

can see many things that are beyond what people who have not opened their third eye can see. This is the stage of enlightenment in Daoism and Buddhism. The third eye or heaven eye is called Yintang (M-HN-3) (印堂) (i.e., Seal Hall) in acupuncture. This place is at the end of the valley, which allows the echo or resonant energy to exit and enter.

In order to re-open the third eye, you must first bring the resonant energy level in the spiritual valley to a higher stage. When this energy reaches to a good level (i.e., threshold energy), the third eye can be re-opened. It is believed that through opening the third eye, you can regain the capability of telepathy.

> *The first step of regulating the spirit is to raise up the spirit. The next step it is to abide the spirit, and to firm the spirit, to stabilize the spirit, and finally to condense the spirit. This is what Lao Zi said in Chapter 10 (of* Dao De Jing*): "To carry and operate the vigorous spirit (Po), can it be (staying) without separation?" If the spirit can be condensed, then it will be firmed automatically. When the spirit can be firmly residing (in its residence), then there is longevity. In Chapter 6 of Lao Zi (i.e.,* Dao De Jing*) it says: "If the Valley Spirit does not decease, it is called 'Xuan Pin'; the door of the 'Xuan Pin' is called 'the root of heaven and earth.' Slender and continuous as if existing, when used, there is no ending (i.e., unlimited)." From the spirit's condensation, the electric potential*

difference can be increased. Consequently, the third eye can be re-opened and reach the highest cultivation goal of heaven-human unification.

調神之首步在於提神，之後，為守神，繼之為固神，定神，爾後凝神。此亦即老子第十章所謂之〝載營魄抱一，能無離乎？〞神能凝，則自固。神固守則長生。老子第六章云：〝谷神不死，是謂玄牝；玄牝之門，是謂天地根。綿綿若存，用之不勤。〞此即是道家調神之長生功夫。不但如此，由凝神可增進腦部之電位差，由之可開啟第三眼而達天人合一之最高修養境地。

The first step in cultivation is to lead the Qi upward through the Thrusting Vessel (Chong Mai, 衝脈) (i.e., Spinal Cord) to nourish the brain and thus raise up the brain's resonant level and also widen the vibration frequency band. However, even if you can lead the Qi up, if you do not know how to keep it and protect it, the high energy status of the brain cannot be controlled. Therefore, you must learn how to keep the spirit there (Shou Shen, 守神), and then how to firm it (Gu Shen, 固神). Only then are you able to condense your spirit intensely (Ning Shen, 凝神), which allows you to re-open the third eye.

Literally, "Xuan Pin" (玄牝) means "Concealed Female" or "Mysterious Female." Female gives birth to new life. It is the root and origin of reincarnation. Therefore, the "Valley Spirit" is this 'concealed or mysterious female' (Xuan Pin). When this Xuan Pin is kept alive, we can unify ourselves with heaven and earth (i.e., nature). The gate of the Xuan Pin is the third eye; as if existing, and as if not. However, if you know how to use it, its utility is unlimited.

2. Thesis of the Unification of Spirit and Qi 神氣相合論

One of the Daoist classics said: "Shen is the master of Qi, and it moves and stops with the Qi. Breathing is the secret key to the Qi's forward and backward. The secret key must have the master (Shen), and the master must have the Yi. Three things (Shen, breathing, and Yi) must be used at the same time. That will produce the really marvelous and tricky Gongfu of heavenly circulation (i.e., Small and Grand Circulations). When one is missing, it is hard to achieve the final goal." This saying has already told us clearly that Shen, breathing, and Yi (i.e., wisdom mind), are mutually related and cannot be separated. It also says that Shen and Qi are in the same position and move or stop together. This means the Shen and Qi are unified. The classic again said: "Shen and Qi move and stop together and not separately. The Yi stays at the center palace like a cart's axle. The wheels (Shen and Qi) and the axle (Yi) (provide) mutual support. The axle does not move, but lets the wheels turn by themselves." From this, it is known that Shen and Qi mutually coordinate with each other and do not separate. From the unification of Shen and Qi, and also from the Embryonic Breathing's conceiving, the holy spiritual embryo can be produced. Li, Qing-An's poetry said: "Shen and Qi combine to originate the super spiritual quality, Xin (i.e., mind) and breath are mutually dependent to generate the holy embryo." From this, it is known that if the Shen and Qi are not unified, the spiritual embryo will not be generated. Even if (you) have mastered the Gongfu of regulating the Xin and breathing, it is still difficult to conceive the holy embryo and achieve the final goal (i.e., spiritual enlightenment).

道經云：〝神是與氣同行同住之主宰，息是進氣退氣之機關，機不可少主，主不可少意，三物並用，方為真正玄妙周天之功夫，缺一難成正果。〞此言已明顯的告訴我等，神、息、與意三者互相關連，不可分離。並言之，神與氣之同位，必須同行同住，即神氣相合也。經再云：〝神氣同行同住而不離，其意主中宮如軸心，輪軸互用，軸不動而任輪之自轉也。〞從此可知，神氣互相為用，而不分離。由神氣之相合，與胎息之蘊化，聖胎可望產生矣。李清庵詩云：〝神氣和合生靈質，心息相依結聖胎。〞由此可知神氣未合，靈胎不生。即使有了調心與調息之功夫，仍難蘊結聖胎，而成正果也。

The Shen (i.e., Spirit) (神) is the master of the Qi and moves together with it. Though the secret for controlling the movement of the Qi is the breathing, the most important of all is what is behind, the Shen. It is the Yi (意) which ultimately controls the entire training. Shen and Qi move together like wheels. However, these wheels are directed and controlled by the axle. This axle is your mind (Yi). The mind keeps to the center so that it can direct what is happening, but it should not get involved in the turning of the wheels. This is the stage of regulating without regulating. When this happens, your mind will reach a profound meditative state and Shen and Qi can move freely without any disturbance. When you have reached this stage, the Spiritual Embryo (Sheng Tai, 聖胎) will be conceived. This is the seed of reaching the goal of enlightenment.

When you practice Taijiquan, the final stage of cultivation is spiritual enlightenment. Therefore, you must know how to raise up your Spirit of Vitality. When this spirit is raised, the Qi's circulation will be smooth, natural, and can be led efficiently. When this happens, the Qi can be manifested into physical power (i.e., Jin, 勁) for martial purposes. This Qi can also be led upward following the Thrusting Vessel (i.e., Chong Mai, 衝脈) (Spinal Cord) to the brain to nourish it for enlightenment.

3. Thesis of the Mutual Dependence of Spirit and Breathing 神息相依論

From the previous article, it is known that in order to generate a holy embryo, (you) must be able to unify the Shen and Qi. However, without a proficient level of Gongfu in Embryonic Breathing, Qi still cannot be stored in the Real Dan Tian. Without an abundant level of bioelectricity (i.e., Qi's) storage, the spiritual embryo cannot be conceived effectively, and then led upward following the Thrusting Vessel to achieve the goal of 'returning the essence to nourish the brain' and 'training the Qi for sublimation.' In this case, the vibration band of resonant frequencies of the brain will be narrow and the Shen cannot be raised to a higher level. Therefore, when (you) train Shen, (you) must first start from regulating the breathing. When (you) have reached the stage of regulating without regulating, then the spiritual embryo has already been generated. When this spiritual embryo has been led upward to the Spiritual Valley (i.e., space between the two hemispheres of the brain), then (you) have reached the stage of regulating the spirit. When (you) regulate the spirit until no regulating is necessary, then everything is natural, smooth and effortless, and the goal has been achieved. The Complete Book of Principal Contents of Life and Human Nature; Conceiving in Qi Cavity, Marvellous Public Return to Roots *said: "Regulating the breathing should regulate the breathing until it is stopped, training the Shen must train until the Shen of training is no more in Shen." This is what it means.*

由上篇已知，為產聖胎，必須能神氣相合。然而，未能有高度之胎息功夫，氣仍然不能蓄積於真丹田。未能有高度之蓄電量，則不能有效的達到產生靈胎，再由衝脈上引以達返精補腦、練氣昇華之目的。由之，腦之共振量與幅度必低，神亦無法上提。因此，練神必先由調息著手。當達到不調而調之境地時，神胎已孕。在神胎上引至神谷後，即為調神之功夫。當調神調至無神自神時，一切自然，則正果已成矣。《性命圭旨全書‧蟄藏氣穴，眾妙歸根》云：〝調息要調真息息，煉神須煉不神神。〞此即其意也。

The final goal of Daoist spiritual cultivation is to lead the Qi from the Real Dan Tian following the Thrusting Vessel (Chong Mai, 衝脈) (i.e., spinal cord) to the brain to energize the brain cells to a higher state. When this happens, the band of resonance frequencies between the two brain hemispheres will be widened and the spirit can therefore reach a more enlightened level. This practice is called "returning the essence to nourish the brain" (Huan Jing Bu Nao, 還精補腦) and also "training the Qi for sublimation" (Lian Qi Sheng Hua, 練氣昇華) in Daoist alchemy.

However, in order to reach this goal, you must first have an abundant store of Qi in the Real Dan Tian. Activating more brain cells and raising up their energy state to a higher level requires a great amount of Qi. For this reason, in order to reach enlightenment, you must first learn how to generate Qi and then store it in the Real Dan Tian through Embryonic Breathing.

To reach the final goal of spiritual enlightenment, you must learn how to regulate the Embryonic Breathing until no regulating is necessary. In the same way, once you lead the Qi to the brain to nourish the Shen, you must train to a stage where it is unnecessary to keep the Shen focused on regulation. This means everything has become natural.

4. Thesis of Wuji Spirit 無極神論

In the Daoist family, Wuji spirit means to refine the spirit and return it to noth-ingness. This also means the spirit has returned to the great nature of emptiness and is no more bothered and confused by human affairs and emotions. The ulti-mate goal of Taijiquan training is to return to the Wuji (spiritual) state from the two polarities of Yin and Yang. This means through the Dao of Taijiquan, (you are) leading the spirit's Yin and Yang in (your) body back to the stage of Wuji (i.e., no extremity).

無極神者，乃道家所謂之練神返虛也。亦即神返回虛空
之大自然，而不再為人間事物與感情所困擾。練太極拳
之最終目的是由陰陽返回無極。亦即由太極拳之道，導
引人身陰陽之神返回無極之境也。

Taijiquan was created based on the theory of Taiji. Taiji is the pivotal force which makes the Wuji divide into Yin and Yang, and also makes the Yin and Yang reunite and become the Wuji. The ultimate goal of Daoist spiritual cultivation is to reunite the human spirit with the natural spirit and re-enter the Wuji state. In order to do so, we must get rid of emotional disturbances and human affairs.

What is the spirit of Wuji? It is carefree and leisurely, no worries and no distur-bance, nature as it is. In order to reach this stage, (you) must first get rid of the seven emotions and the six desires, the mind must be peaceful and the Qi har-monious. This is to get rid of the obsessions in human society and ask for the ter-mination of human thinking. This aims to the same final goal as Taijiquan prac-tice. From practicing Taijiquan, (you are) searching for the comprehension of human Taiji and Yin and Yang, and from this comprehension to achieve the Dao of Wuji. Therefore, practicing Taijiquan is only a path to lead (us) from Yin and Yang to the Wuji. After reaching the Wuji state, there is no more necessity in the use of Taijiquan.

無極神者，悠悠然然，無牽無掛，自然如是。欲達此境
界，必先去七情六慾，心平氣和。去除塵世之困惱，求
凡念之淨除。此與練習太極拳之最終目的相同。由練研
太極拳，而去領悟人生太極陰陽之理，再由中去尋臻無
極之道。因之，習練太極拳，只不過是一條引陰陽至無
極之路。在達無極之地後，太極拳不復為我所用也。

Taijiquan was created in Daoist monasteries, in which the spiritual cultivation aimed for freedom from emotional spiritual bondage. From this freedom, we can return ourselves to the Wuji state. Taijiquan is only one of the methods which could lead us to comprehend the human life, and finally lead us to a harmonious and peaceful Wuji state. Once we have reached this state, Taijiquan practice is no longer important and will become part of our nature. This is the stage of regulating without regulating in spirit.

5. Thesis of the Spirit of No Spirit 無神之神論

The spirit of no spirit means the stage of unification of heaven and human's spirit. My spirit is also the natural spirit. Heaven and human have been unified as one single body and will not be apart again. I am the heaven and the heaven is I. The human body has already come to naught and human nature is no longer existing; (I) will not enter the cycle of reincarnation and will not be born again. This is the highest level of Daoist spiritual Qigong cultivation, the stage of crushing the emptiness.

無神之神亦即天人合一，我神即自然之神。天人合為一
體，而不再分離。我即是天，天即是我。人體已化，人
性無存。不再輪迴，不再轉世。此是道家氣功修練之最
高程次，粉碎虛空也。

The final stage of Daoist spiritual cultivation is to reach the stage of unification of human spirit and natural spirit (Tian Ren He Yi, 天人合一). In this case, no more reincarnation is necessary. Individual spirit becomes part of the natural spirit and contaminated human thoughts have been cleansed and purified. In this case, there is no longer the stage of emptiness, but a reunion with nature.

PART VII

About Jin 論勁

1. Thesis of Jin 勁論

What is Jin? It is Li-Qi or Qi-Li. From the word, it can be interpreted as 'using the Yi to lead the Li (i.e., muscular power) to the (precise) path'. In order to increase the ability to use the Yi to lead the Qi to a higher level and thus be available for you to use, (your) Yi must be concentrated. When the Yi is used to lead, the Qi will follow (naturally). When the Qi follows (the Yi for manifestation), the internal Li can be strengthened. You should know that (all) the (physical) movements are initiated from the Yi. From the Yi's leading, the Qi will reach to the desired part of the physical body. When the nerves are stimulated by the Qi (i.e., bioelectricity), the muscles will withdraw and expand, initiating the movement.

勁者，力氣或氣力也。從字意上解，乃由‘意’引
‘力’入‘徑’之謂也。為能以意引氣至一較高程度，
為我所用，意必專也。意引之，而氣隨之。氣隨之，而
內力增強之。吾須知動始于意，由意引氣而達身體部位，
神經受氣導至肌肉之收縮與伸張，動由是生也。

If you try to find the definition of Jin (勁) in a Chinese dictionary, you will soon see the definition is Li-Qi (力氣) or Qi-Li (氣力). Qi is the bio-energy or bioelectricity, while Li is the muscular power manifested physically. From this, you can see that the definition of Jin should be "the manifestation of Qi into muscular power."

In addition, from the structure of the Chinese word, Jin (勁) can be divided into two words: "巠" (i.e., path) and "力" (i.e., muscular force). From this, you can see that the meaning of Jin (勁) is actually "direct the muscular force into the precise path." In order to direct the muscular force into the right path, the mind (i.e., Yi, 意) must be concentrated. When the Yi is concentrated, the Qi that is led will be strong. When this strong Qi is manifested into physical action, the manifestation can be powerful and penetrating.

In Chinese martial Qigong, it is said: "use the Yi to lead the Qi, and from the Qi, the power is thus manifested" (以意引氣，由氣生力). This clearly implies that it is your mind (i.e., Yi) that initiates the action. When this Yi is initiated, the Qi is led to the physical body for action. From this, you can see that in order to have strong Jin manifestation, you will need a high level of mental concentration.

When the Yi is not concentrated and not strong, the Qi (led) will also be weak. When the Qi is weak, then the power manifested from the physical body will be shallow. In general physical movement, the concentration of the Yi does not have to be high, and the actions can be carried out as wished. Consequently, the Jin's manifestation is not apparent. However, if there is a need to enhance your physical strength to do some special tasks, then the Yi must be concentrated to a higher level. Consequently, the Qi's circulation can also be reinforced and thus the Li's manifestation will be more clear (i.e., stronger), which means the Jin's manifestation is more obvious.

$$Yi \xrightarrow[\textit{Internal Jin}]{\hspace{3cm}} Qi \xrightarrow[\textit{External Jin}]{\hspace{4cm}} Action$$

意不專、不強，氣則弱。氣弱，則身體部位之力顯微。
普通動作，意不用專，即能隨心所欲，因此勁不顯著。
然如須增強體力以行特別之功，則意必較專，氣行因而
能增強，力因而能顯明，勁亦能突出。

$$意 \longrightarrow 氣 \longrightarrow 行動$$
$$\quad\;\; 內勁 \qquad\; 外勁$$

Jin can be distinguished as "internal Jin" (Nei Jin, 內勁) and "external Jin" (Wai Jin, 外勁). The Yi that leads the Qi with the coordination of correct breathing is called "internal Jin." The correct body movement that allows the Qi to be manifested into physical action effectively is called "external Jin." When the internal Jin and external Jin can be coordinated and harmonized with each other efficiently, it is called "unification of internal and external" (Nei Wai Xiang He, 內外相合).

From the above discussion, it can be seen that Jin can be discriminated as 'internal Jin' and 'external Jin.' What is 'internal Jin'? It refers to using the Yi to lead the Qi. It is related to the Yi's concentration and abundance of the Qi's circulation. We will discuss this from the scientific perspective in the next thesis. What is 'external Jin'? It refers to the external manifestation of the Jin. It is related to the conditions of the physical body and the way the Jins are manifested. From different ways of Jin's manifestation, Jin can be classified as hard Jin, soft-hard Jin, and soft Jin. These are emphasized in different styles. We will discuss this in the following thesis.

由上可知，勁可分內勁與外勁。內勁者，以意引氣也。
其有關乎於意之專與氣行之沛否。下篇將由科學上之觀
點討論之。外勁者，勁顯與外也。其有關乎於物理身體
之情況與顯勁之法也。由於勁顯之異，勁可再分為硬勁、
軟硬勁、軟勁。不同門派因之而分也。下將專篇討論之。

Different Chinese martial styles have different ways to express Jin. For example, Tiger Claw style pays more attention to hard Jin, White Crane focuses more on soft-hard Jin, while Taijiquan concentrates more on soft Jin. However, the basic theory of using the Yi to lead the Qi and then manifest externally remains the same. If you wish to know more about the theory of different Jins' manifestation, please refer to the book: *"The Essence of Shaolin White Crane"* published by YMAA.

> *From different applications, Jin can be classified as offensive Jins, defensive Jins, and non-offensive and non-defensive Jins. Offensive Jins are classified as Yang which focus on emitting Jin, as seen in Wardoff Jin (Peng Jin) and Bump Jin (Kao Jin). Defensive Jins are also Neutralizing Jins and are classified as Yin. They neutralize the coming Jins from the opponent, as seen in Rollback Jin (Lu Jin) and Leading Jin (Yin Jin). Non-offensive and non-defensive Jins are used to train the body's feeling, such as Listening Jin (Ting Jin) and Understanding Jin (Dong Jin). However, some Jins can be used both for offense and defense. For instance, though the main purpose of Wardoff Jin is for offense, when the opportunity is appropriate, it is often used for defense. From this it can be seen that the creation of an advantageous opportunity is decided by you, and all the applications depend on you. It is alive and not dead. The learners should ponder this carefully.*

由不同之應用，勁可再分為攻勁、守勁、與不攻不守勁
之分。攻勁者，陽也，專行於勁之發放，譬如掤勁與靠
勁等。守勁者，化勁也，陰也，專用於化解彼之來勁，
譬如攦勁與引勁等。不攻不守勁者，專用於訓練己身之
感覺，譬如聽勁與懂勁等然。雖然，有些勁卻是攻守兩
用，依不同之用法而定。譬如掤勁，雖主用於攻，然而
時機適宜，卻常用於守。由此可知，造機造勢在我，應
用也在我。是活用的，而不是死板的。學者須慎思之。

Generally, depending on the applications, we can classify the Jin into offensive and defensive categories, and also those that are neither, you should not be restricted by these classifications. Application of the Jin depends on the situation. It is alive. If you are interested in more discussion of Taijiquan Jins, please refer to the book: *Tai Chi Theory and Martial Power* by YMAA.

2. Theory of Internal Jin 內勁篇

What is Internal Jin (Nei Jin)? It is the energy source of the power. What is Qi? It is bioelectricity. What is the Yi? It is the electromotive force (EMF) (i.e., electric potential difference). When the Yi is strong, the EMF will also be strong (i.e., greater electric potential difference). When the EMF is strong, the flow of bioelectricity will be strong. When the flow of bioelectricity is strong, the energy flow will also be strong. This the theory of Internal Jin. When the energy flow is strong, the Jin manifested will be powerful. As mentioned earlier, from Ohm's Law it is known that:

$$V = I \times R$$

V=Electric Potential Difference
I=Current
R=Resistance

From this formula, it is known that the potential difference is proportional to the current. That means, when the electric potential difference is bigger, the current is also bigger. That is, when the EMF is strong, the current is strong. EMF (in Taijiquan) is the Yi. That means, when Yi is strong, the bioelectricity is strong. In order to have strong Yi, (you) should start from still meditation. From still meditation, the Gongfu of the Yi's concentration can be trained. When the Yi is concentrated, the Spirit of Vitality is high and the EMF is strong; this is the first secret key to Internal Jin.

內勁者，動力能源也。氣者，生化電也。意者，電動勢也。意強，電動勢強（亦即電位差大）。電動勢強，生化電流則強矣。生化電流強，則動力能量大。此為內勁之理。動力能量大，則其外勁顯現力強。前已題及，由歐姆定律知：

$$V = I \times R$$

V: 電位差（電動勢）
I: 電流
R: 電阻

由此公式知，電位差與電流成正比。此即電位差大，電流亦大。這也就是說，當電動勢強，電流則強。電動勢者，意也。亦即意強，則生化電流強。求意強，當由靜坐著手。在靜坐中，訓練意專之功夫。意專，則精神高，電動勢強。此為內勁之一竅。

Though the bioelectric network in the human body is much more complicated than a regular electric network, Ohm's Law can still be adopted to interpret the manifestation of Jin. When the mind is strong, the power manifested is more powerful and concentrated.

You should always remember that when the theory of Taiji is applied into Taijiquan, Taiji is your mind. This mind is "Grand Ultimate" (i.e., Taiji, 太極). The mind can travel beyond the limits of space and time. This mind is creative and powerful. It is this mind that makes us different from other animals. Therefore, in Taijiquan, the cultivation of mind is always the first priority of training. The key to increasing the mind's power and concentration is through still meditation.

In addition, it is known from the formula that resistance is inversely proportional to current. That means when the resistance is high, the current is small and when the resistance is low, the current is large. The resistance in human is related to whether the body is loose or tight. If it is tight and tensed, the resistance is high and the current is weak. If it is loose and soft, then the resistance is low and the current is strong. From this, it is seen that the second secret key to manifesting Internal Jin is to keep the physical body loose and soft.

再者，由公式可知電阻與電流成反比。亦即電阻高，電流小。電阻低，電流大。人身電阻者，有關身體之鬆緊也。繃緊之，則電阻高而電流弱。鬆軟之，則電阻低而電流強。由此可知，保持身體鬆軟乃是內勁之二竅。

Taijiquan is commonly called "moving meditation" in Western society. The reason for this is that when you practice Taijiquan, you are using your concentrated mind with a sense of enemy (i.e., imaginary opponent) to lead the Qi to the arms and legs for the Jin's manifestation. In order to lead the Qi efficiently and effectively with the mind, the body must be relaxed, loose, and soft. Only then can the Qi circulate without stagnation. The key to keeping the body loose and soft is maintaining movement and agility in the joints. Only then can the Jin be initiated by the legs, controlled by the waist, shaped by the chest and spine, and finally manifested at the hands. From this, we can see that without of a relaxed and soft body, Taijiquan will lose its meaning and basic principles, and the action cannot be called Taijiquan any more.

Furthermore, even if the Yi is strong, (you) must still know the method of using the Yi to lead the Qi. If (you) do not obtain this method, even though the Qi is strong, you still cannot use it effectively and the level of achievement will not be great. (In order to) learn the method of using the Yi to lead the Qi, (you) must start from Taiji Qigong. In Taiji Qigong practice, train with an imaginary opponent, also with coordination with the 'Reversed Abdominal Breathing,' using the

Yi to lead the Qi. After practicing for a long time, it will become a habit. If those learners know the method of 'Grand Circulation,' then its effectiveness will be marvelous. This is the secret of Internal Jin through the use if the Yi to lead the Qi and coordination of the breathing. Those practitioners who are serious martial applications of Taijiquan must not proceed without knowing this theory and methods of practice.

甚者，意雖強，仍須知如何以意引氣之法。如不得法，
氣雖強，但不能有效之引用，其功效仍不大矣。以意引
氣之法，須由太極氣功著手。由太極氣功之練習中，練
習假想之目標，再配合逆式腹呼吸之法，以意引氣，久
而久之，自成習慣也。學者如能知曉大周天運氣之法，
則其效用大矣！此由意配合呼吸以意引氣之法，即內勁
之訣。學者重於太極武學應用者，不可不知此理與練習
方法也。

As explained earlier, "Reverse Abdominal Breathing" (Ni Fu Hu Xi, 逆腹呼吸) is the natural way for us to manifest power physically. Whenever you wish to manifest your energy into physical power, to push a car or lift a weight for example, without thinking you change your breathing manner from "Normal Breathing" (Zheng Hu Xi, 正呼吸) to "Reverse Abdominal Breathing." If you wish to enhance the power manifestation to a higher level, you must also know how to open the Mingmen (Gv-4) (命門) cavity and lead the Qi upward along the spine and then lead it out to the arms through the Dazhui (Gv-14) (大椎) cavity. This is what is called "Qi circulates along the spine" (Qi Yan Ji Xing, 氣沿脊行) in *Taijiquan Classic*. If you are interested in Taiji Qigong, please refer to the book: *The Essence of Taiji Qigong*, by YMAA. You should also review Part V for Grand Circulation Breathing.

3. Theory of External Jin 外勁篇

What is External Jin? It is the external manifestation of Internal Jin. (The effectiveness of) manifesting external Jin is not only affected by the strength or weakness of the Internal Jin, but also by the physical structure and the skills of manifestation. The efficiency of the external Jin's manifestation depends on how the hands act, the eyes' manner, how the body moves, actual fighting skills, and stepping methods. Consequently, Jin can be categorized as hard Jin, soft-hard Jin, and soft Jin. There are some (styles) whose external Jins are initiated from the legs, such as Long Fist and Taijiquan. There are some (styles) whose external Jins are initiated from the waist, such as White Crane. Furthermore, there are some (styles) whose external short Jins are initiated from the four limbs. The emitting of external Jin depends on how (the Jin) is stored in the bows and emits from them. It is said there are five bows in Taijiquan. These five bows are the two arm bows, the two leg bows, and the body bow (i.e., torso). Other styles such as White Crane, which is specialized in soft-hard Jin, say the body is equipped with six bows. For six bows, other than the four bows of the arms and legs, the body (i.e., torso) includes two bows: the chest bow and spine bow. The spine bow is vertical and the chest bow is horizontal.

外勁者，內勁顯現於外者也。外勁之表現，不僅取決與內勁之強弱，亦取決於身體物理之造化與技巧之顯現。外勁之顯現效率取決於手法、眼法、身法、技法、與步法。因而勁分別有硬勁、軟硬勁、與軟勁。有外勁之勁發於腿如長拳、太極拳者，有外勁之勁發於腰如白鶴拳者，更有些硬短勁者，勁發於四肢。外勁之發，取決於如何蓄弓與放弓。大極拳謂身備五弓。五弓者，兩臂弓、兩腿弓、與身弓也。其他有專軟硬勁之門派者，如白鶴拳然，謂身備六弓。六弓者，除臂、腿四弓外，身俱有兩弓，胸弓與脊弓也。

There are five basic elements that influence how the Jin is manifested and how the fighting skills are carried out. These five elements are: hands (Shou, 手), eyes (Yan, 眼), body (Shen, 身), techniques (Fa, 法), and stepping (Bu, 步). In other words, achievement depends on how the Jin is manifested in your hands, the level of alertness and awareness of your being (which usually corresponds to the eyes), how your body stores the Jin in its structure, how the techniques are executed, and your skill and firmness in stepping. From all of these factors, thousands of styles were created and developed and discriminated into hard, soft-hard, and soft styles. Consequently, the manifestation of Jin is also distinct from one style to another.

> *Opening the bow stores the Jin; releasing the bow emits the Jin. The effectiveness of releasing the bow depends on how skillfully the bows are opened. The storage of Internal Jin depends on the Yi, Qi, and breathing. The storage of External Jin is decided on when the root is firmed and also how the six bows are opened. This means the body's skills (i.e., postures of storage). The efficacy of the External Jin's expression depends on the sharpness of the Jin-Li (i.e., focus) and the speed. Therefore, all styles have their own training methods to strengthen (the storing power of) their bows so as to increase the speed and to improve the sharpness of the Jin-Li. (Because) Jin is the key in winning and losing, every style keeps its training methods secret and will not reveal them to the outside. However, the most important key to the Jin's emitting and neutralization is the unification of internal and external. That means that through harmonious coordination of internal and external Jins, (the Jins) are manifested from internal to external.*

開弓者，蓄勁也。放弓者，勁發也。放弓之效取決於開
弓之巧。內勁之蓄在於意，在於氣，在於息。外勁之蓄
在於根之穩度，在於開弓於六弓之巧。此亦即身法也。
外勁之發取決於勁力之脆然與速度之快慢否。由是，各
各門派都有其專練之法以強其弓，以增其速，以提高其
勁力之脆然。勁乃勝負之關要。由之，各門派都以其訓
練方法為秘而不輕易外傳。雖然，勁發、化之最要者，
乃是內外合一。亦即內、外勁之諧調，由內而顯現於外
也。

In order to manifest Jin powerfully, you must first have a firm root. This is especially true for those styles that use the root to initiate the Jin. You must also know how to draw the bows properly so the Jin's storage can reach its highest level. This is no different from throwing a javelin in an Olympic competition. If you know how to store the Jin in all six bows efficiently, the spear you throw will go far. It is because of this that all Chinese martial arts styles have their own training methods in storing the Jin, and this is usually kept top secret. A good method of training can not only make your Jin's manifestation more powerful, but can also shorten the training time. Naturally, though the training methods are different, the Dao (i.e., basic theory and principle) remains the same for all styles. This Dao is the unification of internal and external.

4. Theory of Hard Jin, Soft-Hard Jin, and Soft Jin 硬勁、軟硬勁、軟勁篇

From different Jin manifestation, Jin can be classified as hard Jin, soft-hard Jin, and soft Jin. Hard Jin belongs to Yang and its characteristics are more towards the manifestation of the external Jin, just like the manifestation of a hard staff. Soft-hard Jins are first soft and then hard, and are like rattan in their manifestation. With soft Jins, Yi and Qi are primary, the body is soft, and the Jin is expressed like a whip.

根據不同顯勁之方法，勁可分硬勁、軟硬勁、軟勁也。
硬勁者，陽也，較趨於外勁之顯現，其顯現如棍然。軟
硬勁者，先軟後硬也，其勁之顯現如藤然。軟勁者，身
體柔軟如軟鞭也。意氣為先，勁之發如軟鞭然。

Hard Jins (Ying Jin, 硬勁) focus on the training of external Jin. The strength of the physical body and manifesting this strength externally are the major concerns. With soft-hard Jins (Ruan Ying Jin, 軟硬勁), in order to execute the Jin to its highest level, you must have a concentrated mind which can lead the Qi strongly to the arms or legs for the Jin's manifestation. When you execute the soft Jins (Ruan Jin, 軟勁), your mind must reach to a maximum level of concentration so the Qi can be led more strongly than in the other two Jins. Therefore, the power manifested from the soft-whip Jin can focus on a tiny spot for cavity attacks (Dian Xue, 點穴).

> With hard Jins, the body is tensed and not loose. Though the Li (i.e., muscular power) is strong, the Jins are clumsy, dull, and shallow. This is because, though the Yi is concentrated and the Qi can be strong, due to the tightness of the body, the Qi's circulation is stagnant. Consequently, the Qi cannot reach to the correct place and be manifested efficiently. When using this Jin to strike a sand bag, the sand bag can be bounced very far. If (you) are attacked by these kinds of Jins, though the Jins are shallow, they can bounce you many meters away. It is as if (you are) struck by a truck. When (you) are struck, the sound of "Ouch" can be uttered.

硬勁者，身緊而不鬆。力雖大，然勁拙、鈍、淺。此因為意雖專、氣強，但由於身繃，氣行滯，因而氣未能充分達到部位。以此勁擊打沙包，可將沙包彈出甚遠之地。如為此勁所擊，勁雖淺鈍，卻可將敵彈出丈遠。恰如被卡車所撞然。被擊之，哎聲而發。

When you perform a hard Jin, even if you have good concentration, the tension of your physical body will cause the Qi's circulation to be stagnant, the speed will be low, and the focus area will be big. In this case, the power will not penetrate. If you are struck with hard Jin, you may be bounced many meters away, but you will not be injured internally. It is because of this that, when you are struck, the sound of pain can be uttered.

> With soft-hard Jins, at the beginning, the Yi is strong and the body is relaxed so the Qi can be led to the manifesting place (smoothly). However, when the Qi has reached the intended place, the body immediately turns hard. The Yi remains strong and leads the Jin to the target. When using this Jin to strike a sand bag, though the sand bag can be bounced away, it will not bounce too far. This is because half of the Jin has entered the target and penetrated, while the other half is stagnant in the sand bag. This Jin can penetrate into the body and injure the internal organs. When struck, though the sound of "Ouch" can be uttered, it cannot come out completely.

軟硬勁者，初始意強、身鬆以引氣至所須部位。然當氣達到部位後，身即轉硬，意仍強並將勁引入標的。以此勁擊打沙包，雖可將沙包彈出，然不甚遠。其因乃一半之勁入標的而穿出，另一半卻滯於沙包矣。此勁可透入身體，傷及內臟。被擊之，哎聲雖發，然難盡出。

When you execute a soft-hard Jin (Figure 41), you must first remain relaxed while using your concentrated Yi to lead the Qi to the arms or legs. Once the Qi has reached these places, then you tense up and continue to use your concentrated mind to lead the Jin into the target. This Jin is more penetrating than the hard Jin. It is said that half of the Jin can enter the body and injure the internal organs, while the other half can damage the external structure of the physical body. Since the concentration of the Yi is stronger and the target can be smaller, soft-hard Jins can be used for some cavity strikes.

> In soft Jin, the Yi is strong, the Qi is abundant, and the body has reached its maximum level of softness and relaxation. Because the body is soft, the Jin can reach a very high speed and be focused on a tiny point. The Jin is penetrating and deep, and is used specially for attacking cavities. If (your) body has been struck but not the cavity, though the Li is penetrating, (you) will not be bounced away. When using this Jin to strike a sand bag, the Jin penetrates and passes through it. Consequently, the sand bag will vibrate slightly and then stop. According to Chinese acupuncture, there are more than seven hundred acupuncture cavities. Among them, there are one hundred and eight, which include thirty-six vital cavities and seventy-two non-vital cavities, that can be used in martial arts. When those thirty-six vital cavities are attacked, through Jing (i.e., Primary Qi Channels) and Luo (i.e., Secondary Qi Channels), the internal organs can be shocked and injured, and death can even be caused. When struck, it is hard to utter any sound. When the seventy-two non-vital cavities are struck, it can cause fainting or numbness.

軟勁者，意強氣旺，身至軟至鬆也。因身之軟，勁可達高速並集中之一小點。勁透而深，專打穴也。如穴不中，如被軟鞭擊之然。雖力透，然卻不彈出也。以此勁擊打沙包，勁入沙包而穿出。因之沙包微振盪即止。依中醫穴位，全身計七百多穴。其中有一百零八穴，中三十六大穴與七十二小穴可為武學上所用。當三十六大穴被擊之，可由經絡震傷內臟而重傷甚而致命。被擊之，聲難發矣。當七十二小穴被擊之，可使人暈倒或麻痺難以動彈。

Due to the extremely high concentration, the intensely strong Qi, the high speed, the extraordinarily deep penetration, and the intensity of the focus point, soft Jin can be used to attack the cavities and shock the internal organs. However, it is not easy to reach this level. Even in ancient times, only the old, proficient masters ever reached this level.

Due to its dangerous and harmful potential, normally a master will keep the locations of the 108 cavities secret. Moreover, the timing schedule required to attack,

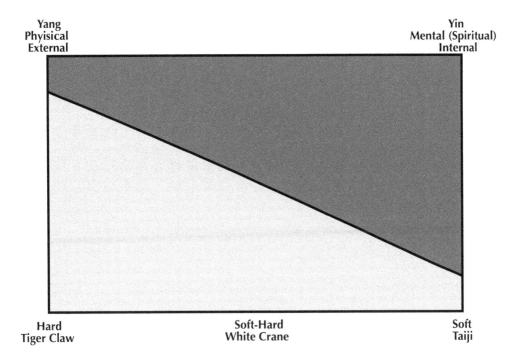

Figure 41. Hard, Soft-Hard, and Soft Jins

and the crucial training methods were also kept highly secret. Usually, only if a student had stayed with a master and earned his whole trust were these secrets revealed to a student.

> *If (you) do not know the correct Jin training methods, the ligaments and the places where the tendons are attached to the bones (i.e., joints) can often be injured. Training hard Jin is the easiest and not dangerous in training. This is because when the Jin is manifested, the limbs are tightened and the joints are locked, thus the ligaments and tendons are protected. It is the same for soft-hard Jin training. Though at the beginning, the Qi is led by the Yi and the body is relaxed and soft, when the Jin is manifested, the limbs are tensed, the joints are locked, and thus the ligaments and tendons are also protected. Therefore, the possibilities of getting injured are minimal. However, the hardest to train and the easiest to produce injury is soft Jin. This is because when the Jin is manifested, the body remains relaxed and soft, so the ligaments and the tendons that attach to the bones can be pulled easily by strong Jin and injured. Therefore, when the Jin has just reached its maximum extension, (you) must know how to bounce it back and protect the ligaments and tendons. If (you) do not know the timing of pulling back, then injury can result. Those who train must be cautious. When (you) train soft Jin, it should not be over twenty to thirty minutes at a time.*

如不懂得勁之練法，往往骨腱與筋骨之交接處，容易遭
遇受傷。硬勁最易練，練之而不危險。其因乃當勁之發
時，肢體繃緊，關節鎖住，骨腱與筋骨交接處被保護之。
軟硬勁者，亦然。雖在初之以意引氣時，身體鬆軟。然
在勁發時，肢體繃緊，關節鎖住，骨腱與筋骨亦被保護
之。受傷性因而減低。然最難練並最易受傷者為軟勁也。
此因軟勁在勁發時，身體仍然鬆軟，骨腱與筋骨之交接
處容易被強勁所拉而受傷。因此在勁將達盡頭時，必懂
得勁往回拉而保護骨腱與筋骨。如不懂得在適時拉回，
則受傷矣。練者須注意之。每次練習軟勁，應不超出二
十分至三十分鐘為限。

From scientific study, we know that the formula of power manifestation is:

$$P = I \times V = I^2 \times R$$

P=Power
V: Potential Difference
I: Current
R: Resistance

In manifesting hard Jins, the resistance R is increased, and the current I is constant due to stagnation; thus the power is increased. In soft Jins' manifestation, the resistance R is decreased since the body is relaxed and soft; however, the current I is increased due to strong Qi circulation. In addition, when Yi (i.e., V) is strong, the current will also be enhanced; therefore, the power is increased. However, in soft-hard Jins' manifestation, at the beginning before the Jin is emitted, the body is kept relaxed and soft and the Yi (i.e., V) is used to lead the Qi to increase the current flow, I. However, at the moment the Jin is emitted, the limbs are tensed to increase the resistance R. Consequently, the power P is increased. From the above discussion, it is seen that the theory of the Jin's manifestation has a scientific root.

由科學上之探討，吾知動力公式為

$$P = I \times V = I^2 \times R$$

P: 動力

V: 電位差

I: 電流

R: 電阻

硬勁者，電阻 R 增強，電流量 I 因滯而保持不變，由之
動力 P 增強。軟勁者，電阻 R 因身體之鬆軟而減少，
然電流量 I 因氣行而增強，再加上意 V 之強勢，電流
量 I 亦隨之更強，動力 P 因而增強。然軟硬勁者，在起
初勁未發時，身體保持鬆軟以意 V 引氣增強電流量 I
，然在勁發時，卻將肢體繃緊以加強電阻 R 之量，動力
P 因而增強。由上可知，勁之來由有其科學根據也。

From this formula, we can see that in order to increase the power P, either the current I should be increased, the resistance R should be increased, or both current I and resistance R should be increased. In hard styles, the body is tensed and therefore, the current is stagnant and becomes constant. However, due to the tension of the physical body, the resistance R is increased, and consequently the power P is increased. In soft styles, due to the mind's concentration, V is increased significantly, consequently the current I is also increased by providing a relaxed body. However, this will reduce the resistance and therefore make the power decrease. Therefore, if you don't have a highly concentrated mind to increase the current significantly, you will lose power. In soft-hard styles, the body is relaxed and soft at the beginning, so the concentrated mind can lead the Qi to the limbs. Once the Qi has arrived, the physical body is tensed, so the R is increased. In this case, the power manifested can reach its maximum level.

5. Theory of Long Jin and Short Jin 長短勁篇

In the offensive and defensive fighting ranges, Jin can be distinguished as long or short. Long Jins are the Jin-Li that are wholly emitted over a long range and are commonly used in long range fighting. Short Jins are the Jin-Li that are not completely emitted and are often used in short range fighting. Hard Jins are specialized in long Jins and long range fighting, and thus are more favored by the northern Long Fist styles. Soft Jins are specialized in short Jins and short range fighting and thus are favored by southern and internal styles. (However,) soft-hard Jins can be used as long and short, soft and hard can be altered according to the opportunity. However, if (you) do not know the key training methods, and do not practice diligently, it is not easy to reach a proficient level and use this as (you) wish.

由攻防之長短，勁可分長短也。長勁者，勁力全部以長
距發出，在通用於長距之攻防。短勁者，勁力不盡然全
部發出，在通用於短距之攻防。硬勁專長於長勁與長距
之攻防，因而較為北派長拳各門派所喜好。軟勁專練短
勁與短距之攻防，因而較為南拳與內家拳各門派所採用。
軟硬勁者，能長能短，軟硬隨機而變。然不懂其竅與勤
練，卻不易達到隨心所欲之境地。

Long Jins (Chang Jin, 長勁) are commonly used for long range fighting and are therefore favored by northern styles, that specialize in long range fighting tactics. Short Jins (Duan Jin, 短勁) focus on short range fighting, which is favored by southern styles and also internal styles, such as Taijiquan. Generally speaking, hard Jins can be adopted into long range fighting much more easily than soft Jins, while soft Jins can be used in short range fighting much more easily than hard Jins. Still, you should not think that soft Jins can't be used for long range fighting. For example, White Ape (Bai Yuan, 白猿) or Taijiquan (太極拳) styles also specialize in long range soft Jins. You should also know that many northern styles also train short Jins heavily.

The best approach is to master both hard and soft and exchange them skillfully following the situations and opportunities. However, only experienced and proficient masters can perform this skillfully. The reason for this is simply that it is not easy to alter the soft and the hard. In order to do so, your mind must easily be able to change according to the strategies, and then the Jins can be manifested accordingly. Normally, this takes many years of fighting experience.

> *When (you) practice long soft Jins, due to the pulling of the ligaments and tendons, injuries can easily occur. Therefore, those who practice soft Jin often begin with short soft Jins. However, it is much harder for short soft Jins to reach a high level of power manifestation. This is because the storage of the Jin bows is not complete. In long soft Jins, though the Jins can be stored and manifested to a peak level, due to the length of range, the accuracy of cavity strike is much lower. Thus, both of them have advantages and disadvantages.*

練長軟勁時，因骨腱與筋之拔拉，較易於受傷。因之，
練軟勁者，皆由短勁著手。然欲達高階段之勁發，短軟
勁卻較難。此乃勁弓未能全蓄也。長軟勁者，雖勁較能
蓄至高峰，然由於勁距之長，打穴準率較低。因之，各
有利弊也。

It is commonly known in Chinese martial arts society that soft Jin training is more difficult and carries a higher risk of injury than hard Jin training. The reason for this is that in order to be soft, you must maintain your muscles and tendons in a soft and flexible state for the Jin's manifestation. Therefore, if you do not know how to tense up the muscles and tendons at the right moment and bounce the Jin backward, the ligaments can be injured easily. It is because of this that a master will let a beginning student train the hard Jins only. Once a student has reached a proficient level, he can train soft Jins.

It is easier to get injured in long soft Jin training than in that for short soft Jins. The reason for this is that when you execute your short soft Jins, before the arm is wholly extended, you pull your muscles and tendons to bounce it back. Consequently, the ligaments are never extended to a degree that can cause injury. Therefore, when you train soft Jin, you should begin with short Jin instead of long Jin.

6. Secret of Jin 勁訣篇

> *The secret of Jin is in the Qi, and the circulation of Qi depends on the breath. Qi and the breath's fast and slow determine the Jin's long and short; full or deficient gauge Jin's strong and weak.*

勁之訣在氣，氣之行決於息。氣息之快緩，定勁之長短、
沛濂，測勁之猛蹶。

Efficient and powerful Jin manifestation depends on how you coordinate the expression with your breathing. In Chinese Qigong practice, breathing is considered a strategy that enables you to use your Yi to lead the Qi in a more efficient and smooth way. When the breathing is fast and focused, the power can be sharp and fast. When the breathing is soft and calm, the Jin manifested can also be soft and controlled.

Oxygen is required for the biochemical combustion processes in the body that convert the food essence into energy. When the oxygen supply is abundant, the Qi produced will be abundant. For example, when you push a car or lift a weight, in order to generate strong power, you must first inhale deeply. This will provide plenty of oxygen so that energy (i.e., Qi) can be abundantly produced. When the Qi is abundant and is led by the Yi efficiently, the Jin manifested will also be powerful.

In a battle, in order to conserve your physical strength, in addition to correct breathing methods, you must also know how to relax your body. Whenever you tense up your body, you are consuming oxygen and also Qi. This is also true for swimming and jogging and other physical/athletic endeavours. If you know how to regulate your breathing and relax your body, you can last for a long time. In ancient times, since a battle usually lasted for several hours, knowing how to conserve your energy with correct breathing was crucial to survival.

Modulate breath properly, Qi will be smooth and exchangeable, and Jin can be round and alive. If breath is held or sealed, Qi will be stagnant and accumulate, and Jin will be dull and stiff.

息調得宜，氣則順轉，勁能圓活。息如閉塞，氣則滯積，勁必呆死。

Wu, Yu-Xiang said: "Yi (Mind) and Qi must exchange skillfully, then you have gained the marvelous trick of roundness and aliveness. This means the substantial and the insubstantial can vary and exchange."[13] In order to reach this goal, the breathing must be regulated correctly. This is the crucial key to roundness and agility. If you are holding your breath, the Jin manifested will be stagnant.

At the beginning of training, Yi is on the breathing, and Qi will then follow. Later, Yi is not on the breathing (Qi) but on the opponent. Yi is forming, Qi will grow, Jin will be emitted naturally, and reach the point where, when Yi arrives, Jin arrives also.

初行之，意在息，氣隨之。爾後，意不在氣，而在彼。意孕而氣生，勁自然而發。而終於意到勁亦到之功效。

In the beginning practice of regulating the breathing, the mind is on the breathing and the Qi will follow naturally. However, after you have reached a stage of regulating without regulating, you should keep your mind on the opponent. When this sense of enemy is established, your Yi will have a target and the Qi can be led efficiently. In addition, when your mind is on your opponent, your spirit can be raised to a higher level. When the spirit is raised, the Qi's manifestation into physical action will be more effective.

The Qi of the Hen-Ha sounds is determined by breathing. When the breathing is right, then the Spirit of Vitality rises, and the Qi will be full, and emitting and withdrawing Jins can reach their highest levels.

哼哈之氣制於息。息正則精神振，氣可沛然。收發之勁亦可達峰。

In addition to the correct breathing method, if you also know how to coordinate the sounds of Hen and Ha, the Qi can be condensed deeply into the bone marrow and stored for the Jin's manifestation, and can also be manifested physically with the highest efficiency.

7. Theory of Storing Jin 蓄勁篇

Taijiquan ancestors said: "The body provides five bows in Taijiquan." What are the five bows? The body (i.e., torso) is the major bow while the two arms and two legs are four minor bows. The bow is the equipment that stores the Jin. The White Crane style talks about six bows provided by the body. (This is because) there are two major bows in the body (i.e., torso): the spine bow and chest bow. Therefore it is known that it does not matter which (Chinese) style, they all talk about (i.e., study) the bows and the methods of storing.

太極拳先哲謂：〝太極拳身備五弓。〞五弓者，身體主弓也，兩臂、兩腿四副弓也。弓者，蓄勁之器也。白鶴拳者亦謂身備六弓。身體主弓計有兩主弓：脊弓與胸弓也。由是可知，不論何者門派，都論弓與蓄勁之法。

It does not matter which Chinese style you study, all discuss how to manifest Jin externally to its maximum. In order to reach this goal, all include studying how to store external Jin into the body's structure. There is no exception for Taijiquan. The Taijiquan ancestor, Wu, Yu-Xiang said: "Single body with five bows that are ready to emit, spread, cover, match, and swallow should be pondered and studied carefully."[14] This means that Taijiquan recognizes the five bows in the body that can store the Jin and then emit it. Other than the four limbs that can bend and shoot, the torso is the major bow. This is what Chinese martial society called "the body skills" (Shen Fa, 身法). If any style does not study how to use the torso and limbs to store and manifest the Jin, then the style is considered shallow.

Some styles are even more specific, such as White Crane, which teaches that there are actually two bows in the torso—the spine and the chest. If you can coordinate all six bows and store the external Jin to its maximum, the power manifested will be marvelously strong and fast. Wang, Zong-Yue said: "Accumulate Jin like drawing a bow, emit Jin like (a bow) shooting an arrow."[15] He also said: "Power is emitted from the spine; steps change following the body."[16] All of this explains how to store the Jin efficiently.

The Jin in Taijiquan is initiated from the leg bows, controlled by the waist, with the coordination of the spine bow and chest, then enhanced by the arm bow and finally manifested at the fingers. Taijiquan classic said: "The root is at the feet, (Jin or movement is) generated from the legs, mastered (i.e., controlled) by the waist and manifested (i.e., expressed) from the fingers. From the feet to the legs to the waist must be integrated, and one unified Qi developed. When moving forward or backward, (you can) seize the opportunity and gain the superior position." It again said: "Once in motion, the entire body must be light (Qing) and agile (Ling), (it) especially should (be) threaded together." From this, it is known that the Jin in Taijiquan is soft Jin that is manifested just like a soft whip.

太極拳之勁，由腿弓發，主宰於腰，與脊弓、胸弓配合，再而由臂弓加強而現於手指。太極拳經云：〝其根在腳，發於腿，主宰於腰，形於手指。由腳而腿而腰，總須完整一氣。向前退後，乃能得機得勢。〞又云：〝一舉動，週身俱要輕靈，尤須貫穿。〞由此可知，太極拳之勁，軟勁也，如軟鞭然。

Taijiquan emphasizes the Jins of listening (Ting, 聽), understanding (Dong, 懂), attaching (Zhan, 沾), sticking (Nian, 黏), connecting (Lian, 連), and following (Sui, 隨). In order to execute all of these Jins effectively, the movements of your joints must be agile and the contact with your opponent must be light. The action of the entire body is just like a stack of ancient coins that have been threaded together by a cord. All of the joints, from the ankles, knees, hips, waist, vertebrae, shoulders, elbows, and wrists, to the fingers, are all threaded together and act like a soft whip. When this happens, the entire body will act as a unified whipping unit. This means Taijiquan specializes in the manifestation of soft Jins.

> *The key location for storing Jins are, Mingmen on the spine, Jiuwei (i.e., lower sternum) on the chest, elbows at the arms, and knees on the legs. These are the places where the force must be applied when opening the bows. When the forces are applied adequately, the Jins (manifested) will be powerful, the target will be accurately aimed at, and the percentage of success in cavity strikes will be high. Therefore, when all styles practice the Jin-Li Gongfu, they all begin from these six places. It is the same in Taijiquan practice. In order to have proper body movements, (you) must know how to coordinate the chest bow by "drawing in the chest and arcing the back" with the bow of the spine. In order to have the joints threaded together (as a single unit), (you) must know the theory of opening and closing. In this case, the Jin-Li can be initiated from the spine. Together with the coordination with the bows on the legs and the arms, you can choose either long or short Jins and you can also decide if you want to execute emitting or neutralizing Jins, extend or withdraw, or be soft or hard (as wished).*

蓄勁之樞紐，於脊在命門，於胸在鳩尾，於臂在肘，於腿在膝。此些處乃開弓之著力點也。著力恰到好處，勁猛，準確度、打穴率高。因而各門派練習勁力功夫，無不由此六處著手。太極拳亦然。為求身法，必知含胸拔背與脊弓之配合。為求貫穿，必知一開一合之理。如此，才能力由脊發。再加上腿、臂四弓之配合，長勁、短勁由我取決，發、化依我本意。能伸能縮，能軟能硬。

Jin (勁) is sometimes replaced by Jin-Li (勁力). The reason for this is simply that Jin is the manifestation of muscular power (i.e., Li) with the Yi and Qi's internal support. Often, it is also simply called Li.

Even though Taijiquan emphasizes soft Jins, a proficient Taijiquan practitioner must also know how to be hard. Wŭ, Yu-Xiang said: "When using Jin, (it is) just like steel refined 100 times, no solid (strong opposition) can resist destruction."[17] He also said: (Fist) extremely soft, then extremely hard. If able to breathe (properly), then (you) can be agile and alive."[18] This means that to become a proficient Taijiquan martial artist, you must know how to be soft and also to be hard when necessary. When this happens, you can exchange the insubstantial and substantial skillfully, which will confuse your opponent. In order to reach a proficient level, you must begin with softness. It is easier to be soft and then hard. If you are hard and have established a habit of hardness, it is difficult to become soft.

In order to manifest your Jin efficiently, you must know how to coordinate all of the six bows. Initiate the movement from the leg bow, control by the waist, store at the spine bow and chest bow, and finally manifest with the arm bows to the target. Wŭ, Yu-Xiang said: "Power is emitted from the spine"(Li You Ji Fa, 力由脊發). In order to store the Jin efficiently in the chest and spine, you must know how to "drawing in the chest and arc the back" (Han Xiong Ba Bei, 含胸拔背).

> *However, the most important of all is knowing how to reach high efficiency in using the waist to control (the Jins). The waist is just like the steering wheel of a car and also like the handle of a soft whip. In order to be light and agile, and also effectively control the Li-Jin, the waist must be soft and alive. The coordination of the Yi and the body must be highly efficient, otherwise, even though the body is soft, the Jins will not be directed effectively.*

然，最要者，是懂得如何達主宰於腰之效。腰者，開車之轉盤也，軟鞭之握把也。為能輕靈，為能有效的主宰力勁，腰身必軟、必活。意與身之調配與合作必至高效率，否則身雖軟，導勁必無成效。

In order to have a high level of Jin control, you must know how to effectively use your Yi to direct the body's function. The key is to know the feeling of the body precisely. Feeling is the language between your mind and body. The more sensitive you can feel your body, the more highly refined the control of your body's action will be. This feeling will also provide good listening and understanding between you and your opponent.

In addition, in order to control the Jin efficiently, your Yi must be able to control the waist area effectively. The waist area must be soft and easily moveable. If not, it will be just like a stuck steering wheel that hinders the control of a car. In order to have a loose and soft waist, you must first have loose and soft hip joints (Kua, 胯). The hips are the places where the body connects to your root. Whenever the hip joints are stiff, your root will be shallow and the movement of the waist will be dull. This will influence the effectiveness of your Jin's steering.

8. Secret of Hen and Ha, Two Qis 哼哈二氣訣

Emitting or storing the Jin depends on the Yi's response to the opportunity. When the Yi is strong, the fighting morale is high, and the Qi is also abundant. However, most important of all is the manifestation of the Spirit of Vitality. When the Spirit of Vitality is high, then every action can be carried out as desired. When the Spirit of Vitality is low, even if the Yi is strong, the fighting morale will still be weak.

勁之發與蓄取決於意對時機之反應。意高，鬥志強，氣亦強。然而最重要者乃精神之顯現。精神高昂，則一切隨心應手。精神低落，即使意高，鬥志必弱。

Generally speaking, when your mind is strong, the Qi that it leads will be strong. The Jin manifested will then be efficient and powerful. However, even if you have strong Yi and abundant Qi circulation, if you do not have a highly motivated fighting spirit, the power manifested will not be effective. This means that the quality of the Jin's manifestation will not be high. Consequently, you can still be defeated. In order to win a battle, you must raise up your fighting morale. When this fighting spirit is high, the Yi can lead the Qi for power manifestation effectively and efficiently.

In order to reach this goal, you must know how to condense your spirit and keep it from scattering. That is why it says in *Taijiquan Classic* that: "Spirit should be retained internally" (Shen Yi Nei Lian, 神宜內斂). It is also said: "An insubstantial energy leads the head upward" (Xu Ling Ding Jin, 虛領頂勁). This means that the practitioner or student should raise up the Spirit of Vitality. Wang, Zong-Yue said: "(If) the Spirit of Vitality can be raised, then (there is) no delay or heaviness (i.e., clumsiness). That means the head is suspended."[19] This also underscores the importance of raising up the spirit. When the spirit is raised, then your response and action will be light and agile. He also said: "(Throughout your) entire body, the mind is on the Spirit of Vitality, not on the Qi."[20] This means when your spirit is raised up to a high level, the Qi will flow naturally and strongly. In addition, Li, Yi-Yu also said: "Spirit condenses. All in all, (if) the above four items (are) totally acquired, it comes down to condensing Shen (i.e., spirit). When Shen condenses, then one Qi (can be) formed, like a drum. Training Qi belongs to Shen. Qi appears activated (i.e., abundant) and smooth. The Spirit of Vitality is threaded and concentrated. Opening and closing have numbers (degrees of fineness). Insubstantial and substantial are clearly distinguished..."[21]

Hen and Ha two sounds are the keys to making the spirit high or low. The Hen sound is classified as Yin and is the sound of sorrow. The Ha sound is classified as Yang and is the sound of cheer. When a person is sad and cries or gets depressed, the sound of Hen is often uttered, inhalation is longer than the exhalation. At this time, the Guardian Qi (Wei Qi) condenses into the bone marrow and the entire body feels chilly. But when a person is happy, the laughing sound of Ha is often uttered and exhalation is longer than the inhalation. At this time, the Guardian Qi expands and the entire body is hot and sweating. From this it is known that when the inhalation is longer than the exhalation with the sound of Hen, the Qi can be condensed into the bone marrow (i.e., Marrow Qi) (Sui Qi). This is the secret key to storing the Qi and Jin. Conversely, when exhalation is longer than inhalation while making the Ha sound, the Qi can expand outward and the muscles can be energized to a higher energy state. This is the secret key to emitting the Qi and Jin. This is especially effective if the Ha sound's uttering is short, the Jin is condensed and the spirit is raised up; then, the emitting of the Jin can reach its peak.

哼哈二聲二氣乃決定精神高低之竅。哼者，陰也，悲傷
之聲也。哈者，陽也，快樂之聲也。當人悲傷哭泣或沮
喪之時，常發哼聲，同時吸氣較長而呼氣較短。此時衛
氣內斂入骨髓，全身發冷。反之，當人興奮快樂之時，
常發哈笑聲，同時呼氣較長而吸氣較短。此時衛氣闊張，
全身發熱發汗。由此可知當吸氣較長同時發出哼聲，能
引氣內斂入骨髓。此乃蓄氣蓄勁之竅訣。反之，當呼氣
較長同時發出哈聲，能引氣外張並激發肌肉展力之能量。
此乃放氣發勁之竅訣。尤其如發哈聲短暫，勁之發必集
中，精神上提，勁發之效可達頂峰。

It is said in *Taijiquan Classic*: "Grasp and hold the Dan Tian to train internal Gongfu. Hen, Ha, two Qis are marvelous and infinite. Move open, calmly close, bend and extend following (your opponent). Slow responds to (slow), fast follows (fast), the principles must be understood thoroughly."[22] This implies that when the Hen and Ha sounds are used skillfully, the spirit can be raised to a high level. When this happens, all of the fighting strategies and skills can be carried out successfully.

The key to storing the Qi and Jin is to inhale and make the sound of Hen, then the abdomen is withdrawn and the Huiyin (Co-1) (會陰) (i.e., perineum) is held up. When you exhale to emit the Qi and Jin, the abdomen is pushed outward while the perineum is pushed downward. That means the use of Reverse Abdominal Breathing (Fan Hu Xi or Ni Hu Xi, 反呼吸．逆呼吸) is adopted.

PART VIII

About Pushing Hands
論推手

1. Practicing Methods of the Four Directions and Four Corners 四方四隅練法 (Eight Doors, Eight Trigrams) 〔八門、八卦〕

What are the four directions and four corners? They are the eight doors. It is also the theory of Eight Trigrams in Taijiquan. What are the four directions? They are Peng (i.e., Wardoff), Lu (i.e., Rollback), Ji (i.e., Squeeze or Press), and An (i.e., Push or Press Down). What are the four corners? They are Cai (i.e., Pluck), Lie (i.e., Split), Zhou (i.e., Elbow), and Kao (i.e., Bump). The four directions are the four main supporting posts (in a building), the major generals (in a battle), and are the major Jin patterns of Taijiquan. The four corners are the four assistant posts and are the four assistant Jin patterns in Taijiquan and are the deputy generals.

四方四隅者，八門也。亦即太極拳八卦之理也。四方者，
掤、攦、擠、按，四隅者，採、挒、肘、靠。四方者，
四主撐支柱也，主將也。乃太極拳之主要勁勢。四隅者，
四輔助支柱也。乃太極拳之四輔助勁勢，副將也。

Taijiquan is also called "Thirteen Postures" or "Thirteen Patterns" (Shi San Shi, 十三勢), which includes "Eight Jin Patterns," commonly called "Eight Doors" (Ba Men, 八門) and "Five Strategic Steppings" (Wu Bu, 五步). According to *Taijiquan Classic*, the actions of the eight Jin patterns correspond to the eight trigrams (Bagua, 八卦) while the five steppings correspond to the "Five Elements" (Wu Xing, 五行). The eight trigrams are: Qian (乾) (Heaven), Kun (坤) (Earth), Kan (坎) (Water), Li (離) (Fire), which correspond to the four main sides, and Xun (巽) (Wind), Zhen (震) (Thunder), Dui (兌) (Lake), and Gen (艮) (Mountain), which correspond to the four diagonal corners. The five elements are: metal (Jin, 金), wood (Mu, 木), water (Shui, 水), fire (Huo, 火), and earth (Tu, 土).

Peng (掤), Lu (攦), Ji (擠), and An (按) are the four major Jin patterns that have become the four major crucial foundations of the Taijiquan art. Cai (採), Lie (挒), Zhou (肘), and Kao (靠) are the four assistant Jin patterns that make the art more complete. With the five strategic steppings, the art of Taijiquan becomes a complete fighting art.

> *Peng is constructed from the two arms, shaped as two crescent moons and is called "drawing in the chest and arcing the back" which can be used as yielding to neutralize the coming Jin. Arcing stores the Jin in the body's two bows. These two bows are the chest bow and the spine bow. These two places are the most important Jin storing places in the body. If (you) know Peng, then (you) will know how to store. If (you) know how to store, then (you) will know how to emit. Peng Jin exists everywhere in Taijiquan. Not only Lu, Ji, and An have Peng included within, but it is also included in Cai, Lie, Zhou, and Kao.*

掤者，雙月以手臂拱之，稱曰含胸拔背，乃用於讓以化
來勁，用於拱，以蓄勁於身上兩弓。兩弓者，胸弓、脊
弓也。此兩弓乃全身最要蓄勁之所。懂得掤，即懂得蓄。
懂得蓄，即懂得發。掤勁在太極拳中，處處皆是。不但
攦、擠、按中有掤，採、挒、肘、靠中亦有掤。

The word Peng (掤) was created in Taijiquan society and does not exist in regular dictionaries. This word is constructed from three words: hand (才) and two moons (月). The moon is single and therefore implies loneliness in Chinese culture. When two moons are put together, it means friends (朋) in Chinese language. Since they are friends, they mutually support, help, and harmonize with each other. This indicates that the word Peng means to arc both arms like two moons and to coordinate them with each other. In Taijiquan, in order to make the arcing harmonious, the chest is drawn in while the back is rounded backward. This is an important oral secret for storing the Jin and is called "Han Xiong Ba Bei" (含胸拔背) which means "draw in the chest and arc the back." When this happens, the body can be used to yield and neutralize the incoming force, and can simultaneously be used to store the Jin in the body's two bows for emitting.

As mentioned earlier, the body includes six bows. The two arms and two legs are four bows that allow you to store Jin in the posture and then release it. The torso has two bows—the chest bow (Xiong Gong, 胸弓) and the spine bow (Ji Gong, 脊弓). The force-exerting point for the chest bow is the lower part of the sternum (Jiuwei, 鳩尾) (Co-15) while the exerting point for the spine is the Mingmen (Gv-4) (命門). From these two points the body can be shaped as a bow and Jin can be stored for emitting (Figure 42).

Peng Jin is the first and the most important Jin pattern in Taijiquan. In fact, it can be said that unless you know the essence of Peng Jin, you really don't know Tai-

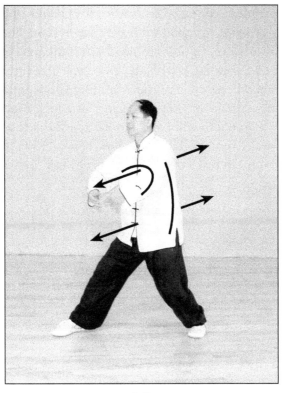

Figure 42. Wardoff Jin (Peng Jin)

jiquan. In order to make the storage of all other Jins effective, Peng Jin can be found in almost every Taijiquan posture.

> *To train Peng Jin, (you) allow your training partner to control your elbows and use any possible technique to push you. His intention is to destroy your central equilibrium. You use Peng Jin, which is initiated from your legs, controlled by (your) waist, and then you draw in the chest and arc your back to manifest it in your arms. Turn your waist to neutralize, to arc outward, and to yield. Repeat the practice until the action has become natural. After you have practiced for a long time, you will be able to use Peng Jin everywhere.*

> 掤勁練法，任由友伴拿我肘，而採取任何方法以推我，
> 意欲損我之中定。我以掤勁由腳而發，主宰於腰，而含
> 胸拔背拱於手臂，由腰轉以化之，拱之，讓之。反覆練
> 習而至自然之境地。久而久之，自然無處不存掤勁矣！

There are many ways of training Peng Jin in all Taijiquan styles. However, one of the most effective ways for a beginner to build up a firm foundation and sound habits is through elbow controlling practice. In this practice, allow your opponent to use both of his hands to control (i.e., Na Jin, 拿勁) your elbows. Since the elbow is very close to the center of your body, it is easy for your opponent to find your center and push you off balance. In order to neutralize, you must turn and also draw in your chest, and round your back with the two arms arced outward. When this is done, your opponent will have a hard time locating your center. Naturally, it is not easy at the beginning. However, after practicing for a long time, it will become easier and more natural. You also will have familiarized yourself with the body's structure, rooting, and waist control. This will allow you to be softer and softer in your actions and finally you can reach the target of using "four ounces to repel one thousand pounds" (Si Liang Po Qian Jin, 四兩破千斤).

> *Lu involves using the hands to rollback and neutralize (the coming force). That means using Peng Jin as the major (Jin) to yield, lead, and neutralize the coming force to the left or to the right. Lu Jin can be classified as Small Rollback (Xiao Lu) and Large Rollback (Da Lu). In small rollback, the circle of coiling and neutralizing Jin is smaller. In large rollback, the action is larger, the stepping is bigger, and the circle of coiling and neutralizing is also on a larger scale. When practicing, Lu Jin is used together with Ji Jin (i.e., Press or Squeeze Jin) and Kao Jin (i.e., Bump Jin). After Lu, immediately follow with Ji or Kao. After Ji or Kao, immediately Lu. Repeat as such.*

攦者，用手攦化之意也。以掤勁為主，將來勢讓之、引之、而左右帶化之。攦勁可分為小攦與大攦。小攦者，纏化勁圈小，步子亦較小。大攦者，圈大、步大、纏化勁之圈亦較大。練習時，攦勁與擠勁、靠勁並用。攦後即擠或靠，擠靠後再攦，反覆而行。

Lu Jin includes Yielding Jin (Rang Jin, 讓勁), Leading Jin (Yin Jin, 引勁), and Neutralizing Jin (Hua Jin, 化勁) (Figure 43). For effective execution, these three Jins all include Wardoff Jin (Peng Jin, 掤勁). The ancient oral key implies Lu is "leading the Jin into emptiness" (Yin Jin Luo Kong, 引勁落空). In order to do this, you must lead the Jin to your side, so you can neutralize it by leading the incoming force into emptiness.

In practice, there are two skills of Rollback; they can be classified as "Small Rollback" (Xiao Lu, 小攦) (Figure 44) and "Large Rollback" (Da Lu, 大攦) (Figure 45). In the execution of Small Rollback, the action of coiling, leading, and neutralizing is smaller and the techniques are different from those of Large Rollback. Theoretically and practically speaking, to be effective in action, Rollback is always used together either with Press Jin (Ji Jin, 擠勁) or Bump Jin (Kao Jin, 靠勁).

> *Ji (Press) is used for small range offense and defense. It can be done by overlapping both hands and then pressing forward. It can be done by using one hand to press the other hand's wrist and then press forward. It can also be done by using*

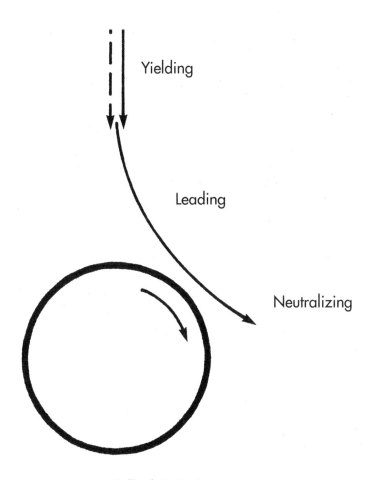

Figure 43. Rollback Jin (Lu Jin)

one hand to press the other forearm and then press forward. All the above Jis are used for offense and are used to press the opponent's upper body to destroy his central equilibrium. In addition, Ji can also be done by squeezing two hands or two arms toward each other. This kind of Ji is mostly used to squeeze the opponent's elbows to close off and hinder his Ji Jin (Press Jin), An Jin (Push Jin), or to seal off his arms' function. Squeezing can also be used to press the opponent's chest (i.e., solar plexus) to make the opponent's Qi float.

擠者，小圈攻防也。可施於雙手互疊前擠，可一手擠壓
另一手之腕而前擠，亦可以一手擠壓另一手臂而前擠。
以上之擠為攻勢，用以擠對方知上身部位，以損其中定。
再者，擠亦可由兩手或兩臂對擠。對擠者，大都用於擠
敵之雙肘，以封挫其之擠勁、按勁、或封鎖其臂之活動。
對擠亦可用之於擠彼之前胸，以浮其氣。

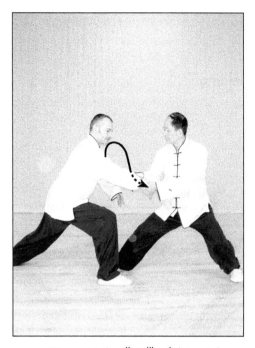

Figure 44. Small Rollback (Xiao Lu)

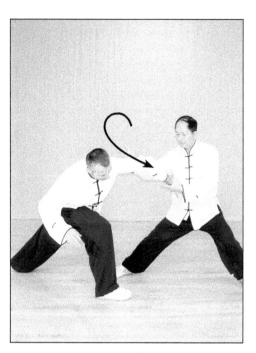

Figure 45. Large Rollback (Da Lu)

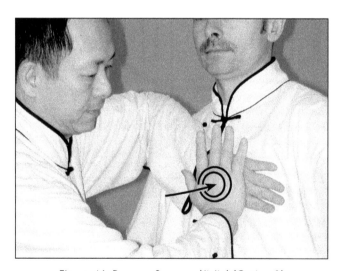

Figure 46. Press or Squeeze (Ji Jin) (Option 1)

Ji is a Jin pattern that is designed to be used in short range fighting. Ji can be done in different ways, such as with both hands overlapping each other and then pressing forward (Figure 46), one hand pressing the other wrist and then pressing forward (Figure 47) or one hand pressing the other forearm and then pressing for-

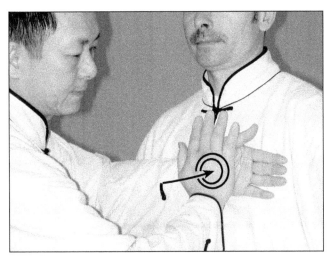

Figure 47. Press or Squeeze (Ji Jin) (Option 2)

ward (Figure 48). When the Ji Jin is applied as such, usually it is used for offense and aims to destroy the opponent's central equilibrium. This kind of Ji can also be used to press-strike the solar plexus to inflict pain or injury on the opponent's stomach and make his Qi float (Figure 49).

Ji can also be done by squeezing both hands or arms toward each other. This Ji can effectively be used for defense and against an opponent's Ji or An (Figure 50). The hands are used to squeeze the opponent's elbows to hinder his intention. Occasionally, this kind of Ji can be used to upset the solar plexus area as well (Figure 51).

An (Press or Push Down) means to settle the wrist. It is executed by using the base of the palm, either one palm or both palms can press and push. An can be divided into offensive An and defensive An. In offensive An, the base of the palm is used to push upward to the chin to destroy the opponent's central equilibrium; to the throat to seal the opponent's breath; to push forward to Xinkan (Jiuwei) (i.e., solar plexus area) to seal the breath as well as destroy the opponent's central equilibrium or shock his heart; to push downward to the abdominal area to destroy the stability of the lower part of his body or to seal his breath. Defensive An is used to seal off the coming Jin from the opponent. This is commonly done by pressing-pushing down the opponent's shoulders or elbows, which will cause the opponent to lean forward and will seal off his coming Jin.

按者，坐腕也。亦即以單掌或雙掌根按壓之謂也。按者，
可分攻按與守按兩者。攻按者，以掌根上按下巴，以損
彼之中定。按喉，以閉其氣。中按心坎（鳩尾）以閉其
氣，以損其中定，或震盪彼之心臟。下按腹部以損敵之
下定或閉其氣。守按者，用之封化敵之來勁也。通常下
帶按敵之肩或肘使敵前傾而挫敵之來勁。

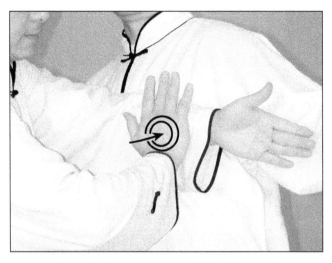

Figure 48. Press or Squeeze (Ji Jin) (Option 3)

The secret of "An" that has been passed down by oral tradition is to "settle the wrist" (Zuo Wan, 坐腕). That means to press the base of the palm forward (Figure 52). An Jin can be used either offensively or defensively. When it is used for upward attack, the target can be the chin to upset the opponent's central equilibrium (Figure 53) or the throat to seal the breath (Figure 54). When it is used for forward attack, the target is the solar plexus area (Xinkan, 心坎) (Jiuwei, Co-15, 鳩尾). Xinkan is a martial name, while Jiuwei is a Chinese medical name. When this place is attacked, you can seal the opponent's breath or even shock his heart (Figure 55). Naturally, you can also use it to destroy the opponent's central equilibrium. When An is used for downward attack, the abdominal area is the main target (Figure 56). When this area is attacked correctly, the muscles can be contracted and will seal the breath.

An is also commonly used for defense, allowing you to seal incoming attacks such as Ji or An. When it is applied for this purpose, the shoulders or elbows are pressed downward to hinder the incoming attack (Figure 57).

Cai means, to pluck and then take away. Cai does not mean, to grab. When (you) grab, you tighten up and the Jin will be dull and not alive, and can be used by the opponent. If (you) use Grabbing Jin, the body must be stiff and the upper body will be tight. When the upper body is tightened, the opponent can take this opportunity (to defeat you). Cai means to use the thumb and index finger or middle finger to pluck and pull away. Pluck also means to press the cavities, and pull away means, to destroy the opponent's central equilibrium. Generally speaking, the places for plucking and pulling are shoulders, elbows, and wrists. When it is used for the shoulders, it is used to control the Jianjing or Jianneiling cavity. When it is used for the elbows, it is to pluck and press the Quchi and Shaohai two cavities and then pull downward and sideways. When it is used for the wrists, it is to pluck the Neiguan cavity and then pull it downward and

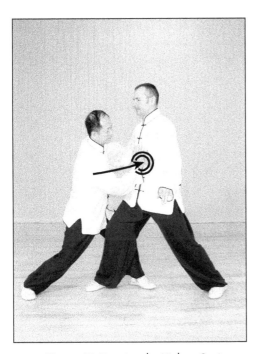

Figure 49. Pressing the Xinkan Cavity

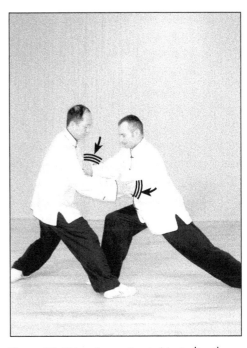

Figure 50. Using Squeezing to Neutralize the
Opponent's Push

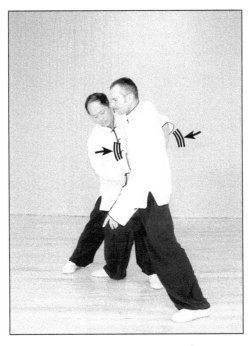

Figure 51. Using Squeezing to Press
the Xinkan Cavity

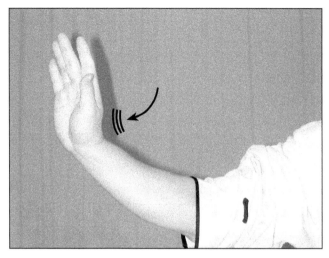

Figure 52. Settle the Wrist (Zuo Wan)

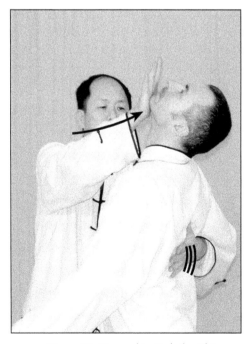

Figure 53. Upward to Push the Chin

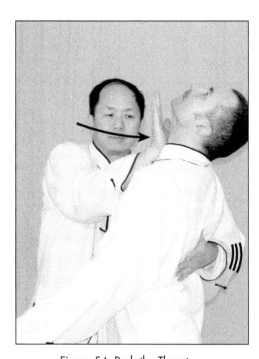

Figure 54. Push the Throat

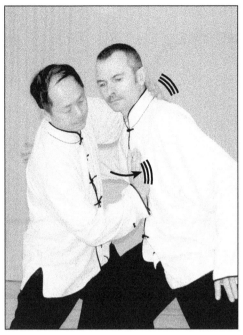

Figure 55. Push the Xinkan Cavity

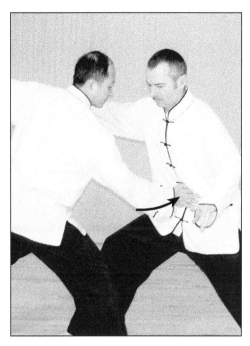

Figure 56. Push the Abdominal Area

sideways. If the situation allows, (you) may use both hands to pluck and press any two places. When (you) use Cai, (you) must pluck and lead the opponent until he loses his central equilibrium. If (you) stop midway, the opponent can easily use his Zhou (Elbow) or Kao (Bump) to counterattack you. Those students must be very careful about this. Additionally, the pluck must be fast. If slow, it can also be used by the opponent.

採者，採帶之謂也。採非抓也。抓之則緊，勁呆死不活，
易為敵所用。況乎，抓勁身必硬而上身繃。上身繃緊，
敵可乘之。採之，亦即以姆指與食指或中指扣帶之也。
扣者，扣其穴也。帶之，損其中定也。一般言之，扣帶
之所為肩、為肘、為腕。採肩，扣其肩井或肩內陵穴也。
採肘者，扣其曲池與少海兩穴而側下帶之者也。採腕者，
扣其內關穴而下帶也。如情勢可，可雙手扣採任何兩處
矣。應用時，採化必採至敵失其中定。如採至半途而廢，
則敵易以肘或靠而反擊之。習者，必特別防意也。不但
如此，採勁必速。緩採，亦為敵所防所乘也。

When you use Cai Jin, you should not grab. If you grab, the arm will be tensed and the body will be stiff. This will provide a good opportunity for your opponent to find

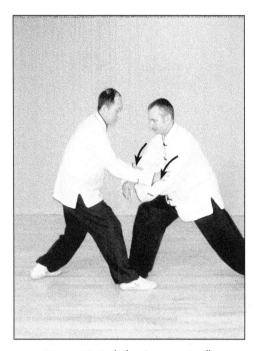

Figure 57. Push the Opponent's Elbow
to Neutralize Press

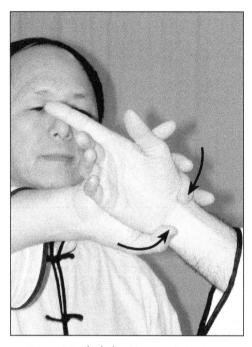

Figure 58. Pluck the Opponent's Wrist

your center. When you pluck, normally you use your thumb and index or middle finger (Figure 58). It is common that when you pluck, you press the cavities as well. When cavities are pressed, it can cause numbness and this will prevent the opponent from getting away. Common cavities for this on the shoulder are Jianjing (GB-21) (肩井) and Jianneiling (M-UE-48) (肩內陵), on the elbow are Quchi (LI-11) (曲池) and Shaohai (H-3) (少海), and on the wrist is Neiguan (P-6) (內關) (Figures 59 and 60).

When you apply Cai Jin in combat, once you have plucked the opponent and begin pulling to destroy his central equilibrium, you must continue your pulling until he has lost balance, otherwise he can use his elbow or shoulder to bump you (Figure 61). In addition, pluck is used in a fast action. If you are slow and your intention is sensed by your opponent, he can easily create an advantageous opportunity for his attack.

> *Lie means to split both of (your) arms in opposite directions and use the front arm to attack diagonally. The two arms are opposite divided and become mutual Yin and Yang. When there is a Yin and Yang balance, the central equilibrium can be maintained during attacking. Taijiquan postures such as Grasp the Sparrow's Tail, Diagonal Flying, and Wild Horse Parts Its Mane contain patterns of Lie Jin (Split Jin). When (you) execute Lie Jin, (you) must first know Peng Jin. Without knowing Peng Jin, the Lie Jin will be ineffective. Additionally, the central equilibrium can be lost easily. Lie Jin is often used against the opponent's Zhou and Kao Jins (i.e., Elbow and Bump Jins). When applying Lie*

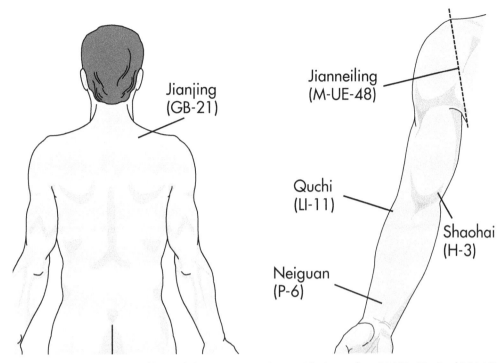

Figure 59. Jianjing (GB-21) Cavity

Figure 60. Jianneiling (M-UE-48), Quchi (LI-11), Shaohai (H-3), and Neiguan (P-6) Cavities

Jin, (you) must first pluck the opponent's wrist or elbow. If (you) don't know how to pluck the opponent and apply (your) Lie Jin, then (your) opponent can easily use this opportunity and attack you with his elbow.

挒者，兩臂反向分開而以前臂側攻也。兩臂反向，互為陰陽也。一陰一陽，攻勢可持中定也。太極拳中，攬雀尾、斜飛勢、野馬分鬃者，乃挒勁之勢也。施挒勁必知掤勁。不知掤勁，挒勁難期其效，亦易失其中定也。挒勁遍用於防敵之肘與靠。施挒勁，必先採敵之腕或肘，不知採而施挒勁，必為敵之肘所乘。

Lie (挒) means to split. In order to generate a split action, you will need two forces executed in opposite directions (Figure 62). One is used to attack the opponent while the other is used to balance the attacking force. In this case, you can maintain your balance and center. When you use Lie Jin, you must have Peng Jin within. Without Peng Jin, the spine and chest bows will not be able to store the Jin in the posture. In addition, with Peng Jin, you can protect your center easily. In order to make Lie Jin effective and place yourself in a secure position, you must first pluck

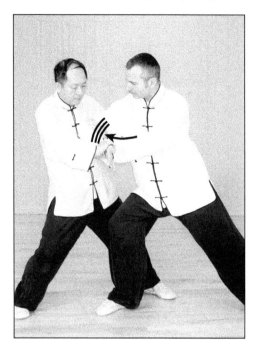

Figure 61. Opponent Uses Bump (Kao)
Against my Pluck (Cai)

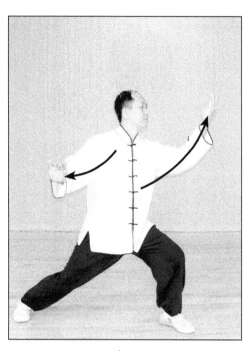

Figure 62. Split Jin (Lie Jin)

your opponent's elbow or wrist. If you do not do this, your opponent can easily use his elbow to attack you.

Zhou means to use the elbow to neutralize, to attack, or to coil. The neutralization of Zhou prevents your elbows from being plucked or squeezed by the opponent. If your elbows are plucked, controlled, sealed, or squeezed, then you must use the Zhou Jin with the coordination of Peng Jin to neutralize it. The attack of the elbow must be executed in short range fighting (i.e., small circle). To execute Zhou Jin, you must have entered the central door or have occupied the opponent's empty door, so Zhou Jin can be used. If you have already plucked the opponent's wrist, you can use your elbow to press his elbow upward to control his arm. When you execute your Zhou Jin, you must be very cautious to guard yourself against the opponent's Lu Jin (i.e., Rollback Jin). If your opponent is good at using Lu Jin, (he) can pull your root and destroy your central equilibrium. Therefore, (you) must be very careful to prevent this from happening.

肘者，以肘化、攻、纏之謂也。肘之化，在防我之雙肘
為敵所扣、所擠也。如我之肘被扣、被拿、被封、被擠，
我必以肘配合掤勁轉化之。肘之攻，必在短距（小
圈）。欲施肘勁，我必已入中門或已搶佔敵之空門，肘
可用矣。如我已扣敵之腕，我可以肘上頂其肘以擒其臂。
我施肘勁，必慎防敵之攟勁。敵如善用攟勁，可拔我根，
損我中定，不可不防也。

The skill of Zhou Jin can be used for neutralization, stroke, or even to coil the opponent's arm for control. When it is used for neutralization, it is commonly used to prevent your opponent from plucking, controlling, sealing, or squeezing your elbows. Through circling your elbows with Peng Jin, you will be able to re-direct the opponent's force and neutralize it. This will prevent him from locating your center and destroying it (Figure 63). When you and your opponent are in a short range fighting situation, if the opportunity allows, you should use your elbow to strike the opponent's vital areas. When you execute your strikes, you must have already taken an advantageous position, such as occupying the central door or entering his empty door. If you have not placed him into this urgent position, he can easily counter you by controlling your shoulder or elbow and destroying your balance (Figure 64). The elbow can also be used in Qin Na techniques. For example, if you have grabbed your opponent's wrist with one hand, you can use the elbow of the other arm to coil his elbow and lock him up (Figure 65). When you apply Elbow, you must be alert to prevent your opponent from using Lu Jin (i.e., Rollback Jin) to counter.

> *Kao means to use part of your own body to bump the opponent's body to make him lose his central equilibrium. Kao Jin can be divided into shoulder Kao, chest Kao, back Kao, hip Kao, and knee Kao, etc. Kao Jin is the same as Zhou Jin, which must be applied when the opponent is near. Therefore, the skills of how to occupy the central door and enter the empty door must be expert and alive; (you) can then create an advantageous opportunity and establish a desirable position. As with Zhou Jin, when (you) apply Kao Jin, (you) must be cautious to guard yourself against the opponent's Lu Jin. If the opponent is good at using Lu Jin, (he) can pull (your) root and destroy (your) central equilibrium. Therefore, (you) must be careful to prevent this from happening.*

靠者，以己身之部位靠撞敵身使之失其中定也。靠勁可
分肩靠、胸靠、背靠、臀靠、膝靠等種種。靠勁，如同
肘勁者，必施於近身。因此搶中門、入空門之技必先善
活，才能創機立勢。如同肘勁之施，施靠勁，必慎防敵
之攄勁。敵如善用攄勁，可拔我根，損我中定，不可不
防也。

Kao and Zhou Jins specialize in short range fighting situations. To apply Kao, you may use any part of your body to bump your opponent out of balance. For example, you may use your shoulders, chest, back, hips, knees, etc. to bump your opponent off. Since Kao is a short range fighting technique, you must already have an advantageous position when you use it to avoid your opponent's attack. Only when your opponent is in an urgent situation can you get closer to his body without taking too much of a risk. If you are interested in knowing more about these Taijiquan eight basic Jin patterns, please refer to the books: *Taiji Chin Na* or *Taijiquan-Classical Yang Style* by YMAA.

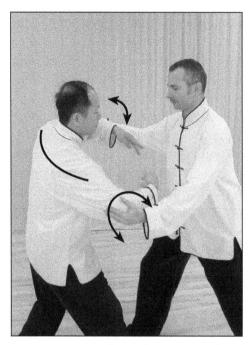

Figure 63. Using Elbow (Zhou) to Neutralize the Opponent's Pluck (Cai)

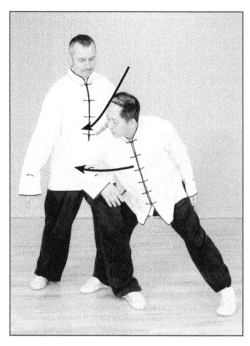

Figure 64. Opponent Applies Control (Na) to my Elbow to Neutralize my Bump (Kao)

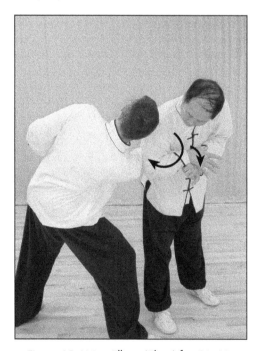

Figure 65. Using Elbow (Zhou) for Qin Na

2. Practicing Methods of the Five Steppings 五步練法 (Five Elements) 〔五行〕

What are the five steppings? They are advancing, retreating, beware of the left, look to the right, and central equilibrium. The eight doors are the Jin patterns for eight directions and the five steppings are the stepping actions of the four sides. However, in order to keep a steady and firm (center and root) in the stepping action, (you) must first try for central equilibrium. This has been discussed in detail earlier. Taijiquan Classic *said: "The root is at the feet, (Jin or movement is) generated from the legs, mastered (i.e., controlled) by the waist and manifested (i.e., expressed) through the fingers." "To generate Jin from the legs" during stationary or moving situations, you search for the legs' rooting and stability and the body's central equilibrium. In the stepping movements, the legs' actions are light and agile and the Jin can be manifested as wished. When (you) practice the five steppings, (you) should begin from a stationary position. Train to keep (the body and mind's) central equilibrium and to comprehend the body's emitting and neutralization. After that, begin the practice of stepping movements.*

五步者，前進、後退、左顧、右盼、中定也。八門勁勢
為八方之勢，而五步為四面步動之勢。然為持步動穩定
之勢，必先求中定，前已詳述之。經云：〝其根在腳，
發於腿，主宰於腰，形於手指。〞其發之於腿即在定步
與動步中，腿之根能紮穩，身能持中定之勢。動步中，
腿之移步輕巧，勁能隨心所欲而發化。練習五步，須從
定步練起。由定步中去持中定、去懂身體之發、化。之
後，才能步入動步矣。

Even though the five strategic steppings are considered stepping actions, most Taijiquan practitioners realize that the strategic actions of advance, retreat, beware of the left, look to the right, and central equilibrium should also be applied in stationary pushing hands. From stationary training, a practitioner will be able to build up his awareness, alertness, and strategic body actions, such as shifting the body forward, yielding backward, turning to the left, and neutralizing to the right. In addition, a student will learn how to coordinate these five strategic body actions with the eight strategic Jin patterns harmoniously and smoothly. Naturally, in order to execute these four body actions, you must first have a firm and stable central equilibrium. It is because of this that most Taijiquan teachers will teach a student how to apply these five strategic actions in stationary pushing hands first.

Central equilibrium, advance forward, retreat backward, beware of the left, and look to the right should be practiced in stationary pushing hands. Central Equilibrium involves balance, rooting, and making sure "the head is suspended." Advance and retreat involves the upper body's advance and retreat. This advance and retreat can be accomplished from the exchange of the Climbing Mountain Stance (i.e., Bow and Arrow Stance) and Four-Six Stance. Mountain Climbing Stance is mainly used for advancing, offense, and sealing, while Four-Six Stance is mainly used for retreating, defense, and yielding. Beware of the left and look to the right are carried out from the upper body's turning and mainly used for leading, neutralizing, and controlling.

定步中定之勢與定步之進、退、顧、盼由定步推手練起。
中定者，平衡、紮根、頂勁之謂也。進、退者，由腰而
上身體之進與退也。此進退由蹬山步（弓箭步）與四六
步之轉換而成。蹬山步主進、主攻、主封，四六步主退、
主守、主讓。顧、盼者，由腰而上身體之輾轉而成，主
引、主化、主拿也。

The first step in practicing stationary pushing hands is learning how to protect your center and keep it in a state of equilibrium. In order to reach this goal, you must be able to firm your root, maintain your center, and keep your body in balance. That means the torso is upright and the head is suspended. In order to reach all of these goals, you must know how to be relaxed and soft. Without these two criteria, your body will be tensed and the mind will be scattered. Naturally, the root will be shallow and your listening and understanding Jins will be dull.

Stationary advancing forward and retreating back are done by changing the stance from Climbing Mountain Stance (Deng Shan Bu, 蹬山步) into Four-Six Stance (Si Liu Bu, 四六步) and vice versa. When you are in Climbing Mountain Stance, you enter the central door and occupy the advantageous position for attacking and sealing (Figure 66). Once you change into Four-Six Stance, you are yielding and become defensive (Figure 67). You should remember that it does not matter if you advance forward or retreat back, your torso should be kept upright, your head suspended, and the tailbone tucked in at all times. The strategic body actions of beware of the left and look to the right in stationary pushing hands are accomplished by the body's turning and are used for coiling, turning, and controlling (Figure 68).

From the fundamental practice of single pushing hands, advancing into double pushing hands, (you learn) to listen, understand, advance forward, retreat backward, beware of the left, and look to the right. When (you) have reached a natural reactive stage of using the Yi without the Yi, then (you) may enter the practice of moving pushing hands. (However, you should know that) in moving pushing hands training, the practice of advance forward, retreat backward, beware of the left, look to the right, and central equilibrium also start from single pushing hands. Its main goal is to train central equilibrium so it can harmonize the criteria of advance forward, retreat backward, beware of the left, look to the right. After the hands, the eyes, the body movements, the techniques, and the stepping can be coordinated and harmonized with each other, then (you can) enter the practice of double pushing hands, large rollback, and small rollback of stepping moving pushing hands. Afterward, (you can) enter the practice of Taijiquan

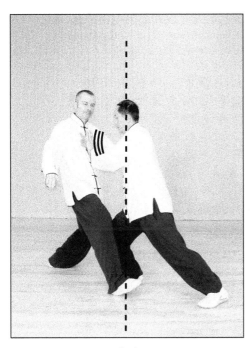

Figure 66. Using Climbing Mountain Stance (Deng Shan Bu) to Occupy the Central Door

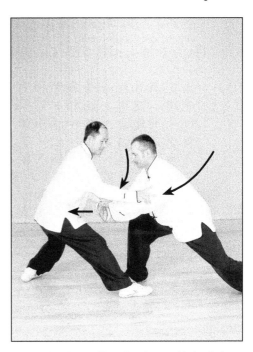

Figure 67. Using Four-Six Stance (Si Liu Bu) to Neutralize the Coming Press (Ji)

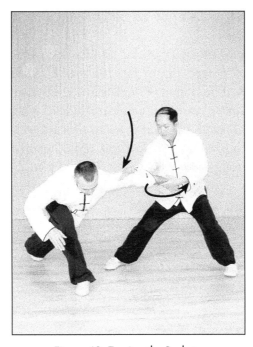

Figure 68. Turning the Body to Neutralize the Coming Force

sparring. From the practice of sparring, (you) should continue to search deeper for profound understanding, experience, and applications. After a long period of practice, the moving of the five steppings can be carried out as wished.

由定步單推手晉為雙推手之基本練習中，而聽、而懂、
而進、而退、而顧、而盼。在達乎意不為意之自然反應
後，即能步入動步推手練習。動步之進、退、顧、盼、
與中定亦由單推手始。其主要目的在訓練行步中之中定
與步伐之進、退、顧、盼也。在手、眼、身、法、步能
合諧調配得宜後，即步入雙推手與大、小履之動步練習。
之後，即可步入太極散手之練習。在由散手對練中去尋
求更深之瞭解、經驗、與應用。久而久之，五步之行隨
心所欲也。

After you have mastered all of the basic skills for your body's strategic actions and are familiar with the techniques of applying the eight basic Jin patterns in stationary pushing hands, then you can start your moving pushing hands. If you have not mastered the basic stationary pushing hands skills, but rush into moving pushing, your body will be tense and stiff. The central equilibrium will not be maintained, the stepping root will be shallow, and the techniques will not be highly effective. Building up good habits and basic skills is the key to reaching a profound level of Taijiquan pushing hands.

When you advance to moving pushing hands, again you must start from single moving pushing hands, progressing to moving double pushing hands. From these practices, you learn how to maintain your central equilibrium while you are stepping and turning. After you have reached a comfortable level where the Yi does not have to be there (i.e., natural reaction), then you can proceed to large and small rollback training. Gradually, you proceed into sparring and other advanced Jin skills such as spiraling, coiling, controlling, borrowing, etc. (Figure 69).

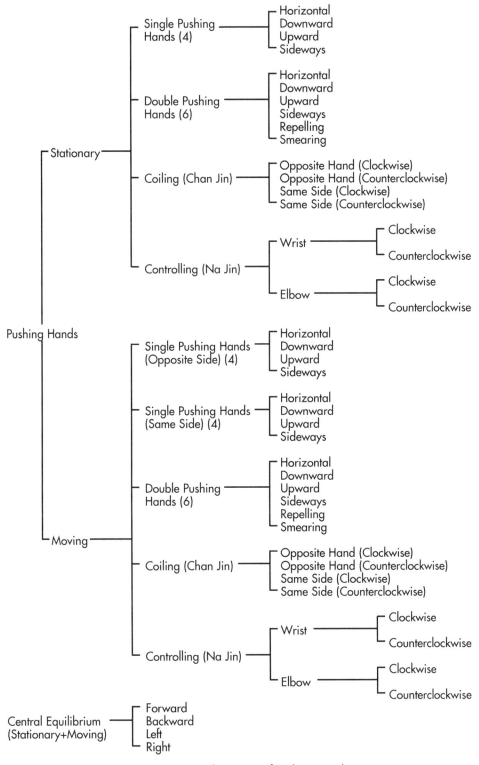

Figure 69. General Contents of Pushing Hands Practice

3. Practicing Methods of Central Equilibrium 中定練法

Central equilibrium is the most important in the Five Steppings. Central equilibrium is needed (when you are) in a stationary position. It is also needed (when you are) in moving situations. If central equilibrium is not kept, then (you) lose balance. Once you have lost (your) balance, then (you are in) an urgent situation. Your opponent can easily take advantage of this opportunity. Central equilibrium refers to the equilibrium of the physical body. The Yi is kept at the Real Dan Tian, and the Qi residence is protected. This is the posture of Wuji state. Taijiquan Classic said: "If there is a top, there is a bottom; if there is a front, there is a back; if there is a left, there is a right." In summary, it is a single point. That means the central equilibrium of the Real Dan Tian.

中定者，五步中之最要者也。定步須中定，動步亦須中
定。中不定，則失平衡也。失平衡，則急迫也。易為敵
所乘矣。中定，乃身體物理之中定，乃意守真丹田，氣
舍之守之定也。此乃無極之勢。經云：〝有上即有下，
有前必有後，有左必有右。〞歸納之，乃一點之定，亦
即真丹田之定也。

Central equilibrium requires the balance and stability of the Real Dan Tian (Zhen Dan Tian, 真丹田), which is located at the center of gravity or physical center. Therefore, it is a point instead of a line. If you can keep this point in equipoise either in stationary or moving position, your opponent will have a hard time finding your center and destroying your root.

In order to keep the central equilibrium of the physical center, steadiness of the Qi's entrance and exit, and stability of the Xin (i.e., emotional mind) and Yi (i.e., wisdom mind). The most important thing is to keep the waist and Kua (thighs and hip joints area) loose. The waist is the connecting place of the upper body and the lower body. When the waist is loose, the root can be firm and the top and the bottom can be harmonized with each other. When the waist is loose, the body will naturally be loose. When the body can be loose, then the Yi can be concentrated. When the Yi can be concentrated, the Xin will be peaceful. When the Xin is peaceful, then the spirit will have its center. When the spirit has its center, then the body and the mind are all steady.

為持身體物理中心之定，氣能進出丹田自如之定，心與
意之定，其首要在於鬆腰鬆胯也。腰為上身下體關連之
所，腰鬆則根穩，上下相合。腰能鬆，則身能鬆，身能
鬆，則意專，意專則心安，心安則神有主矣。神有主，
則身心均定矣。

In order to keep yourself in a good state of central equilibrium, the first requirement is to keep this central place (i.e., Real Dan Tian) loose and comfortable. When this central place is loose and comfortable, the Qi can flow in and out easily, and the mind can be sensitive in this place and steady. In this case, you can protect your center and keep the equilibrium. In order to keep this center loose and comfortable, you must first learn how to keep your waist and the hip joint area loose. When these places are loose, you will be able to protect your root. When your root is firmed, the center can be protected.

> *The practicing method for maintaining central equilibrium is to allow your partner to control your elbows and find your center. His intention is to destroy your central equilibrium. You will only be defensive. Use Peng Jin and turn (your) waist and legs to neutralize the coming Jin. Taijiquan Classic said: "If you fail to catch the opportunity and gain the superior position, (your) body will be disordered. To solve this problem, (you) must look to the waist and legs." Use the waist and the legs to find the neutralizing Jin. Use the posture of Peng to find central equilibrium. After long practice, the root will be firmed and the central equilibrium is established.*

> 其練法，由練伴拿我肘並尋我之中心，其意欲損我之中
> 定也。我僅防守而不攻，以掤勁與腰腿轉化來勁。經云：
> "有不得機得勢處，身便散亂。其病必於腰腿求之。"
> 此即其意也。由腰腿上，求化勁。由掤勁勢上，尋中定。
> 久而久之，根紮矣！中定矣！

The way to protect your central equilibrium is to keep the waist and hips loose and to also know how to turn the waist to re-direct the incoming force to the sides to neutralize. The way of training this is to let your opponent control your elbows and put you in an urgent situation. Then you can use your waist and legs to neutralize the urgent situation, rolling and directing the attack into emptiness.

4. Method of Rooting 紮根法

> Taijiquan Classic *said: "The root is at the feet, (Jin or movement is) generated from the legs, mastered (i.e., controlled) by the waist and manifested (i.e., expressed) from the fingers. From the feet to the legs to the waist must be integrated, into one unified Qi. When moving forward or backward, (you can) then catch the opportunity and gain the superior position. If (you) fail to catch the opportunity and gain the superior position, (your) body will be disordered. To solve this problem, (you) must look to the waist and legs. Up and down, forward and backward, left and right, it's all the same. All of this is done with the Yi (mind), not externally." This has clearly implied that the rooting is the most important (point) in Taijiquan's offense and defense. When the root is firmed, the*

central equilibrium will be steady and the Jin can be emitted (effectively). If the root is floating, then the central equilibrium will be damaged, the mind will be scattered, and this can be taken advantage of by an opponent.

太極拳經謂：「其根在腳，發於腿，主宰於腰，形於手指。由腳而腿而腰，總須完整一氣。向前退後，乃能得機得勢。有不得機得勢處，身便散亂。其病必於腰腿求之。上下前後左右皆然。凡此皆是意，不在外面。」此即意繫根乃太極拳攻防之首要。根穩，中定定，而勁能發。根浮，則中定損，意亂，為敵所乘，置我於不得機之境地。

Taijiquan is a martial style that specializes in middle and short range fighting distances. Because of this, the most important concern in a fight is how to maintain your center and root. If you have lost your root and center, your mind will be scattered and your body will lose its balance, and also the Jin you manifest will be shallow. That means you have lost. *Taijiquan Classic* points out three important things: 1. The root is the origin of Jin. 2. When you have lost balance and root, your mind and body will be scattered. You should re-establish your rooting and stability through the waist and legs. 3. All of this balance and rooting must be accomplished through internal (i.e., Yi) understanding and feeling, as well as external understanding and feeling.

The most important thing in the training of firming the root is that all the joints must threaded together and function as a single Qi (i.e., single unit). In order to thread the joint together, (you) must first know how to keep the joints light and agile. According to theory, the entire body can be divided into upper, middle, and lower sections. From the knees and below is the lower section, from the knees to Xinkan (i.e., Jiuwei) is the middle section, and from Xinkan to the neck and head is the upper section. When the root of the lower section is firmed, the middle section can be relaxed, and the Jin manifested from the upper level can be strong. To reach the steadiness and firmness of the root in the lower section, (you) must begin (your training) from ankles, knees, and hips, these three joint places. If these three places can be loosened, soft, agile, and alive, then the root can be firmed. However, the most important of all is to keep the waist area soft. When the waist is soft, you can control the Jin, and emitting or neutralizing can be swift and natural. In that case, it will be hard for (your) opponent's Jin to reach your center and pull your root.

紫根之首要，在於節節貫穿，全身完整一氣。為求貫穿，
必先懂得關節之輕靈。依理而言，全身可分為上、中、
下三盤。由膝而下為之下盤，由膝至心坎為中盤，由心
坎至頭頂為上盤。下盤跟穩，中盤能鬆，上盤之勁顯必
強。為求下盤之根穩，必先由踝、膝、胯三處關節著手。
若此三關節能鬆，能軟，能靈，能活，則根可定。然最
重者，乃是鬆腰。腰鬆則勁可為我主宰，發、化靈活自
然。如此，敵之勁必難達於我之中心，並拔其根。

The entire body is connected by joints. Through these joints, your opponent's power can reach your root and destroy it. In Taijiquan, the body acts as a single soft whipping unit. Jin is initiated from the root, is controlled by the waist and manifested in the fingers. In order to make this happen, the joints must be soft and relaxed (i.e., light) and activated. These conditions are required not just for the Jin's manifestation, but also to prevent the opponent's power from reaching your root.

As mentioned in Part I, the entire body can be divided into three sections (San Pan, 三盤); from the knees down, from the knees to Xinkan (心坎) (or Jiuwei, Co-15) (鳩尾), and from Xinkan to the crown. Xinkan is a martial arts term for the cavity named Jiuwei in Chinese medicine (Figure 70). Xinkan is the lower part of the sternum. In Chinese martial arts training, the lower section (from the knees down) is considered the most important since it is related to your root and stability. If you do not have a firm root and good stability, your mind and physical body will float, and your concentration and spirit will be shallow. In this case, your power cannot be manifested effectively, and you have provided your opponent with an advantageous position from which to destroy your center and take you down.

In order to have firm root and stability, you must first have strong legs, especially the joints in the ankles, knees, and hips. You must also be able to control them efficiently so they can be soft and loose as well. You must have a waist that can be controlled by your mind efficiently. For all of this, you must also learn precision of control so that when it is necessary to be hard, the joints can be hard, and when they must be soft, they can be soft. When this happens, your mind will be able to govern the middle and the lower section of the body effectively for any defensive or offensive situation.

Generally, the distance between your physical center (i.e., gravity) and the ground registered in your subconscious mind was constantly adjusted as you grew taller. From this subconscious mind, we can pull our root any time and walk. If this distance in our subconscious mind is too long, then the root will be too deep and it will be hard to step. If this distance in our subconscious mind is too short, then the root is floating and you can fall. Normally, in order to increase the level

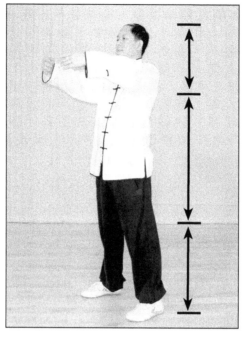

Upper Section

Middle Section

Lower Section

Figure 70. Three Sections of the Body (San Pan)

of stability (i.e., rooting) we sink down to lower the physical center. Consequently, the distance between the gravity center and the ground is extended into the ground. Thus, we are rooted.

人體物理中心與地面之距離，一般人之潛意識，隨身體
之成長而調節。由此潛意識，吾等可隨時拔根而步行。
如此潛意識之距離太長，則根沈而難行。如此潛意識之
距離太短，則根浮而易傾。平時，為增加身體之穩度，
我們下蹲身勢以降低身體之物理中心，同時潛意識理物
理中心與地面之距離，往地裡伸展。由此，根紮矣。

Theoretically, since the day you learned how to walk, your mind has been registering the distance between your physical gravity center and the ground (Figure 71). This distance was adjusted during the course of your growth. It is from the recognition of this distance that you can walk. If the distance in your mind is longer than this distance and sinks into the ground, then you cannot walk. On the contrary, if the distance in your mind is shorter than this distance, then your mind is above the ground and you are not rooted in walking. In this case, you will be floating and awkward. Generally, in order to build up a stronger root, you squat down to lower your physical center of gravity and in addition to the physical strength built, this allows your mind to go underneath the ground to establish a firm root (Figure 72).

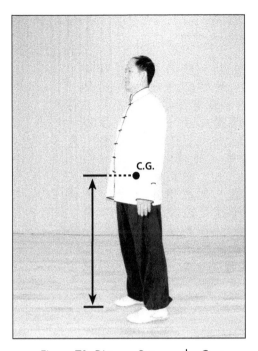

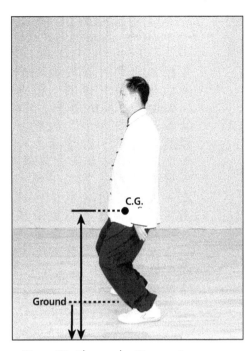

Figure 71. Distance Between the Center
of Gravity and the Ground

Figure 72. Shorten the Distance Between
the Center of Gravity and the Ground

In Chinese martial arts training, there are two ways of establishing a stronger root, one is through the physical stances and the other is through breathing and mental training that allows you to extend the distance from physical gravity center into the ground. Both kinds of training are required.

The next important thing in rooting practice is the endurance and strength of the legs. When the legs are strong and the endurance is high, then the root and stability can be maintained. Otherwise, the root can be pulled easily. To train the legs' endurance and strength, generally (you can) begin from doing basic stances on stakes. Generally, the stances are: Horse Stance, Mountain Climbing Stance (Bow and Arrow Stance), Four-Six Stance, Tame the Tiger Stance, Golden Rooster Stand with One Leg Stance, False Stance, Swallow Stance, and Unicorn Stance. Beginners should (first) stand on the ground for about five minutes (in each stance). After a long period of practice, (you) should be able to stand for thirty minutes without feeling tired. This is the time to begin the practice of standing on stakes. You may use wood stakes or even masonry bricks. Stand on the stakes while the mind is under the stakes. After a long time, the mind can be a few inches under the feet. To make the root even deeper, (you) may follow the same method by increasing the height of the stakes. After (you) step down from the stakes, the root can be a few feet under your feet. In this case, the root is really deep. In order to have lightness and agility of the ankles, knees, and hips, (you) may circle (your) lower section as wished while standing in Horse Stance or Mountain Climbing Stance, etc. In this case, the feeling on the bottom of the feet will be enhanced and the Root Jin can be established. The depth of the root depends on the level of sen-

sitivity feeling on the bottom of your feet. If the sensitivity level is high, the root is deep and if the sensitivity level is low, the root is shallow.

紮根之次要，在於腿之耐力與強勁。腿力強，耐力高，
則根穩可持。否則，根易被拔。練習腿之耐力與強勁，
一般由基本站樁著手。站樁庄勢一般有馬步、蹬山步（弓
箭步）、四六步、伏虎步、金雞獨立步、虛步、吞步、
麒麟步等等。初學者，站於平地上，以五分鐘為度。久
而久之，可站至三十分鐘而不勞累。此時即可步入站樁。
可用木樁或平常之磚塊。站於樁上，意於樁下。久而久
之，意可達足底數寸。欲達更深之紮根境地，可加高樁
高，依法練習。在樁去後，根可達足底數尺，根深矣。
為求踝、膝、胯之輕靈與鬆軟，可在馬步、蹬山步等站
庄時，下盤轉圈自如。如此，增強腳底之感覺並樹立根
勁。根之深淺，由足底之敏感度而定。敏感度高，根深，
敏感度低，根淺。

There are many ways to train your legs and make them strong. One of the most common ways in Chinese martial arts training is through fundamental stance training. From fundamental stance training, you gradually build up strength in your legs (Figure 73). You should stand for a few minutes first until the endurance and strength develops. Then you can extend the time. You should later start to stand on some wood stakes or even bricks (Figure 74). In order to maintain your stability, you gradually train your mind and extend it downward to the bottom of the bricks. After long practice, your mind can register this distance anytime you wish. When this happens, once you have removed yourself from the bricks, your mind will be a few inches under the ground, and you are rooted.

In order to allow your mind to control your legs efficiently during this tense standing, you should also train using a circling motion (Figure 75). This will gradually allow you to control the muscles, tendons, and ligaments required for maneuvering actions. Through this training, you will be able to build up higher sensitivity on your soles. This is also a key to rooting.

Rooting practice with a partner through the game of tug of war. That means you and your partner stand in Mountain Climbing Stance and face each other, the front hands holding each other (like a handshake). During competition, both sides try their best to pull the opponent off balance (in any direction). When there is any shift in rooting, then the one who shifts his root loses. From this practice, (you) can master the skills of leading and neutralizing the coming Jin, to see clearly and to feel the opponent's central equilibrium and root. After practicing for a long time, the root can be firmed. The students should ponder, comprehend, and practice this game and catch its key tricks.

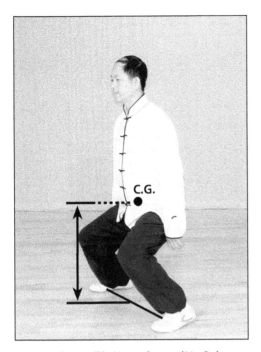

Figure 73. Horse Stance (Ma Bu)

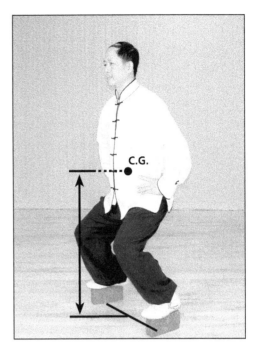

Figure 74. Standing on Bricks

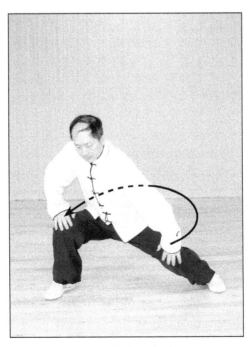

Figure 75. Circling the Knees

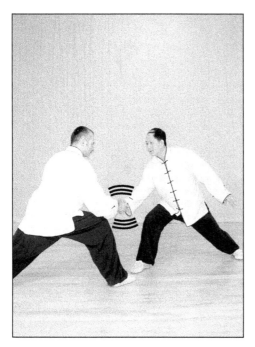 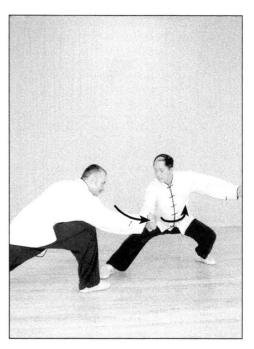

Figure 76. Centering Competition with a Partner   Figure 77. Centering Competition with a Partner

與友伴練習紮根之法，可以拉拒戰行之。亦即與友伴蹬
山步對立，前手相握。比賽時，盡力想將對方拉倒。根
一動即敗。在此練習下，可熟悉如何將來勁引化，可洞
悉感覺對方之中定與根源，久而久之，根定矣。學者當
自習之以悟其竅。

Rooting can easily be trained with a partner. Simply face each other and squat down in Mountain Climbing Stance with the front hands holding each other (Figure 76). Then, both parties try their best to pull the opponent either sideways, forward, or back with the intent to pull the opponent off balance. Naturally, both partners must be rooted and very sensitive and alert about the opponent's intention and power so the incoming attacks can be neutralized. In order to neutralize the attacking force, you must know how to change your Mountain Climbing Stance into Four-Six Stance and also how to use your waist to turn your body skillfully (Figure 77). Both partners must be able to feel and sense the opportunity of this advantage and take it without hesitation. After you have practiced this for a while, you will see how fast this will help you build up your root and center.

5. Method of Uprooting 拔根法

Uprooting is used against the opponent, to destroy his root, and to put him at a disadvantage. In order to pull his root, (you) must first destroy his central equilibrium. When the central equilibrium is disrupted, his mind will be disordered and his Qi will float. Seize this opportunity and pull his root off. In order to destroy his central equilibrium, (you) must know Listening, Following, Attaching, and Adhering Jins. Attach to his center and adhere to his skin and muscles, Yin and Yang mutually exchange, capture his central door, and occupy his empty door to confuse his mind. In this case, (you) will put (your) opponent into a disadvantageous position that can be used by you to destroy his central equilibrium. When the central equilibrium is destroyed, the root can be easily pulled.

拔根乃我對待敵人，以損其根，並置敵於不利之地。欲
拔敵根，必先損其中定。中定損，其意必亂，其氣必浮，
趁此良機，拔其根也。欲損其中定，必懂聽、隨、沾、
黏之勁。沾其中心，黏其肌膚，陰陽交替，搶其中門，
佔其空門，以亂其心。如此，必置敵於不利，為我所用
並損其中定。中定損，根易拔矣。

In order to create an opportunity for your attack, first you must put your opponent into a defensive and urgent situation. One of the most common ways is to destroy his balance and root. When this happens, your opponent must pay attention to his balance and root and try to re-establish it. In this case, you will have created an advantageous situation for your attack. However, in order to reach this goal, you must first be good in the skills of Listening, Understanding, Following, Attaching, and Adhering Jins. With the skillfulness and effectiveness of these Jins, you will be able to place your opponent into a defensive situation. You must also be an expert in using the exchangeable Yin-Yang strategies to confuse your opponent. Once you have created these advantageous opportunities, you should then immediately occupy the central door (Zhong Men, 中門) or reposition yourself and enter his empty door (Kong Men, 空門). The central door is the mid-way position between you and your opponent (Figure 78). Once you have occupied this position, you will have put your opponent into an urgent position. Empty door means the door is opened that allows you to step in for an attack. For example, if your opponent's right leg is forward, then his left hand side is one of the empty doors (Figure 79). Once you have seized this door, your opponent will feel naked and exposed to your attack.

Taijiquan Classic said: "If there is a top, there is a bottom; if there is a front, there is a back; if there is a left, there is a right. If Yi (wisdom mind) wants to go upward, this implies considering downward. (This means) if (you) want to lift and defeat an opponent, you must first consider his root. When the opponent's root is broken, he will inevitably be defeated quickly and certainly." This can be

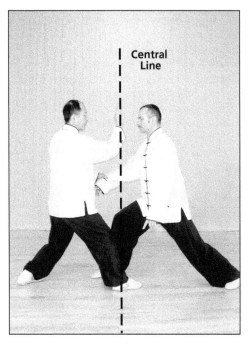

Figure 78. Central Door (Zhong Men)

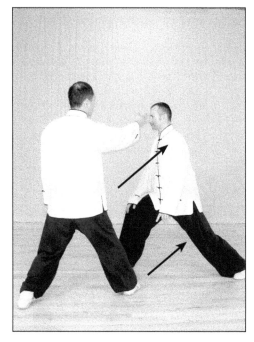

Figure 79. Empty Door (Kong Men)

done through the application of Yin and Yang strategies of exchange. When the opponent's mind is disordered, the root can be pulled. In order to pull his root, (you) must first trick him with downward tactics to entice his mind upward. When his mind is upward, you immediately take this opportunity to pull his root. Knowing is easier than actually executing it; therefore, learners should keep practicing until the skills can be carried out effectively.

經云：「有上即有下，有前即有後，有左即有右。如意
要向上，即寓下意。若將物掀起，而加以挫之之意。斯
其根自斷，乃壞之速而無疑。」此即意陰陽交替而用，
敵心一亂，根可拔矣。欲拔其根，必先寓下意，以引敵
上提之意。敵意一上提，我即趁機拔其根也。知易行難，
學者必多習之以為效。

In order to pull the opponent's root, strategically, you must know how to use insubstantial (i.e., Yin) and substantial (i.e., Yang) tactics skillfully. This will confuse your opponent. For example, in order to pull up, you must first pull down. When the opponent resists with upward intention and action, then you follow his action and immediately pull up. In order to make him fall to the left, first you apply pressure to his left (your right). Once he has initiated a reactive action against your force, then you immediately change your force to your left and make him lose balance. Through these on-off and off-on actions, you will put your opponent into a defensive and disorienting position that you control.

6. Practicing Methods for Listening, Following, Attaching, and Adhering 聽、隨、粘、黏練法

What is listening? It is the consciousness and the feeling before and after contact with the opponent. What is following? It is a moving action in which you follow the opponent's will with a connection. What is attaching? It is the intercepting action — a bridge between no contact and contact. It also refers to attaching and connecting action onto the opponent's center while already in contact, so (you are) able to pull his root. Adhering means after attaching, you stick with the opponent without separation, listening to his Yi and following his movements, connect and adhere like glue and like lacquer.

聽者，對敵接觸前與接觸後之意識和感覺也。隨者，跟從連隨敵意而動之意也。粘者，未接觸而至接觸之截接也，亦為已接觸進而粘連敵中心以拔其根之謂也。黏者，粘之後，緊連而不離也。聽彼之意，隨彼之動，連黏如膠如漆也。

Listening Jin (Ting Jin, 聽勁) in Taijiquan implies sensitivity and alertness to the opponent's intention and action before contact, and also implies the perception of the opponent's attempts to manifest Jin after making contact. Follow (i.e., Following Jin) (Sui Jin, 隨勁) is done without double weighting (Shuang Zhong, 雙重) (i.e., mutual resistance) — simply follow the opponent's action. When this happens, you can yield (i.e., Yielding Jin) (Rang Jin, 讓勁) and this will allow you to lead (i.e., Leading Jin) (Yin Jin, 引勁).

Attaching Jin (Zhan Jin, 粘勁) has a double meaning. One is to attach to the opponent's incoming attack just as he initiates it. The skills of this attachment are very important in combat, since your opponent will not make contact with you right at the beginning. Therefore, you must first attach to his incoming attack and then you can follow and adhere. The other application of attaching Jin is to attach to the opponent's center after you have already made contact. Naturally, this is a higher level of attaching. Once you can attach to his center and affect his central equilibrium, you will make his mind confused, destroy his balance, pull his root, and make his Qi float. When this happens, you may put him into an awkward and defensive situation.

Adhering (i.e., Nian Jin, 黏勁) means to connect to the opponent without separation. You must first be able to follow, then you can adhere. Once you can follow and adhere, you can connect (Lian Jin, 連勁) your thought to your opponent's thought. When this happens, you can establish a very sensitive understanding and reach a stage of "when the opponent does not move, you will not move; when the opponent slightly moves, you move first."[24]

> *As said above, to listen is to sense and to feel the opponent's mind either before contact or right after contact. First, (you) must listen, so you can then understand. It is just like learning a language. (You) must practice with different training partners. This is because everyone's offensive and defensive techniques and habits are different. If (you) practice with many people, (you) can avoid building up the habit of using the same techniques so (you) can handle different situations. When (you) practice listening and understanding before contact with a partner, (both of you) can use different attacking methods to charge each other. After a long time of practice, (you) can then interpret (the opponent's) intentions. When you begin this practice, it is appropriate to move slowly. Only after (you are) familiar with the (opponent's) coming attacks, can you then increase the speed. In order to attach (to the attacks) and adhere to them, (your) eyes' reaction must be fast and the hands' action must be quick. Therefore, (you) must practice keeping your eyes opened without blinking for at least five minutes. Next comes the practice of listening and understanding. This must be achieved in pushing hands. For the same reasons, start slowly first and after (you) are familiar with the coming Jins, increase the speed. After practicing for a long time, (you) will surely be able to listen and understand as wished and as an enlightened being.*

如上所言，聽者，在查覺敵勁接觸我身前後之來意。聽之，而後懂之。其如習語言然。其練習必與不同之練伴練習。其因不外乎每人之攻防手法與習性皆不同。與不同多人練習，可避免慣於同樣攻防手法而能應付不同之情況矣。練習未接觸之聽、懂，可彼此以不同之攻擊手法互相攻擊。久之，必懂其來勢。如習語言然，初開始練時，以慢為宜，在習慣於來勢後，即可漸漸加快。為能粘接，眼必明手必快。因而須練眼睛而不閉之能至少五分鐘餘。練接觸以後之聽與懂，須由推手練習著手。同理之，以慢為先。在熟悉來勁後，始漸加快。久之，必能隨心所欲，聽懂如神。

After listening, you can have an understanding (Dong Jin, 懂勁) of your opponent's intention and know how to deal with the situation. In order to listen to the opponent's attempts continuously, you must know how to follow his action so you can adhere with him without separation (Sui Jin, 隨勁).

Developing a high level of Understanding Jin is the same as learning a language. You must keep practicing until it becomes natural. You must practice with different partners. If you do this, you will not build up a routine habit from a single partner.

Since Listening Jin can be divided into situations before contact and after contact, Understanding Jin can also be divided into two situations. To train Understanding Jin before contact/until contact, you must ask different partners to attack you with different options and learn how to intercept the incoming attack by attaching and following. To train Understanding Jin after contact, you must practice pushing hands with different partners. All of these aim for high alertness and sensitivity through sensing and feeling. Once you have reached a high level, you will recognize any slight intention and movement initiated by your opponent.

What is following? It means to move by following the coming force. In order to follow, there must not be double weighting (i.e., mutual resistance). If there is double weighting, then there is stagnation and you cannot follow. If (you) can follow, then (you) are able to attach and adhere. If (you) can attach and adhere, then (you) can connect and stick. If (you) can connect and stick, then (you) can lead the coming force into the emptiness, neutralize the coming Jin, and use four ounces to neutralize one thousand pounds. All of these important points must be gained from experience and pondering of Taijiquan pushing hands practice. From stationary single pushing hands practice, establish a firm foundation; from stationary double pushing hands, search for the offense and defense opportunity; from moving pushing hands and large and small rollback practice, learn how to coordinate with the five steppings. To comprehend the keys of listening, understanding, attaching, and adhering when the entire body is in the actions of advancing, retreating, beware of the left, and looking to the right, practice following the schedule and do not advance too fast. If you advance too quickly, your learning will not be deep. If you advance gradually, not only can (your) feeling be deep and can the Yi be strategic, but in addition the Qi's circulation will also be natural. After a long period of practice, every action can follow (your) wish in (your) heart, and reach a stage of action without Yi, regulating without regulating.

隨者，隨敵之來勢而動也。為能隨，必不能雙重。雙重
則滯而不能隨也。能隨，才能沾粘。能沾粘，才能連黏。
能連黏，才能引進落空，能化解來勢，能四兩破千斤。
此些要目，皆由太極推手中去體驗，去思索。由定步單
推手奠基，由定步雙推手中求攻守，由動步推手與大、
小擺練習中去配合五步，去瞭解全身進、退、顧、盼之
聽、隨、粘、黏之竅。按步練之，不可速進。速進者不
深。漸進者，不但覺深意玄，氣之行亦能順然。久之而
隨心所欲，無意而動，不調而調也。

This paragraph has summarized the theoretical concepts and basic requirements of pushing hands. You must first listen (i.e., sense and feel) and understand the opponent's intention. Then you must attach to the opponent's incoming attack (i.e., intercept). In order to attach skillfully, you must know how to follow and then attach. Once you have attached to the opponent's body, then you adhere and connect with him without separation. In order to reach all of this, you must not commit the common mistake of double weighting (Shuang Zhong, 雙重) (i.e., mutual resistance). If you commit this mistake, you will be in a situation of competing forces with your opponent. In this case, you have lost the basic principle of using four ounces to repel one thousand pounds.

7. The Practice of Yin-Yang Taiji Circle 陰陽太極圈之練習

Yin-Yang Taiji Circle Coiling Practice is a fundamental training Gong of Taijiquan's pushing hands, Jin's emitting and neutralization, and free sparring. Those who practice the martial aspects of Taijiquan must know this training. (This training) is called "Chan Si Jin" (i.e., Silk Reeling Jin) in Chen style and is called "Yin-Yang Taiji Circle Sticking Hands" in Yang style. This is because the Taiji circle can be classified as Yin and Yang, two different circles. The Yang circle emphasizes offense, seal, advance, and is circling clockwise. The Yin circle emphasizes defense, neutralization, withdrawing, and circling counterclockwise.

陰陽太極圈纏手練習，乃太極拳推手、勁之發化、與自由散手之基本功。習太極拳武學者必須知之。在陳氏太極拳稱之為纏絲勁，楊氏卻稱之為陰陽太極圈纏手也。其因為太極圈之練習分為陰、陽兩手。陽手主攻、主封、主進，以右旋為主。陰手主守、主化、主退，以左旋為主。

In order to train a beginner in how to use the waist to lead the Jin and then manifest it into the extremities, almost all soft martial styles have developed their own ways of training. This training has four goals: 1. to improve the communication of the mind and the waist so the mind can control the waist efficiently; 2. to keep the joints soft so the Jin can be led from the waist to the extremities without stagnation; 3. to manifest the Jin as a soft whip; and 4. to use the mind to lead the Qi from the Real Dan Tian to the extremities so the Jin can be manifested with maximum efficiency.

Since Taijiquan is a soft style and its Jins act like a soft whip with the waist as a controlling handle, it also emphasizes the above training so the Jin can be manifested efficiently. Chen style called it "Chan Si Jin" (纏絲勁), which means "Silk Reeling Jin." From this training, a practitioner learns how to use the mind to lead the Qi from the Real Dan Tian to the extremities and also how to use the waist to direct the Jin to the desired target without stagnation. A similar training has also been used in Yang style and is called "Yin-Yang Taiji Circle Coiling and Spiraling Training" (陰陽太極圈纏手練習) or "Yin-Yang Taiji Symbol Sticking Hands Training" (陰陽太極圈粘手練習).

In the Taiji symbol, clockwise is classified as Yang, while counterclockwise is classified as Yin. In the practice of the Taiji Circle, the hand moves following the symbol and circles, rotates, coils, and spirals. The motion is initiated from the bottom of the feet, is controlled from the waist, and is then manifested into the fingers. From the bottom of the feet to the fingers, every section of each joint follows the symbol and circles, rotates, coils, and spirals. This is to train the entire body to be threaded as a single Qi (i.e., single unit). From the bottom of the feet to the fingers acts as a soft whip. From the circling, rotating, coiling, and spiraling in the Taiji symbol, (we also) search for the root of the Jin's emitting and neutralization through the entire body. Furthermore, from practice, (we are) aiming for the regulating uniformity of the breathing and the smoothness of the Qi's circulation. From the last stage of Bagua Taiji stepping training, (we) learn how to comprehend, familiarize, and experience the secret keys to the Five Phases steppings.

太極圖者，右旋為陽，左旋為陰。太極圈之練法，手依圖而輾轉、纏繞而行。圈由腳底起，控制於腰，而形於手指。由腳底至手指，節節關節有圖輾轉纏繞之。此練習全身關節之貫串一氣，由腳底至手指如軟鞭然。亦由太極圈之輾轉纏中，去求全身勁發、化之根由。更從練習中，去調合呼吸之均勻和運氣之通順。不但如此，在最終雙人之八卦太極行步練習中，去瞭解、熟悉，體驗五行步伐之訣竅。

In this training, the Yin and Yang aspects of the Taiji symbols are classified. When performed on the right hand side, the Yang Taiji symbol rotates clockwise and is used for offense (Figure 80) while the Yin Taiji symbol rotates counterclockwise and is mainly used for defense (Figure 81). In the Yang symbol, the Jin is originated from the legs, the coiling is initiated from the center of the waist (i.e., Real Dan Tian) and then gradually expands outward with circling, rotating, coiling, and spiraling motions until it reaches an imaginary opponent's body. From this training, a practitioner learns how to use the mind to lead the Qi from the Real Dan Tian to the extremities and also how to use the waist to direct the motion from the center to the target. In the Yin symbol, again the Jin is originated from the legs, the coiling is initiated from the opponent's body, and through circling, rotating, coiling, and spiraling motions, the circle is gradually reduced toward the center until it reaches the Real Dan Tian. This symbol is used to neutralize and is mainly for defense.

There are many stages of Taiji symbol training. From solo to matching, from stationary to moving, and from straight line to Bagua circle stepping (Figures 82-84). Through rotation, the circle can be vertical, horizontal, large, and small. From this, you can see that the entire action is alive and variable. The final stage of two person Bagua circle stepping training is used to train the practitioner to step correctly with

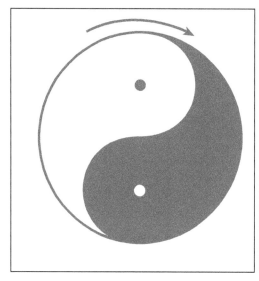 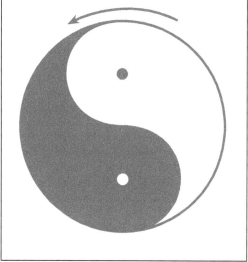

Figure 80. Yang Taiji Yin-Yang
Symbol (Right Hand)

Figure 81. Yin Taiji Yin-Yang
Symbol (Right Hand)

the Taijiquan's five strategic stepping techniques that coordinate with the Five Phases (Wuxing, 五行) (i.e., metal, wood, water, fire, and earth).

> *At the beginning of training, one hand moves following the pattern of the clockwise Yang Taiji symbol. First practice solo, follow the Taiji symbol to circle and coil. After becoming familiar with the symbol pattern, (you) can enter two-person practice. Two-person practice can be classified as stationary, advance and retreat moving, advance and retreat parallel moving, and finally Bagua Taiji circle stepping practice. After (you have) mastered the movement of clockwise Yang Taiji symbol, then (you can) start in the practice of the counterclockwise Yin Taiji symbol. Its practice procedures are the same as those of Yang Taiji symbol, from solo to the two-person Bagua Taiji circle stepping. After (you) have practiced enough to reach a proficient level and all of the movements have become natural, then mix the clockwise and counterclockwise pattern in your practice. This will lead to the practice of free style Yin-Yang Taiji symbols matching. In this stage, Yin and Yang, insubstantial and substantial strategies can be varied; sealing, emitting, neutralizing, and controlling as you wish. The opponent does not know you but you know the opponent.*

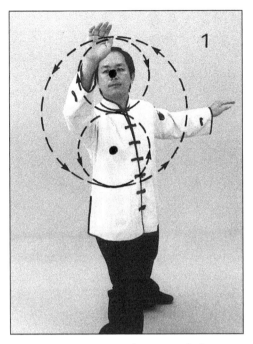

Figure 82. Solo Taiji Symbol
Sticking Hand Training

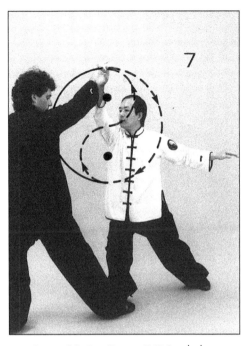

Figure 83. Two-Person Taiji Symbol
Sticking Hand Training

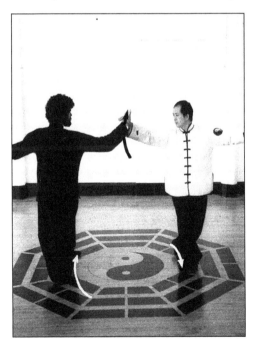

Figure 84. Bagua Circle Taiji
Symbol Sticking Hand Training

初練時，手依右旋陽式太極圖之型為主而動。先由各人
獨自練習，依太極圖輾轉而動。在熟悉圖型後，即可步
入雙人練習。雙人練習，可分定步，前進與後退動步，
前進與後退平行動步，最終為八卦太極行步之練習。在
熟悉右旋陽式太極圖之動後，即可步入左旋陰式太極圖
之動。練習程序與右旋陽式太極圖之練法同。由各人之
練習，而終至雙人八卦太極行步之練習。在練到一切動
作成自然後，右旋陽式與左旋陰式即混合著練，而成為
自由陰陽太極圖對練。到此程度，陰陽、虛實由我變，
封發化拿隨我意，敵不知我，我卻知敵。

Once you have mastered both Yang and Yin Taiji symbol sticking hands train-ing from solo until Bagua Taiji circle, then you begin to mix them up. Through these Yin-Yang interactions, hundreds of techniques are derived. In this case, Yin and Yang can be exchanged, and the insubstantial and substantial strategies are alive and con-trolled. When this happens, you will put your opponent into an urgent and disad-vantageous situation and under your control. You will know your opponent but your opponent will not know you. From this, you can see that Taiji symbol sticking hands training is the essence and the root of Taijiquan fighting arts. That is the reason it has always been kept secret in the past.

8. Six Turning Secrets of Taijiquan 太極拳之六轉訣

Eight Doors and Five Steppings are the main essence and fundamental structures of Taijiquan. From these thirteen postures, it (i.e., Taijiquan) further evolved and resulted in the derivation of six living turning skills. They have since become the most important (essence) of Taijiquan's pushing hands and sparring applica-tions. If those who learn Taijiquan can ponder and comprehend these six turn-ing secrets thoroughly and apply them skillfully and with liveliness, then their achievement in Taijiquan will surely reach the peak (of the art).

八門五步乃太極拳之主要精髓與基本結構。由此十三勢
進而演繹出六個活用之轉動技巧，為太極拳推手與散打
應用中之首要。學太極拳者，如能參透與澈底的去領悟
此六轉訣並活用之，則其太極拳之造詣，必能登峰。

The entire art of Taijiquan is constructed from thirteen basic actions. These thirteen actions are commonly called "Thirteen Postures" (Shi San Shi, 十三勢) which are constructed from the eight basic Jin (勁) (i.e., power manifestation) pat-terns and five basic stepping strategies. Therefore, the "Thirteen Postures" are also

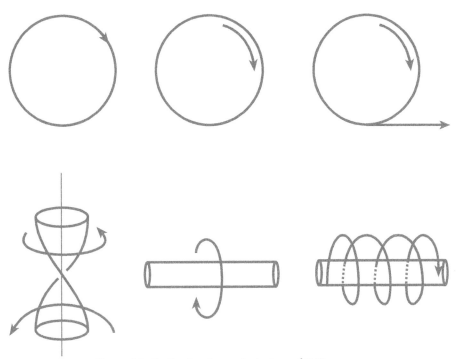

Figure 85. Six Turning Strategic Actions of Taijiquan

commonly called the "Eight Doors" (Ba Men, 八門) and "Five Steppings" (Wu Bu, 五步). "Eight Doors" is used simply because from these basic eight Jin patterns, the eight directions including the four formal directions of front, rear, left, and right, and also the four diagonal corners can be effectively protected and techniques can be executed.

In addition, the development of Taijiquan is built upon the concepts of "round" and "circling" actions. With the thirteen postures and the concept of roundness, six turning secrets can be discerned (Figure 85). In fact, these six turning secrets are the most important fundamentals of Taijiquan's pushing hands and free fighting applications. Taijiquan practitioners who are interested in Taijiquan pushing hands and free sparring and who ponder, study, and practice these six turning secrets diligently can achieve a profound level of skill.

> *What are the six turning secrets? They are circling, spinning, rotating, twisting, coiling, and spiraling. When circling is applied in the stepping, it is the living application of "Five Steppings." From the steadiness of "Central Equilibrium" (Zhong Ding), with the coordination of advancing forward, retreating backward, beware of the left, and looking to the right, the circle is formed through stepping. When the circling is used in the body's maneuvering, it is the circling (or half circling) of the touching hands which can thus be used to lead and neutralize (the coming power).*

六轉訣者，圈轉、自轉、旋轉、扭轉、纏轉、與螺旋轉
也。圈轉之用於步伐，乃五步之活用。由中定之定，配
合前進，後退、左顧、右盼而成步圈。圈轉之用於身法，
為八門搭手之輾轉〔半轉圈〕與引化。

Of the six turnings, circling is the largest action, and can be used for stepping or the body's maneuvering actions. From stepping-circling, you can enter the opponent's empty door (Kong Men, 空門) which can provide you with an opportunity for attack. In addition, through stepping-circling, you can evade the opponent's aggressive forward or sideways attack. In a fight, if you step in a straight line, it is easier for your opponent to follow you and to corner you. However, if you know how to step with a circling action skillfully, then it will be very difficult for your opponent to trap you in a corner.

When the circling action is used in the body, it initiates the arms' circling action. From the arms' circling, you can yield, lead, and then neutralize. In fact, the success of using "four ounces to repel a thousand pounds" relies on how skillfully you are able to circle your arms.

> *What is spinning? Under the conditions of "Central Equilibrium" and also the stillness of the axle, the body spins so as to neutralize the coming force. Spinning is just like the steering wheel of a car. Under the condition of stillness in the axle, the steering wheel can be turned clockwise or counterclockwise as wished. Consequently, the car wheel can be orientated in the desired direction. Where is the body's axle? It is our body's gravity center, the Lower Dan Tian, the central (area) of the waist, and is the root of Central Equilibrium. From the stillness and equilibrium of this center, the waist is able to spin as wished, and (then the Jin) can be manifested at the fingers. Taijiquan Classic says: "The root is at the feet, (Jin or movement is) generated from the legs, mastered (i.e., controlled) by the waist and manifested (i.e., expressed) from the fingers."*

自轉者，乃在中定不變之下，由軸心不動之前題下，身
體自轉以引化來勢。自轉者，如開車之轉盤也。在軸心
位置不移動之下，而轉盤可順時、逆時針而轉動，車輪
因而轉向自如。身體之軸心者，身體之重心也，下丹田
也，腰之中心也，中定之本根也。由此中定，腰之自轉
如意，而顯現於手指。太極拳經云：〝其根在腳，發於
腿，主宰於腰，形於手指。〞即此意也。

Spinning takes place without any movement of the center or axle—the edge is turning. In the human body, this center is the center of gravity where the Real Dan Tian (Zhen Dan Tian, 真丹田) is located. If you can stabilize this center, you will be able to reach the goal of Central Equilibrium (Zhong Ding, 中定) in Taijiquan. In order to maintain this equilibrium, your waist area must be exceedingly soft, relaxed, and mobile. To reach this goal, your Kua (胯) (i.e., hip joint area) must also be loose and soft. If your Kua area is tensed, your waist will also be tensed and stiff.

The body's spinning is controlled by the waist and is the most important key to neutralizing incoming power, and for Jin manifestation. Those who know how to keep the waist area soft and use it efficiently should be able to lead and direct the incoming power easily.

> *What is rotating? It is turning while shifting position. That is, the body spins while the center of the body is moving. It is just like the wheels' spinning and the axle's moving. Thus, (the car) is able to roll forward, roll backward, roll to the left, and roll to the right. In Taijiquan, under the condition of Central Equilibrium, the body rotates with the coordination of forward, backward, left, and right stepping actions. Consequently, the body is able to roll forward, roll backward, roll to the left, and roll to the right so as to lead and neutralize the coming force and also to set up tactics and maneuvers.*

旋轉者，移轉也，亦即身體中心移動中之自轉也。如車
輪之旋轉與輪軸心之移動，因而可轉進、轉退、滾左、
滾右。太極拳中，在中定之下，身體之旋轉與進、退、
左、右步伐之配合行動也。由此身體之轉進、轉退、滾
左、滾右，以引化來勢，以定玄機也。

Rotating is different from spinning. In spinning, the center or the axle does not move. However, in rotating, the center or the axle is also moving while spinning. Since there is a shifting of the center, you can yield while at the same time neutralizing the incoming force through spinning. In fact, rotating is one of the keys to neutralizing and repositioning yourself in moving pushing hands and sparring. Rotating is also a key to neutralizing the opponent's elbow stroke (Zhou, 肘) or the opponent's bumping (Kao, 靠) techniques.

> *Twisting refers to the twisting of the joints. From the twisting of the ankles, knees, and hips, the upper body can be spun and rotated, and can therefore lead and neutralize the coming force. From the twisting of the opponent's wrists, elbows, and shoulders, you can seize and control his joints. Furthermore, from the twisting of my joints, you can store your Jin and be ready to emit.*

扭轉者，關節之扭轉也。由足、膝、胯關節之扭轉產生
上身之自轉與旋轉，因而可引化彼之來勢。由腕、肘、
肩關節之扭轉，我可擒拿扣制彼方之關節。更由我關節
之扭轉，我勁得以蓄積，待之而發。

Most of the twisting actions in Taijiquan are in the joint areas. The body's spinning and rotating actions are initiated from the twisting of the three leg joints. If these three joints can be twisted and controlled carefully and efficiently, you will be able to keep your upper body upright and centered. In addition, the firmness of the root is determined by how soft and how flexible you keep these three joints as well. From this, you can see that the neutralization efficacy of the body is decided by the flexibility and mobility of your leg joints. Not only that, many Jins are stored through the legs twisting position. Note that you should train the knee areas especially with extreme care. Your goal is to encourage opening, strength and flexibility of the joint, and not to push it to its limits.

When you apply the twisting action to the three joints of your arms, you can seize and control (i.e., Qin Na, 擒拿) the opponent's joints. In the same manner as with the leg's joints, through twisting, you can store Jin in the arms.

In coiling, you use (your) hands to coil around the opponent's arm so as to exchange the Yin and Yang (maneuvers). Consequently, the opponent's joints can be positioned under your palms for your control. Furthermore, from coiling, you can open your opponent's skylight (Tian Chuang) and ground window (Di Hu) for your use. What is spiraling? It means coiling forward or backward. From spiraling, you can coil the opponent's arm and move from one joint to another joint, which could therefore prevent the opponent from escaping. This is the proficient level of Na Jin (i.e., Controlling Jin) in Taijiquan pushing hands training.

纏轉者，以手纏繞彼臂，以變陰、陽。因而，彼之關節
可在我掌下，而為我所拿。甚之，由纏轉中，我可開彼
之天窗、地戶而為我所趁。螺旋轉者，在纏轉中而進、
退也。由螺旋轉，我可由纏轉彼臂自一關節而至另一關
節，而不讓彼輕易逃脫。此為太極推手拿勁訓練之高層
次也。

Coiling in Taijiquan means to coil your hand around the opponent's arm like a snake coiling around a branch. This coiling action is two-dimensional, and allows you to change the Yin to Yang and vice versa. For example, if your wrist is under the opponent's palm, you will be in a defensive and disadvantageous situation (i.e., Yin situation). If you know the skill of coiling, you will be able to coil around his wrist and position your hand above his wrist and thus change your defensive and disadvantageous situation into a favorable one (i.e., Yang situation). In addition, through coiling action, you will be able to open the area above his arms (i.e., sky window) (Tian Chuang, 天窗) or under his armpit area (i.e., ground wicket) (i.e., Di Hu, 地戶) for attack.

Spiraling is slightly different from coiling. Spiraling refers to moving forward or backward while coiling. It is just like a snake that wraps around a branch and moves forward. In Taijiquan, this skill allows you to move from one joint to another. In fact, coiling and spiraling are the two major keys of the Na Jin (拿勁) (i.e., Controlling Jin) in Taijiquan pushing hands and sparring.

With the above six turning secrets, Yin and Yang can be exchanged skillfully in three dimensions. This is the crucial secret in pushing hands and sparring (training). They allow (you) to change a disadvantageous situation into an advantageous situation, to attack or defend as wished, and to put the opponent in a confused and dazed condition. The opponent does not know you, however, you know the opponent. To reach the proficiency of these six turning secrets, (you) must practice Yin-Yang Taiji Circle Coiling, searching for clear comprehension, skillfulness, and their living applications. Those who practice Taijiquan should ponder them carefully.

由上六轉訣，陰陽可互變在三度空間中，為推手、散打之要訣。可轉逆勢於順勢，可攻、可守如意自由，可置敵於恍惚之中。敵不知我，我卻知敵。此六轉訣，為能順手，必由太極圈纏手中去練習，求慎解、熟練、與活用。習太極拳者，應慎思之。

If Taijiquan practitioners wish to seriously study and understand the essence of Taijiquan martial applications, they must first ponder, comprehend, and practice the skills of these six turning secrets in three dimensions. The ancient Taijiquan master, Li, Yi-Yu (李亦畬), said: "In the insubstantial, (the techniques) vary following the opportunity (i.e., situation). The marvelous (tricks) are found in the round."[23] Round is the key to the six turning secrets.

PART IX

About Sparring 論散手

1. Taijiquan's Kicking, Striking, Wrestling, and Na 太極拳之踢、打、摔、拿

Taijiquan is an internal style of Chinese martial arts. All Chinese martial styles, after a thousand years of practice and experience, understand that in order to have an effective way of fighting, they must acquire the four skills of kicking, striking, wrestling, and Qin Na. The skills of kicking and striking are good for subduing Qin Na, wrestling is good to conquer kicking and striking, and Qin Na can be used against wrestling. Four of them mutually compensate and support each other. If there is one missing, then the art is not complete. It is for this reason that every Chinese martial style emphasizes the practice of the techniques of kicking, striking, wrestling, and Qin Na that are used to match the internal Gong's (i.e., internal Gongfu) practice.

太極拳者，中國之內家武學也。中國之各派武學，經歷
千百年之燻陶與經驗，深知欲達到有效之攻防技巧，必
須俱備踢、打、摔、拿之技。踢打者，善制擒拿手也。
摔跤者，專克踢打也。擒拿者，可敵摔跤也。四者互為
補缺，互為贊助。缺一而不全。由於如是，中國各門各
派皆著重於踢、打、摔、拿之法，以配合內功之修練。

It is commonly known in Chinese martial arts society that every style must acquire four categories of fighting skills. Without all four of these categories, the art will not be complete and can be defeated easily. These four categories are: kicking (Ti, 踢), striking (or punching) (Da, 打), wrestling (Shuai, 摔), and Qin Na (Na, 拿). These four skills mutually compensate, counter, and support each other.

However, these four skills are the external manifestation of the internal understanding (i.e., mind) and Qi. Therefore, all Chinese martial artists must also cultivate internal understanding of the arts and learn how to build up the Qi to an abundant level. When this Qi is led by the mind to the physical body for manifestation, its power can reach to a more highly efficient level. That is why it is said: "Internal and external are unified as one" (Nei Wai He Yi, 內外合一). Gong (功) means Gongfu (功夫). Any study or task that will take a great deal of time and effort to accomplish is called Gongfu.

Kicking, striking, wrestling, and Qin Na are shaped externally. The effectiveness of their applications is a function of the depth of the internal Gong's cultivation. What is internal Gong? It involves using the Yi to lead the Qi, so that it can be manifested externally. Because of this, all styles also emphasize the practice of internal Gong's breathing and using the Yi to lead the Qi. Thus, Taijiquan practitioners should practice both internally and externally; only then can (they) reach the profound understanding of the Taijiquan essence.

踢、打、摔、拿者外形外象也。其之應用效率決之於內
功之涵養。內功者，以意引氣而發於外技也。由是，各
門各派又著重於內功呼吸與以意引氣之氣功練習。因此，
太極學者應內外兼修，才能達到瞭解太極拳精髓之境地。

As mentioned, in order to become a proficient Taijiquan practitioner, you must not just know the external physical actions of the art. You must also practice the internal aspects. These internal aspects include: the cultivation of the Qi until it reaches an abundant level; the use of the mind to lead the Qi so it can circulate in the body smoothly; and the manifestation of the Qi into external physical actions. Furthermore, you must also keep pondering the Taijiquan theory until your comprehension has reached a profound level. Only then can you become a proficient Taijiquan practitioner.

2. Taijiquan's Attaching and Adhering 太極拳之粘黏

To stick means to attach. It means to get contact and then stick and connect. To adhere means to stick together without separating. The most difficult thing in Taijiquan sparring training is the Jin of attaching. If (you) are able to attach, then you are able to adhere, connect, and follow. Attaching can be classified into two kinds: the attaching from the body's not being connected to connecting; and the attaching in that the bodies have already connected and you attach to the opponent's center to upset his root.

粘者，沾也，接觸而粘連之意也。黏者，緊接而不分離。
太極拳散手練習中最難者，即是沾粘之勁。能沾粘，才
能黏連而隨。沾粘可分兩款：由身體未接觸而接觸之沾
與身體已接觸由粘連敵中心而提拔之粘。

Attach (Zhan, 粘) and then Adhere (Nian, 黏) are two different Jins. These two Jins are considered two of the most difficult Jins to understand and practice for Taijiquan practitioners. Attaching is an action of contacting and then connecting. Adhering means after contacting, then you stick together. In order to do so, you must maintain your contact and follow your opponent's movement. It is just like fly paper that sticks on your opponent's hands and cannot be separated.

Attaching can be distinguished into two kinds. The first kind of attaching is to get in touch with the opponent's body and then connect. Naturally, this is to build up a connection from a separated original position. The second kind of attaching is after you and your opponent's bodies have connected, then you find the attachment of your Jin to his center and root. Normally, in Taijiquan pushing hands training, both parties are constantly searching for each other's center so the opponent's center can be damaged and the root can be pulled. Once you have attached to this center, you will stick with it, and keep connecting and following. This will place your opponent in an urgent and defensive position at all times. Therefore, this kind of attaching Jin is always associated with Growing Jin (Zhang Jin, 長勁). Growing Jin is a continuous Jin through which you can attach to the opponent's center and grow into it until it can be destroyed.

> *At the beginning of a fight, the opponent and you do not have any contact. (In this case), even if you have special expertise in pushing hands skills, you still cannot use it. (Therefore), in order to use your pushing hands skills to defeat the opponent, you must first understand how to connect with the opponent with Attaching Jin. (After attaching), then (you) immediately follow with the Jins of Adhering, Connecting, Listening, and Following, thus placing the opponent into a position that allows neither advance nor withdrawal. To apply this Jin, (you) must wait for the opponent's first attack, then following (his/her) coming posture and attach with it. If the opponent does not attack first, then you must use a false attacking posture to induce (his/her attack). When he emits his hands, immediately attach with them.*

初應敵之際，敵我尚未接觸。即使我有特高之推手技能，
亦無從應用。為求以己推手之技以侮敵人之強，我必先
懂觸接沾粘之勁。緊接著黏連聽隨，以置敵於進退不得
之地。此勁之用可候敵之首攻，再隨來勢以沾粘之。如
敵不主攻，我必以虛勢引之。待其手發之際，再沾粘之。

When you first encounter an opponent, you are not in a connecting position that allows you to apply your pushing hands expertise. Therefore, you must first attach to your opponent's arms so you can place him into the disadvantageous position for your further attack. The best way to build up this attachment is waiting for the opponent's attack and then following it and attaching to it. However, if the opponent does not attack first, then you must present a false opportunity, or use a faking action to induce his attack.

This kind of training exists in almost every style and is commonly called Intercepting (Jie, 截). However, the difference is that once a proficient Taijiquan fighter attaches to an opponent, he will not separate.

If your opponent and you have built up a connection and his pushing hands skills are not worse than yours, and if the opponent's Xin is peaceful and his Qi is harmonious, if his Qi moves naturally with the Yi, and if his Jin emits following the Yi, then it will be hard to defeat him. In order to win, you must be able to find his center and connect with it with Attaching Jin to damage his central equilibrium, pull his root, irritate his Xin, and to make his Qi float. However, in order to execute this Jin efficiently, (your) sensitivity exercises of attaching, adhering, connecting, and following must have reached a profound level.

如敵我已接觸而敵推手之技與我不相上下，敵心平氣和，
氣隨意動，勁隨意發。在此之際，必難輸贏。為能致勝，
我必能以沾粘之勁接其中心，以損其中定，以拔其根，
以躁其心，以浮其氣。然為達此勁，粘黏連隨之知覺運
動必達高峰。

In a different situation, in that the attaching Jin is applied after you and your opponent have already connected with each other, and are in the exchange of pushing hands skills. In this case, if you know how to attach your feeling and Jin to his center, follow it, and finally damage his balance; you will find his mind is irritated, his Qi is floating, and his root is shallow. Naturally, you are in a position of winning.

However, if your opponent is also a proficient pushing hands expert, then your sensitivity (i.e., Listening Jin) of attaching, adhering, connecting, and following must be higher. Otherwise, you will be in an awkward situation. Because of this, you must keep practicing your sensitivity in these Jins. In addition, in order to keep the Attaching Jin connected with your opponent, you must also know how to apply Growing Jin (Zhang Jin, 長勁) effectively.

What are the sensitivity exercises of attaching, adhering, connecting, and following? Yang, Ban-Hou said: "What is attaching? It means to raise up and pull to a higher position. What is adhering? It means reluctant to part, and entangled with (the opponent). What is connecting? It means to give up yourself, and without being apart from (the opponent). What is following? It means when the opponent is yielding, you respond (with follow). (You) should know that without clearly understanding attaching, adhering, connecting, and following, a person's conscious feeling (i.e., sensitivity) and movements will not be developed. (In fact), the Gongfu of attaching, adhering, connecting, and following is very refined." What he said is very reasonable.

何謂粘黏連隨之知覺運動？楊班候云：「粘者，提上拔
高之謂也。黏者，留戀繾綣之謂也。連者舍己無離之謂
也。隨者彼走此應之謂也。要知人之知覺運動，非明粘
黏連隨不可。斯粘黏連隨之功夫亦甚細矣。」此言甚合
理也。

This is an excerpt from Yang, Ban-Hou's thesis that describes the importance of the four Jins.

3. Taijiquan's Kicking 太極拳之踢

Kick means to use the feet to kick the opponent's vital places. In the small circle fighting range, kicking is commonly used to trip the opponent, to kick the opponent's lower section or legs, as well as his knees, to destroy his balance. Kicking techniques and hand techniques are classified as one Yin and one Yang, one on the top (i.e., Yang) and one on the bottom (i.e., Yin), mutually supporting each other.

踢者，以足踢擊敵之要害也。在小圈攻防時，踢者亦慣
用之於踔倒敵人或踢擊敵之腿根部與膝以損敵之中定平
衡。腿法與手法一陰一陽，一上一下互為用之。

Kicking (Ti, 踢) is one of the four fighting categories in Chinese martial arts. Kicking is the technique of using the legs to attack the opponent's critical areas. Kicking is also commonly used to trip an opponent who is specialized in the middle and small fighting range. A proficient fighter will use both kicking and hand techniques and know how to exchange them mutually and skillfully. The hand techniques, which can be seen easily, are generally classified as Yang, while the kicking, which cannot be seen easily in middle and short range fighting, is classified as Yin.

Taijiquan is specialized in the middle and small circle fighting ranges and is good at sticking and adhering skills. Therefore, to protect the root's steadiness and avoid the floating of the lower section, which can be used by the opponent, Taijiquan's kicking usually pays more attention to low attack. Furthermore, it is not practical to use a high kick in the middle and short fighting range and also can expose your vital area for an attack easily.

太極拳者，善於中小圈之粘黏技擊也。因之，為防根之
不穩，下盤輕浮，為敵所乘，太極拳之踢均著重於低踢。
況乎中小圈之高踢，不切實際，易暴露己之要害。

When you fight in the middle and short range, it is not easy for you to initiate a high kick. If you do, you can easily lose your balance and root. Furthermore, a high kick in these two fighting ranges will also offer your opponent an advantageous opportunity to attack you. Since Taijiquan is a style that emphasizes the middle and short fighting range, normally, high kicks are not desirable.

When Taijiquan's kicking is used in middle-range fighting, it is commonly used to attack the opponent's abdomen, groin, and knee caps. When Taijiquan's kicking is used in small-range fighting, it is used to kick (the opponent's) shin and the sides of his calf. The hook kick is also commonly used to hook the heel of the opponent to tumble the opponent's center. In the small fighting range, Taijiquan is also good at using the knee to attack the opponent's groin or bump his knee to destroy his root.

太極拳之踢於中圈之用，慣於攻擊敵之腹部、下陰、與膝蓋骨。太極拳之踢於小圈之用，卻慣於踢擊小腿之前脛與側骨。蹺腿亦善被用之以勾提敵之後腿根，以跘倒敵之中定。在小圈之下，太極拳亦善用膝以攻擊敵之下陰或靠敵之膝以拔其根。

Since Taijiquan is good at the middle and short fighting ranges, almost all of the legs' attacks focus on the lower section of the opponent's body. The groin is always the first choice since it is hard to protect, and the attack can be very fast and effective. Other places such as the knee caps, shin, sides of the calf or thighs are all common targets. Therefore, Taijiquan practitioners who are good at using the legs to attack also know how to protect their own vital areas since the opponent will have the equal chance.

Those who are good at using the legs to attack all know how to balance themselves on the top and bottom, as well as the Yin Yang theory of coordination of the hands and legs. Up up and bottom bottom, Yin Yin and Yang Yang, insubstantial insubstantial and substantial substantial, suddenly on the top and suddenly at the bottom, these (maneuvers) make the opponent not know how to handle the situation; the Xin and Yi are floating (i.e., confused), and (therefore) this can be used by you. However, if you do not have a firm root and a good center, then all of the kicking techniques are useless.

善用腿法者，均懂得上下平衡，手法、腿法陰陽相配合之理。上上下下、陰陰陽陽、虛虛實實、忽上忽下，使敵不知所措，心意輕浮，為我所乘。然己無根，中定無成，則腿法之用為虛談矣。

In order to initiate a fast, powerful, and accurate leg attack, you must first have a firm root and good balance by yourself. Without these requirements, the kicking will be slow and ineffective. Furthermore, your body will be tilted backward or sideways and naturally this will provide your opponent with a good opportunity to attack you.

In addition, to make the attack effective and successful, you must also know how to cheat your opponent. The attacks from top and bottom should be skillfully exchanged; the hands and legs coordinate with each other so the attacks can be either insubstantial or substantial. This will make your opponent confused and finally you will prevail.

When encountering an opponent, (you) must be aware of his kicks. Attaching, adhering, listening, and following, the hands are not even a moment separated from the opponent's (body). Whenever (the opponent) just initiates a kicking intention, you immediately push him downward, press him over, bump him off, or pluck and pull him off balance, to subdue his kicking. The effectiveness of this defense (against kicking) is decided by how good your sensitivity exercises are (i.e., alertness and awareness). When the opponent's shoulder just slightly moves, immediately be aware of his kicking. After practicing for a long time, (you) will be able to apply these defensive keys as wished.

應敵時，必防敵之腿法。粘黏聽隨，手不離敵，稍一有腿之動意，我即下按之、擠之、靠之、或扣帶之，以制克敵之腿擊。此防敵之效，取決於己身之知覺運動。敵肩稍一有動，即防其腿。練習久而久之，自然隨心所欲。

In order to prevent a kick from your opponent, the main key is to keep contact and stick with him. With this contact, whenever you sense a kicking attack, immediately destroy his balance and root by pushing, pressing, pulling, or bumping. This will hinder his attack immediately and effectively. Normally, when your opponent is initiating a kick, his shoulder will move slightly backward first. How to apply all of these into the actual situation depends on how sensitive you are. That means your Listening and Understanding Jins must be proficient. Naturally, it will take you a long time of practice to build up this sensitivity and awareness.

4. Taijiquan's Striking 太極拳之打 (Cavity Press) 〔點穴篇〕

Taijiquan's Jin is a soft Jin. Taijiquan's offense and defense belong to the middle and small ranges. Therefore, Taijiquan is good at striking cavities and is also specialized in short Jin's emitting and neutralizing. In order to catch an advantageous opportunity and create a favorable situation, under the conditions of attaching, adhering, connecting, and following, you must find the way to situate your hands either inside or above the opponent's two arms. In this case, (you) will be able to put the opponent into a defensive and disadvantageous situation (for you) to initiate an attack. Not only that, due to the exposure of the opponent's vital cavities, it will provide you with an opportunity to attack. However, in order to create an advantageous opportunity and establish a favorable situation, you must know and be good at Coiling Jin (Chan Jin), thus (you) can vary the situation of Yin (i.e., insubstantial) and Yang (i.e., substantial). In addition, you must have mastered the skills of Control Jin (Na Jin), otherwise, you will lose your opportunity and become defensive.

太極拳之勁，軟勁也。太極拳之攻防，中小圈也。因之，
太極拳善打穴道並善於短勁之發化。為求先機立勢，在
彼我粘黏連隨下，必求己手在於敵手或臂之上或在其內。
如此可置敵於防衛而不利於攻擊之勢。不但如此，敵之
要穴亦暴露於我而為我所打擊。然而，為能創機立勢，
我必懂得並善用纏轉之勁，以易陰陽之勢。甚之，我之
拿勁必已純熟，否則我必失勢而為下風也。

Taijiquan specializes in soft Jin that is manifested as a soft whip. Due to its softness, and the high level of mental concentration, the Jin can be focused onto a tiny point and the speed can reach a very high level. When this soft Jin attacks the vital cavities, through the sudden change of Qi in the meridians, the internal organs can be shocked.

Because of the emphasis on the skills of listening (i.e., touching-feeling), understanding, adhering, connecting, and following, Taijiquan also specializes in the middle and small fighting ranges. Therefore, once you have attached to the opponent's arms, pushing hands skills become critical in determining who will win. During pushing hands, in order to create a favorable situation and establish an advantageous opportunity, you must keep your hands either inside or above his arms. When this happens, you have automatically placed your opponent into a defensive and disadvantageous situation.

In order to create or reverse the situation, you must know two crucial skills: Coiling (Chan Jin, 纏勁) and Controlling Jins (Na Jin, 拿勁). Coiling Jin allows to change Yin to Yang and Yang to Yin; thus insubstantial and substantial strategies can be exchanged smoothly and skillfully. Controlling Na allows you to control the opponent's joints and place him into a defensive and disadvantageous position.

Though you have occupied an advantageous situation, in order to have a high efficiency of attacking, you must know how to create a favorable opportunity. The most common strategy is to destroy the opponent's central equilibrium and balance. When this happens, the opponent must first re-establish his root and maintain his central equilibrium. his mind is confused and Qi is floating. This is the best timing for your attack to his vital cavities. Therefore, how to destroy the opponent's central equilibrium and pull his root are two of the most important subjects in pushing hands training.

雖然我已佔其優勢，然而為求攻擊之效，我必知創機。慣用之機為先損敵之中定與其平衡。此時，敵必先穩其根，持其中定。其意已亂，其氣已浮。此為我進擊其要穴之良機。因之，損敵之中定並拔其根為推手訓練之主要要目。

During pushing hands, even if you have gained the advantageous position, it does not mean that you have an opportunity to initiate your attack. That is because your opponent's hands are also adhering. Whenever you initiate an attack, he will know, through feeling, and easily neutralize your attack. In order to make your attack effective, you must create a favorable situation so that you are able to disturb your opponent's feeling and concentrated mind. To reach this goal, you must destroy his balance and central equilibrium. Once you have put your opponent into an unbalanced situation, he must immediately regain his balance and maintain his central equilibrium. Otherwise, he can be uprooted easily. In this situation, his mind will be disturbed and his Qi will also be floating. This will provide you with an opportunity to attack. It is because of this reason that the training of how to destroy the opponent's balance and central equilibrium is the major training in Taijiquan pushing hands.

In addition, in order to create a favorable opportunity and establish an advantageous situation, you must also know how to occupy the central door, to seize the empty door, to enter the sky window, and to go in the ground window. In this case, (you) can place your opponent into an urgent situation that you can use. In order to make these (tactics) effective, you must know the knack of five steppings, and be familiar with the appropriate opportunities for advancing, retreating, beware of the left, and look to the right. Insubstantial (can be) insubstantial and substantial (can be) substantial, substantial (can be) substantial and insubstantial (can be) insubstantial, the opponent does not know you but you know the opponent. Control (your) opponent as in the center of your palms and defeated by you.

不但如此，為求創機立勢，我亦必懂得搶佔中門，奪其空門，進天窗，入地戶。如此，可置敵於迫急之境，而為我所乘。為求此效，我必知五行步之竅，曉進、退、顧、盼、定之機。虛虛實實，實實虛虛，敵不知我，我惟知敵，置敵於我掌中，為我所算。

As explained earlier, central door (Zhong Men, 中門) means the mid-point between you and your opponent's centers (Figure 86). Once you have placed your opponent into a disadvantageous and defensive position, you should immediately

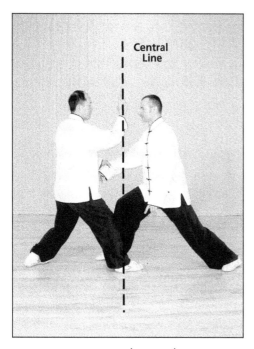

Figure 86. Central Door (Zhong Men)

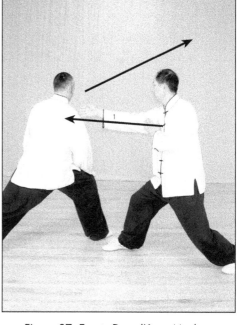

Figure 87. Empty Door (Kong Men)

occupy this central door. This will put your opponent into an urgent position and agitate his mind's concentration and the Qi's natural smooth flowing.

If your opponent stands with his right leg forward, then there are two empty doors (Kong Men, 空門) for your attacks. One is on his left (Figure 79) and the other is on his right (Figure 87). Again, through stepping, if you are able to attack through your opponent's empty doors, you will put him into a defensive and urgent situation.

The empty space above your opponent's arm is a sky window (Tian Chuang, 天窗) (Figure 88), while under the arm is a ground wicket (Di Hu, 地戶) (Figure 89). These two spaces allow you to attack the opponent's vital areas. When you use your hand to seal the opponent's arm down so the area above his arm is exposed for your attack, it is called "open the sky window" (Kai Tian Chuang, 開天窗) and if you push the opponent's arm up to expose the area under his armpit area for your attack, it is called "open the ground wicket" (Kai Di Hu, 開地戶).

In order to occupy the central door and seize the empty door, you must know how to step and reposition yourself to your advantage. In order to open the sky and ground windows, you must also know how to seal, neutralize, coil, and how to use the insubstantial and substantial strategies. These two strategies should be exchanged with skill and liveliness.

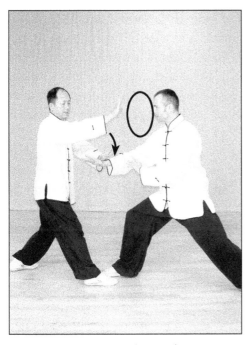

Figure 88. Sky Window

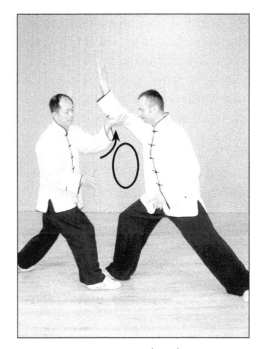

Figure 89. Ground Wicket

The hand techniques for cavity strike can be varied according to different positions of cavities. There are: vertical fist, horizontal fist, phoenix eye fist, Gong-word hand, thumb hand, hammer hand, hand knife, sword secret, and palm press, etc. All applications follow each individual's expertise and mastery. The execution of techniques focuses on the concentration, speed, and accuracy of the power. To be effective, (you) must also know the Qi and blood's major flow according to the timing. In the entire body there are a total of 108 cavities—36 big cavities and 72 small cavities—that can be used for cavity attack. The techniques and the timing for cavity strikes are usually kept secret in every style and not revealed to the outside easily. This is because all of these secrets are related to human life and morality. Those who learn these skills must be very cautious when they use them.

打穴手法依不同穴位而定，有立拳、平拳、鳳眼手，工字手、姆指手、錘手、手刀、劍訣、掌按等等。依各人各派所長、所專而用。打穴之技與勁力，必求力專，快速與準度。不但如此，必懂氣血子午流注之行，才能致效。全身計有一百零八穴，三十六大穴，七十二小穴，可為打穴之用。穴位之打法與時辰，各派皆持密中，不輕易外傳。此因其有關人命道德也。學者知之，不可不慎用之。

According to Chinese martial society, out of more than seven hundred acupuncture cavities, there are one hundred and eight that can be used for martial arts attacks and cavity press massage. Seventy-two of them are not vital when attacked, while the remaining thirty-six will maim or kill. Normally, to be effective, the attacks to those vital cavities must match the time of the day. It is known from acupuncture that the major Qi and blood flows in the body are influenced by the time of the day. This is called "midnight and noon major flow" (Zi Wu Liu Zhu, 子午流注).

In addition, to be effective, a special hand form and skill must be used and trained so that when the cavity is attacked, the power can penetrate to the meridian and shock the organ. Usually, the timing of the major Qi flow and the special attacking skills are kept secret in every style. The reason for this is simply that once anyone knows these skills and the timing, he can easily injure or kill others.

5. Taijiquan's Wrestling 太極拳之摔

Shuai means Shuai Jiao (i.e., wrestling). It is a martial art that uses skills to trip, pull down, and topple the opponent. Because Taijiquan is an art that is specialized in middle-and-short-circle fighting, it is also good at the techniques of Shuai Jiao and Qin Na. Generally speaking, Shuai Jiao is a skill that is specially designed against the skills of kicking and striking in martial arts. However, Taijiquan favors this art due to its theory of using the soft against the hard. When the opponent is hard, the body and the root are all tightened and therefore not solid and rooted. This can be used easily by you. Taijiquan is an art that is primarily good at damaging the opponent's center and destroying his root. When (the opponent's) center and root have been destroyed, (you immediately) follow (i.e., borrow) this advantageous situation to take (the opponent) down.

摔者，摔跤也。乃利用技巧以絆倒、拉倒、推倒敵人之
武術也。太極拳因善於中小圈之攻防，因而亦善於摔跤
與擒拿之技也。摔跤在一般武學上，本專對付於踢打之
術。太極拳卻借重之於以軟制硬。敵硬，身連根皆繃緊
而不實，易為我所乘。太極本善於損敵之中定與拔敵之
根。在中定損與根拔之時，順勢摔倒也。

Shuai is an abbreviation of Shuai Jiao (摔跤) and means wrestling. Generally speaking, there are four categories of fighting skills commonly used in every style of Chinese martial arts. These four categories are: kicking (Ti, 踢), striking (Da, 打), wrestling (Shuai, 摔), and Na (i.e., Qin Na, 擒拿). Wrestling can be used to conquer kicking and striking, Qin Na is capable of subduing wrestling, and kicking and striking can be used against Qin Na. All these categories mutually support each other and can conquer each other.

Though wrestling can be used against kicking and punching effectively, in Taijiquan, due to its expertise in middle and short fighting range, wrestling is used to take the opponent down when his balance and root are destroyed. Thus, Taijiquan wrestling is soft and not hard, is round and not square, and is relaxed and not tensed. Therefore, it is able to put the opponent into a disadvantageous situation during a fight.

> *Wrestling is primarily used as defense, not offense, to find attacking tactics and opportunities from defensive maneuvers. Therefore, it uses the strategy of stillness and waiting for the opponent's action and uses defense as offense. (However,) if the opponent also uses the defensive strategy, then the tactics of wrestling will be hard to execute. In this case, (you) must know how to create an opportunity and establish an advantageous situation. Creating an opportunity and establishing the advantageous situation is derived from the Eight Doors and Five Steppings (i.e., Thirteen Postures). From the skillfulness of Jins in the Eight Doors, create the insubstantial and substantial (opportunities) to entice the opponent to change (his/her) strategy from defense to offense, and then find a way to neutralize it. In addition, (you) must also know how to use the Five Steppings to approach the opponent, to create the opportunity, and to establish the advantageous situation that allows you to use wrestling.*

摔跤本主守而不主攻，而在守中求攻勢與攻機。因而以靜待動，以守為攻。如敵亦採守勢，則摔策難以執行。此時必懂得去造機立勢。造機立勢，概從八門五步中蘊育演繹出來。從八門巧勁中去造虛實，去引敵反守為攻，再求化解。並從五步中去逼身、去造機、去立勢而為我之摔跤所用。

Wrestling is a defensive tactic. Normally, you wait for your opponent's attack and then find the opportunity to take him down. The reason for this is simply in order to take your opponent down, you must approach into short range, and this allows you to grab him or bump him off balance. When you approach your opponent, you enter his punching and kicking range. Therefore, if you use wrestling as offense, you must know how to create an appropriate opportunity and establish an advantageous situation. All of these possibilities depend on how skillfully you are able to apply the eight basic Jin patterns (i.e., Eight Doors) and your ability to step from far to near. Normally, these fighting maneuvers must be learned from an experienced teacher.

> *In order to damage the opponent's centering and destroy his root, your center and balance must first be secured, and your root must be solid and firm. If you do not have this prior condition, then even though the advantageous situation is established, it is hard to execute. This is because you do not have a firm foundation that allows you to take the opponent down; consequently, the opponent does not topple and on the contrary you will be bumped off balance. In order to create the*

opportunity and establish the advantageous situation, you must be familiar with the skillfulness of the Eight Doors and Five Steppings; more importantly, (you) must also know the trick of how to occupy the Central Door, enter the Empty Door, open the opponent's Sky Window and Ground Wicket. Without knowing these, it will be hard to use wrestling to defeat the opponent.

為損敵之中定與拔其根，自己之重心與中心必先穩固，
根必緊實。如我未有此先決條件，則雖機勢已立，必難
成行。此因我無有摔倒敵人之根基，敵人不倒，我反被
彈出也。為能創機造勢，除了我必熟悉八門五步之巧，
更要瞭解如何搶中門、入空門、開其天窗與地窗之竅。
不知此，摔跤制敵，必難行之。

The most important condition for applying wrestling techniques is that you must have good balance and a firm root. Without this prior foundation, you will be in a position of imbalance and you will be floating. Consequently, your body will be tensed and this will offer your opponent an advantageous opportunity to defeat you. Therefore, to become an expert in wrestling, you must first practice your balance and rooting.

In addition, other than knowing how to apply the skills of the Eight Basic Taijiquan Jin patterns and Five Basic Steppings, you must also be familiar with the tactics of occupying the Center Door, entering the Empty Door, and opening the opponent's Sky Window and Ground Wicket. As mentioned earlier, Central Door (Zhong Men, 中門) is the central point between your opponent and you. When you are in an advantageous situation, you should occupy this door immediately and this will put your opponent into an awkward defensive position. Empty door (Kong Men, 空門) means the door that allows you to step in and put the opponent into an urgent situation. If your opponent's right leg is forward, there are two empty doors; one on his left between his legs, and one on his right back shoulder. When you step in the first door, he will lose balance and expose himself/herself for your attack. When you step in the second empty door, you will be able to bump him off balance easily. Sky window (Tian Chuang, 天窗) and ground wicket (Di Chuang, 地窗) mean above and under the opponent's arm.

However, if your opponent has occupied the advantageous opportunity and put you into a disadvantageous position for him to take you down, the first and the most important thing is to stabilize (your) Xin (i.e., emotional mind) and keep (your) Yi (i.e., logical mind) clear, and not be alarmed. Once alarmed, the body will be tensed and tightened and your root will be floating and your central balance will be damaged. This provides the opponent with an opportunity to exploit. To avoid being taken down, other than knowing how to stabilize (your) Xin and clarify (your) Yi, (you) must know how to create the opportunity and establish an advantageous situation to solve your difficult position. The keys are three important skills: Peng Jin (i.e., wardoff), soft and relaxed, and also turning and rotating. If (you) know the skill of 'drawing in the chest and arcing the back' in Peng Jin, then (you are) able to keep (your) center. If (you) know the trick of being soft and relaxed in all of the joints, then you are able to protect your root. If (you are) hard, (your) root will be pulled for sure. If (you are) good at the maneuver of using rotation and turning, then you are able to change the situation and reverse the Qian and Kun (i.e., Yin and Yang), following the opponent's attacking posture and neutralizing and changing it, to re-establish a new situation that can be used by you.

然而，如敵已占先機而置我於被摔之不利境地時，其首要在心定意明，切忌慌張。一慌，則身體繃緊矣，根浮矣，中定損矣。此正中敵計而為其所用。防敵之摔，除先要心定意明外，須知造機立勢以解己之困。其竅在於掤勁，在於鬆軟，在於輾轉三要。懂掤勁含胸拔背之技，則能保中定。能鬆軟骨節連串之巧，則能保吾根，硬必被連根拔起。善於身體之輾轉，則能變其勢，逆轉乾坤。順其勢而化之，轉換之，從新立勢而為我所用。

If you are already in a disadvantageous situation that allows your opponent to use his wrestling on you, you should not be alarmed and tense, and lose your center. The first step is to sink your gravity center downward to firm your root. In order to reach this goal, you must be relaxed and soft. In this case, it will be hard for your opponent to pick you up and destroy your rooting. You must also know how to use wardoff Jin (Peng Jin, 掤勁) to protect your center. Once your chest is drawn in and the back is arced with both of your arms expanded outward, your opponent will have a hard time to find your center. From the above two efforts, you will save yourself from a disadvantageous position into a neutralized situation. Then, if you know how to use the two skills of rotating and turning, you can change the entire situation to one more favorable to you.

Those who know the martial art of Taijiquan must know how to use wrestling and Qin Na together. If (you) are able to Shuai and also Na, then (you) can execute (your) fighting tactics as you wish. If (you) only know how to wrestle, it can be seized easily by Na. If (you) only know how to use Qin Na, then it is hard to apply it and its effectiveness will be low. The two skills of wrestling and Qin Na are both good for the middle and small circle fighting ranges, and they talk about the advantageous angle and the theory of leverage. Both are closely related to each other, which should not be ignored lightly. Therefore, those who know wrestling are also good at Qin Na, and vice versa.

學太極拳武學者，須懂摔、拿並用。能摔能拿，才能隨
心所欲。只懂摔，易被拿。僅知拿，拿無門路，其效必
低。摔跤、擒拿二術，均善於中、小兩圈之戰，講利我
角度與桿竿原理之用。兩者相關甚切，不可忽視。因而，
一般善於摔跤者，亦善於擒拿。反之亦然。

Since both wrestling and Qin Na are specialized in using advantageous angles and leverage, often one who is good at wrestling is also an expert in Qin Na and vice versa. If you are able to apply these two skills mutually, you will be an expert in middle-and-short-range fighting.

6. Taijiquan's Na 太極拳之拿

Na means Qin Na. It includes: dividing the muscles/tendons, misplacing the bones, sealing the breath, blocking the vessels, grabbing the tendons, and grappling the cavities. Qin Na is mainly used when the opponent and you have contacted each other, and in exchanging the techniques of attaching, sticking, connecting, and following. It is the major skill against Shuai Jiao (i.e., wrestling). The skills of dividing the muscles/tendons and misplacing the bones are specialized in controlling the joints. When the joints are locked and controlled, they cannot move. Then follow with Shuai Jiao, kicking, or striking to subdue the opponent. The skill of sealing the breath is done by using the hand to grab and control the opponent's throat to seal the breathing pipe. Alternatively, it can be done by using the hand to press and push the opponent's abdominal area to cause the muscles' contraction (around the lungs), thus sealing the breath. Blocking the vessels is done by sealing the arteries (on the neck) connecting to the brain to stop the oxygen supply to the brain, which results in fainting. Grabbing the tendons is done by grabbing the opponent's large tendons to hinder his movements. Grappling the cavities is to grab the opponent's cavities that cause numbing or fainting.

拿者，擒拿也。包括分筋、錯骨、閉氣、斷脈、抓筋、
與扣穴等技。擒拿主用於敵我已接觸、粘黏連隨，為克
制摔跤之主要技能。分筋錯骨者，專制關節。關節一被
扣鎖，不能動彈，繼之以摔或踢打以制敵。閉氣者，以
手扣制彼之咽喉，以閉其氣管，或以手按壓其腹部收縮
其肺以悶其氣。斷脈者，截其通腦之動脈，以斷其腦氧
氣之供給，而致暈倒。抓筋者，抓其大筋以妨其行動也。
抓穴者，抓其麻穴與暈穴也。

This paragraph summarizes the categories of Qin Na skills and their basic control theories. These categories include: dividing the muscles/tendons, misplacing the bones, sealing the breath, blocking the vessels, grabbing the tendons, and grappling the cavities.

> *Qin Na in Taijiquan applications is good at using the round and turning (tactics). From neutralizing the coming Jin, use round (movements) to lead the opponent into your trap so he can be seized by you. The Jin-Li used in Taijiquan Qin Na are soft. When you look at it, it is hard to figure it out and when you feel it, it is not clear. Consequently, it can place the opponent into a state of mystification (i.e., unclear mind) to be seized by you without being aware. According to the achievement, Qin Na can be distinguished in three levels. In the beginning level, the techniques are executed by the muscular power of the arms. In the middle level, (the power and movements are) executed from the body. In the high level of Qin Na, the Yi is used to lead the Qi, with the coordination of breathing and body movement to execute the techniques. There are more than a hundred Qin Na's used in Taijiquan; however, if (you) wish to reach a highly proficient level, (you) must learn from a renowned teacher.*

太極拳之擒拿，善於圈轉。在化來勁之下，以圈引之，
使敵墜入我之陷阱而為我所擒。太極拳之擒，其勁力也
軟。視之難明，覺之不清，置敵於矇矓之中，在不知不
覺下被擒拿。依程度而言，擒拿之術可分三等級。初級
之拿，以臂力行之。中級之拿，以身法行之。高級之擒
拿則以意引氣，再配合呼吸與身法行之。太極拳之拿計
不下上百之數，然欲達高明熟用之境地，非得名師指導
不可。

Jin is the manifestation of Qi into physical form, while Li is physical strength commonly demonstrated by the muscles. The main difference between Taijiquan Qin Na and those of external styles is that the applications of Taijiquan Qin Na are round and use the body's turning to set up the neutralizing and controlling angles. Moreover, the power used in Taijiquan Qin Na is soft and difficult for your opponent to notice. There are many Qin Na applications. Most people are able to learn some basic applications. However, to reach a proficient level, a qualified teacher is often necessary.

For a Qin Na beginner, the techniques are normally executed from the muscular force of the arms. Therefore, the Jin is clumsy and the skills are forceful. This level of Qin Na can be detected easily by the opponent and defended against. However, when you have mastered Qin Na to a good degree, then you start to use your body, especially the waist and chest, to execute the techniques. When this happens, not only can the power generated be stronger, the techniques can also be executed with round movements. This will make them less detectable by the opponent. However, the highest level of Qin Na is reached from the unification of both internal and external. That means with the coordination of the Yi, Qi, and breathing, the techniques are executed through round body movements.

7. Taijiquan's Long and Short Fighting Strategies 太極拳之長短攻防

Ancestors said: "To use the long to attack the short is to battle with force (i.e., advantage). To use the short to attack the long is a battle (which needs) wisdom. Use the enemy's long to attack the enemy's short and use the enemy's short to attack the enemy's long, then it is called enlightened combat." Taijiquan is good at the middle and small circle fighting ranges. Therefore, those who learn martial Taijiquan must know how to place the opponent into the middle and small circle ranges, thus using the self's long (i.e., advantage) to attack the opponent's short (i.e., disadvantage). (In addition,) Taijiquan also specializes in the skills of using defense as offense, using stillness to subdue movement, and using peace to conquer irritability; when the opponent does not move, you do not move, and when the opponent slightly moves, you move first. Therefore, it is the maneuver of using four ounces to neutralize one thousand pounds. Under the skillfulness of Attaching, Adhering, Listening, and Following, this is the key secret to put the opponent into a condition where (he/she) cannot advance, withdraw, or even quit. This is using the self's long to defeat the opponent's short.

古云：「以長攻短，是為鬥力。以短攻長，是為鬥智。
以敵之長，攻敵之短，以敵之短，攻敵之長，則為鬥之
以神。」太極拳者，善於中小圈之攻防也。因之，習武
學太極拳者，必懂得如何置敵於中小圈內，以己之長，
攻其之短。太極拳亦善於以守為攻，以靜制動，以安克
躁之戰技。因而，敵不動，我不動，敵微動，我先動之
四兩破千斤之法。在粘黏聽隨下，置敵於進退不可，欲
罷不能之訣竅。此為以己之長，攻其所短也。

Here "long" (Chang, 長) means advantage, and "short" (Duan, 短) means disadvantage. For example, if you are strong and use your strength to defeat a weaker person, your strength is called long. Therefore, if you have an advantage, you will naturally use this advantage to defeat the enemy. However, if you are on the disadvantaged side, you will not be able to defeat your enemy through your weakness, so you must use your wisdom in a fight. To use your opponent's advantage to reveal his weakness, and to use his weakness to attack his advantage, is called fighting with enlightenment. For example, if your enemy is strong and muscular, he may be slow, so you must use your speed to defeat his strength. Or if your enemy has a long weapon, he will not be effective in short range defense, so you should specialize in short range attack. If your opponent specializes in high and long kicks, his root must be shallow, so you should attack his root. This is using his short to defeat his long.

You can use his long against his short if, for example, he specializes in long-range kicking. If you stay in the long range you will encourage him to confidently attack. This will give you the opportunity to slip past his attack and attack at short range. If you are able to do all this, it is called enlightened combat.

Taijiquan specializes in a few important things. First, Taijiquan is a martial training that is good at middle and short range fighting. Second, Taijiquan uses defense as offense. Therefore, it specializes in using calmness to react to irritability, using the soft against the hard, and using four ounces to neutralize a thousand pounds. In order to reach this goal, a Taijiquan practitioner must have mastered the skills of Listening, Understanding, Attaching, Following, Sticking, and Connecting Taijiquan Jins. Without good skills in the crucial Jins, the Taijiquan fighting maneuver will almost never succeed. However, if you are skillful in these important trainings, you will adopt all of these skills into your fighting and put the opponent into a disadvantageous situation.

> *Not only that, those who are good at Taijiquan sparring must be aware of the opponent's long range and large circle's offense and defense. (He/She) must pay special attention to the opponent's kicking. These are the self short (i.e., disadvantages) and therefore you should avoid them as much as possible. However, if the opponent is also good at the middle and small circles' offense and defense, then you must know and be expert in using the insubstantial and substantial (strategies), the theory of soft and hard, and good at changing fighting maneuvers; consequently, the opponent does not know your intentions. This is the fighting of (using) wisdom.*

不僅如是，太極拳善戰者，必慎防敵之長距大圈之攻防，
更必嚴防敵之腿法。此乃己之短，應儘量避之。然，如
敵亦善於中小圈之攻防，則我必懂得善用虛實，軟硬之
理，善變戰策，使敵不知我之所向。此為鬥之以智也。

Since Taijiquan is a middle range fighting style, any good Taijiquan fighter must know how to avoid long range fighting, especially with those who are good at long range kicks. These are your disadvantages.

However, if you encounter an opponent who is also good at the middle and short range fighting skills, then not only must you have mastered the skills of Listening, Understanding, Attaching, Following, Sticking, and Connecting, you must also be an expert in using the insubstantial and substantial strategies, applying the soft and the hard interchangeably, and keeping the fighting maneuvers alive. This will confuse your opponent and put him into a defensive position. This means you must fight with your wisdom.

However, the most important thing in sparring is knowing yourself and knowing the opponent. Only under the condition of knowing yourself and the opponent, can (you) play the strategies of using the opponent's long to attack his short and using his short to upset his long. If (you) do not know your opponent and yourself, then this fighting strategy will be hard to execute. Therefore, when encountering the opponent, at the beginning, (you) must first test the opponent and know the opponent. Be extremely cautious and do not explore (your) expertise and allow your opponent to know your root and foundation (i.e., major skills). Once you know the opponent and yourself for sure, then plan your strategies and raise up your fighting spirit to encounter the coming attacks and also to create the advantageous opportunity and establish a favorable situation (for yourself). This is the fighting of enlightenment.

然而，散戰中，最要者，乃是知己知敵。在知敵我之情況下，才能以敵之長攻其之短，以其之短攻其之長。如不知敵我，此策難行也。因此，初逢敵手，必先試敵，識敵。千萬小心，不可儘露身手，令敵知我根基。我一但確知敵我，即佈戰略，提我精神，以應來勢，以創機立勢。如此，即門之以神也。

Sun Zi (557 B.C.) (孫子) said: "Knowing the opponent and knowing yourself, a hundred battles without a loss."[24] This means only if you know your opponent and yourself, can you set up an effective strategy and execute it successfully. Therefore, when you first encounter your opponent, you should test him and see how skilled he is. At this time you must cloak your expertise as much as possible so your opponent will not know you. Once you have a sense of him, then raise up your fighting morale, and bring your alertness and awareness to the highest level. When you do this, not only can you respond to the opponent's actions naturally, but you will also learn to create opportunities for yourself, and maximize any advantages that you discover.

8. Strategy of Attacking Timing 攻時略

(When) the enemy's attacking Yi is forming and his posture has not yet surfaced, you suddenly attack and disturb his Yi, stopping him from forming the posture. (This) is reaching "enlightenment." (This timing) is the best among the best strategies (see 1 of Figure 90).

敵擊意已孕，而勢未現，我驟然反攻以亂其意，挫其勢之孕形，是為通乎神明，乃為上上策。

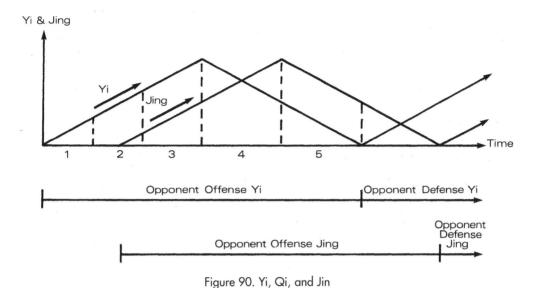

Figure 90. Yi, Qi, and Jin

Remember — Yi is always ahead of Qi, and where the Yi is, there is the Qi also. When you have developed your Qi you can use it to support your Jin as you express it through your posture. Therefore, when you sense the enemy's Qi, it means that his Yi is forming, and his Qi is not yet strong enough to support Jin. If you attack just when you sense his intention and Qi, you can disturb the forming of his Yi and Qi and put him into a passive, vulnerable situation (Figure 90). It takes a great deal of experience to sense the opponent's intention. This is one of the timings used for "Cold Jin" (Leng Jin, 冷勁). When you reach this stage, you have reached "enlightenment." Naturally, this is the best among the best timings in attacking the enemy.

> *(When) the enemy's attacking Yi shows, and his Jin is about to emit but hasn't yet, you borrow this opportunity to stop (his attack) and interrupt his Yi and posture. (It is) normally among the best strategies (see 2 of Figure 90).*

敵擊意已現，而勁將出未出，我借此機，阻其意、其勢，
乃上平策。

When the enemy's Yi is almost complete, his Qi is generated and is ready to support his Jin. If you take this time to interrupt his Yi and stop his Jin, the Jin he generated will bounce back at him. Since his Yi is almost complete it is totally concentrated on attacking, and he will not be able to instantly stop his attacking Yi and withdraw his Qi and Jin. his Jin will therefore be bounced back. This is the first timing of "Borrowing Jin" (Jie Jin, 借勁). Taijiquan ancestor Wǔ, Yu-Xiang (武禹襄) said: "the opponent does not move, you do not move; the opponent moves slightly, you move first."[25] This is the timing of "Borrowing Jin."

> *(When) the enemy's attacking Yi is completed and Jin is emitted, you must first stop his (attacking) posture (and) then counterattack. (This is) the most common strategy (see 3 of Figure 90).*

敵攻意已成，勢亦已發，我必先阻其勢而反擊，乃平策。

When the enemy's Yi is completed and his Jin is emitted, you must intercept or avoid his attack first, and then counterattack. This timing is a common one that most martial artists can perform.

> *(When) the enemy's attacking Yi is weakening and his attacking posture is strongest, you borrow his Jin and reverse (the situation) to check his posture. (This is) difficult but one of the best strategies (see 4 of Figure 90).*

敵攻意漸蹶，攻勢正盛，我借其勁而反挫其勢，是為上
難策。

When the enemy's Jin has reached its maximum, his attacking Yi will be weakening. However, at this time his Jin will be the strongest. If you know how to borrow his Jin at this moment, you will be able to bounce him away. This is the more difficult level of "Borrowing Jin" (Jie Jin, 借勁).

> *(When) the enemy's attacking Yi is ended and his defensive Yi is about to be generated, and his posture moves back for defense, you borrow this opportunity and follow his posture and attack. (It is) the easiest, and one of the best strategies (see 5 of Figure 90).*

敵攻意已盡，守意將生，勢正回守，我借此機而反攻，
是為上易策。

When the enemy's attacking Yi is ended and his Yi is about to withdraw, you should take this opportunity and attack in along his extended limb before he withdraws it. When his Yi is about to withdraw, his defensive capability is weak, and vital areas are exposed because his arm is extended. If you take this moment to attack just as he is starting to withdraw, you will certainly get him unless he is very good in sticking hands.

9. Fighting Strategies of Sun Zi 孫子戰略 Sun Wu (557 B.C.) 孫武

Sun Wu (孫武), also known as Sun Zi (Mister Sun, 孫子), (known in the West as Sun Tzu), was a very famous strategist who lived around 557 B.C. His book *Sun Zi's Fighting Strategies* (Sun Zi Bing Fa, 孫子兵法) (often translated as "*The Art of*

War") has been studied by Chinese soldiers for centuries, and has become required reading in most military schools throughout the world. Although phrased in terms of battles and troop movements, the book applies equally well to individual conflicts.

> *Knowing the opponent and knowing yourself, a hundred battles without a loss. Not knowing the opponent but knowing yourself, one victory one loss. Not knowing the opponent and not knowing yourself, every battle will be lost.*

知彼知己，百戰不殆。不知彼而知己，一勝一負。不知彼，不知己，每戰每敗。

In a battle, if you know your opponent and yourself, you will be able to set up your strategy according to the situation, and win every time. When you know yourself but do not know the enemy, you are at the mercy of chance and have only a fifty-fifty chance of winning. If you know neither yourself nor your opponent, then you will lose for certain.

> *In a battle, use regularity to combine (engage), (but use) surprise to win. The one who is good at using surprise, (his strategy) is limitless like heaven and earth; (his wisdom) is not dry, (it is) like a river or stream. The conduct of battle is nothing but using regularity and surprise. The exchange of surprise and regularity (is) limitless. Surprise and regularity mutually grow, like a cycle with no end. Who can limit it (i.e., figure it out completely)?*

凡戰者，以正合，以奇勝。故善出奇者，無窮如天地，不竭如江河。戰勢不過奇正，奇正之變，不可勝窮也。奇正相生，如循環之無端，孰能窮之？

Regularity (Zheng, 正), in the sense of both fixed organization and standard operating procedures, is Yang. Surprise, or change (Qi, 奇), is Yin. Regularity in organization and operating procedures allows your units to combine and work together for greater strength. Regularity also means developing routines and techniques that allow you to effectively develop and use maximum power. However, if you always follow these routines your opponent can develop ways to defeat them, so you must also use surprise, or alternate the routines, to keep the enemy off balance so he cannot effectively mobilize his strength. In individual training and fighting, you must develop set routines, but you must never be bound by them. You may do something several times so that the opponent expects you to do it again, but then you must change in order to surprise him and win. If you can skillfully alternate regularity and surprise (which can be called substantial and insubstantial), you will be able to respond to the opponent's actions with a limitless variety of actions.

Therefore, when using soldiers, the ultimate shape is to have no shape. If there is no shape, then it is like a deep mountain torrent that cannot be fathomed, and (even) a wise person cannot set up a strategy (against you). Everyone (thinks he) understands how you win the victories from the shape (they can see), but they don't know the shape of how you really win the victory. Therefore (you) do not repeat the tactics of (your) victories, and (your) response to shapes (situations) is unlimited.

故形兵之極，至於無形。無形則深潤不能窺，智者不能
謀。人皆知我所以勝之形，而莫知吾所以制勝之形。故
其戰勝不復，而應形於無窮。

When fighting, the ultimate strategy is to seem to have no strategy. If the opponent cannot determine what your strategy is, or if it seems that you have no strategy, then he will not be able to devise a strategy against you. If the enemy thinks he knows you well, he will be able to set up a good strategy and will seem to be winning. However, because your strategy is actually shapeless, he is basing his actions on illusion, and he will lose in the end. When you attack, he thinks he knows what you plan (your shape), and he can counterattack. But it is only a feint used to draw him out and make him act. Once his plans have taken shape, you base your strategy on that shape and act accordingly. Since your strategy is not tied to any particular form, it can change through an endless number of variations and never repeat itself.

In conclusion, soldiers (strategies) are like water. The shape (nature) of water (is to) avoid the high and flow to the low. The shape (correct disposition) of soldiers (is to) avoid the substantial and attack the insubstantial. Water comes over into a stream due to the shape of the ground, soldiers gain the victory through corresponding to the enemy('s shape). Therefore, soldiers do not have a fixed status (posture, disposition) and water does not have a fixed shape. (Being) able to change in response to the enemy's strategy and win the battle is called Shen (Spiritual Enlightenment).

夫兵象水。水之形，避高而趨下。兵之形，避實而擊虛。
水因地而制流，兵因敵而制勝。故兵無常勢，水無常形。
能因敵變化而取勝者，謂之神。

Water avoids the high and flows to the low. When conducting soldiers or fighting, you must avoid the substantial (i.e., strong points) and attack the insubstantial (i.e., weak points). Just as water can become a powerful stream by following the shape of the land, so too can soldiers become a strong attacking force by responding to and corresponding to the shape of the enemy. Basing your strategy on the strategy of the opponent is the way to victory, and is considered Spiritual Enlightenment. In Taijiquan, this is called giving up yourself and following the opponent. If you do not resist the opponent, and stick to him wherever he moves, he will never be able to find you and effectively attack you, but you will always know where he is and what he is planning. Because of this you are certain to defeat him.

10. Strategy of Hard and Soft 剛柔略

When using the soft to subdue the hard, the soft must be skillful and adaptable. Using soft to control soft is harder than hard. Using hard against hard, skill and Li are (both) stagnant and sluggish. If you use hard to defeat soft, your power and skill will be dull and hard to apply. Hard and soft mutually assisting and cooperating is the best strategy.

以柔克剛，柔必巧熟。以柔制柔，難上加難。以剛應剛，
技力遲鈍。以剛克柔，技死難展。剛柔相濟，乃為上策。

If you use the soft against the hard, you must be skillful in yielding, adhering, and sticking. Like a snake wrapping and coiling around a branch, you must adapt to whatever the opponent does. When you meet an opponent who is also skilled at soft-ness, then it will be extremely difficult to defeat him. You must be more skillful than he is, otherwise you will not be able to apply your techniques. If you use the hard to resist a hard attack, your actions will be stagnant and your power sluggish. If you try to use the hard to subdue the soft, your techniques will be dead and impossible to apply. The best approach is to exchange hard and soft appropriately. This mutual assistance and cooperation will make your techniques alive and useful.

11. Strategy of Fast and Slow 快慢略

When using the slow to defeat the fast, Qi must be emphasized. When using the fast to beat the slow, the Yi goes first. When fast and slow are used at the right time, and Yi and Qi exchange skillfully, it is called light and agile (Qing-Ling).

以慢敵快，以氣為重，以快侮慢，以意為先。快慢應得
時，意氣轉得巧，是為輕靈。

When you use the slow to defeat the fast, you must be calm, and concentrated, so the Qi can be abundant and your sensitivity of alertness can be high. Only when your Qi is abundant and stimulated are you able to generate the power needed for both defense and offense. However, when you intend to use speed to beat the slow, your Yi must always go first. This means that, while you are defending, your Yi is already on attacking, and while you are attacking, your Yi is already aware of the opponent's attack. However, the best fighting strategy is to match his speed so that fast follows fast and slow follows slow. If you can do this while skillfully exchanging your emphasis on Yi and Qi, your movements and thinking will be light and agile.

> *(The success of performing) slow (maneuvers) depends on the two Jins of attaching and adhering. (If you) do not understand attaching and adhering Jins, then slow (maneuvers) cannot be executed. In addition, in order to be slow, (you) must also know the skills of centering and rooting. (If you) do not understand centering and rooting, then the applications of attaching, adhering, connecting, and following will not be effective.*

> 慢重於粘黏二勁。不懂粘黏之勁，慢無以行之。慢亦須懂中定與紮根之巧，不懂中定與紮根之竅，粘黏連隨無以成效。

When you act slowly in a fight, not only must your sensitivity be high and your Qi abundant, but in order to follow and connect with the opponent, you must also be skillful in attaching and adhering Jins. In addition, you must have a balanced center and firmed root so you can neutralize the incoming force or emit your Jin effectively.

> *(The success of performing) fast (maneuvers) depends on agility, deftness, responsiveness and speed. When the Yi moves, the body immediately responds. (In order to be) fast, (you) must be skilled at the two Jins of Listening and Understanding; able to listen and able to understand; able to feel and able to respond; and after listening, immediately respond. All of these depend on the reaction generated from feeling and natural reflexes.*

> 快重於靈活輕巧，決於機靈。意動身動，毫不遲滯。快重於聽懂二勁。能聽能懂，能感能應，隨聽即感，隨懂即應。此乃知覺運動之反應也。

In order to be fast, you must be agile and deft. Furthermore, your decision must be quick and precise. In order to reach this stage, your Listening and Understanding Jins must have reached a proficient level. In this case, your feeling will be sharp, responsive, and the reaction will be fast and accurate.

> *However, those who are skilled at fighting are skilled at using both the fast and the slow maneuvers, and use them appropriately. When it needs to be fast, then they are fast, and when it is necessary to be slow, then they are slow. Fast or slow, (you) should not lose (the capabilities of) Listening, Following, Connecting, and Adhering. Then (you) will be able to establish the situation and create the opportunity to confuse (your) opponent and put (him) in a vulnerable position.*

然，善於較技者，皆善於快慢相稱，調配得宜。該快則
快，該慢則慢。不論快慢，不失聽隨連黏。如此，能造
勢立機，置敵於疑惑之中矣。

A good fighter should be proficient at all skills that allow him to fit in any combat situation. He should also be good at using the fast and slow tactics anytime necessary. When this happens, he will be able to control the entire fight, confusing his opponent and taking advantage of the vulnerability this creates.

12. Strategy of Advancing and Retreating 進退略

An ancient document said: "(If you) use an advance as an advance, the advance will not be defensible. (If you) use a withdrawal as a withdrawal, the withdrawal will be defeated. (If you) use a withdrawal as an advance, the withdrawal will create an advance. (If you) use an advance as a withdrawal, advance two, withdraw one. Advance and withdrawal must be mutually balanced. Especially important is (waiting for the right) opportunity. When the opportunity is missed, then advance and withdrawal are both difficult."

古云：〝以進為進，其進不守。以退為退，其退必敗。
以退為進，退以成進。以進為退，進以成退。進之者二，
退之者一。進退相衡，尤貴機先。機先一失，則進退兩
難矣。〞

This paragraph emphasizes the importance of deception. You must keep the opponent confused so that he never knows if what you seem to be doing is what you actually are doing. If he can see clearly that you are advancing, he may be able to react effectively and defeat you. If he can see clearly that you are retreating, he can press his attack and defeat you. If you want to advance, pretend to withdraw, and your advance will take him by surprise. Likewise, if you want to withdraw you must first advance so that you will be able to safely withdraw. To win a battle it is usually more important to advance than to withdraw, but the two must be balanced in the right proportion. Above all it is most important to act only at the correct time. You must wait for the right opportunity and then act, for if you miss the opportunity, it may not come again, and you will surely lose. The Taiji classics refer to this as grasping the moment and seizing the opportunity. Substantial and insubstantial should exchange skillfully.

The most important keys to successful advancing and withdrawing are a high level of alertness, an understanding the appropriate opportunity, and knowledge of the opponent and yourself. When advancing and withdrawing are appropriate, then (you) can create the opportunity and establish the advantage. Use with-

drawal as an advance, and use advance as a withdrawal. Advance provides the opportunity for withdrawal and withdrawal implies the intention of advancing. Among the strategies of advancing and withdrawing are: enter with insubstantial and attack with substantial, enter with substantial and withdraw with insubstantial. Advance, advance, withdrawal, withdrawal, the opponent does not know you but you know the opponent. You are not only able to create the opportunity, but are also able to create a desirable situation. As a result, you can say that you know the opponent.

進退之要在於警覺，在於悟機，在於知敵知我。進退得宜，乃能造機立勢，以退為進，以進為退。進即是退機，退即是進意。在進退中，虛進實出，實進虛退。進進退退，敵不知我，我卻知敵。先機在我，造勢亦在我。如此可謂知敵矣。

To advance or withdraw successfully require a high level of alertness and awareness. You must know the right opportunity to execute your decision and also know your opponent's capability and yours. Only then are you able to create an advantageous opportunity or situation for your actions. Advance and withdrawal must be used skillfully and exchangeably. Both can be an insubstantial or substantial strategic action. This will make your opponent confused and unable to discern your real intention. In this case, you have already controlled the encounter.

13. Theory of the Fight of No Fight 敵而無敵論

The meaning of the fight of no fight is: when encountering the opponent, there is no opponent; when there is a response (to an action), there is no response; when there is a Xin, there is no Xin; and when there is an Yi, there is no Yi. All of the offensive and defensive is natural. This is the level of reaching enlightenment. The spirit is the master, and the Yi is not on the Yi, so the Qi will circulate automatically and naturally.

敵而無敵者，面敵而無敵，應應而無應，有心而無心，有意而無意，一切攻守反應自然。此乃通乎神明矣。神為主宰，意不在意，氣行自如。

When you have reached a proficient level of fighting skills, you are in the state of fighting without fighting. That means, even if there is an enemy right in front of you, it seems there is none. You are natural and not frightened or nervous at all. When you respond to an action from the opponent, your responses are so natural and automatic, it seems you do not put any effort into the response at all. Your emotions are agitated, yet are under control. When you have an intention, it is so natural that your opponent does not even know there is an intention initiated. In this case, you are the master of the entire conflict and control the situation. You know your opponent but your opponent does not know you. Success depends on the status of your spirit. When your spirit is high, fighting morale will be high, and all of the action will be natural and automatic. Your Yi should not be on the Yi, otherwise, the Qi will be stagnant. Your Yi should be on the sense of enemy (Di Yi, 敵意), then you have high alertness and awareness.

> *To reach this level, (you) must practice a hundred times or even a thousand times diligently and ceaselessly. After practicing for a long time, all of the reactions are natural. At the beginning an encounter with an opponent, the Yi is concentrated and the will is strong. Keep aware of the opponent without any carelessness all the time. Step by step watch the opponent closely, and proceed cautiously. This is fighting with Yi. After you have encountered many opponents many times, your experience will be abundant. (In this case), Yi is no longer necessary in the fight and all of the responses are natural. When the opponent slightly moves, you already know and react responsively. You do not have to think or make any effort. At this time, use the spirit to master the entire situation. Even when there is an enemy, it seems there is none; even where there is a battle, it seems there is no battle. Isn't this reaching the stage of the fight of no fight?*

為達此境地，必須千錘百煉，勤練不息，久而久之，一
切反應自然。初應敵時，意專志強，隨時防敵不懈，步
步釘人，節節慎行。此乃鬥之以意也。應敵久之，經驗
充足，鬥之無意，一切反應自然。敵意微動，我已知之，
反應之。不用思索，不用費心。此時，以神宰之，有敵
似無敵，戰如無戰，此達敵而無敵之境地乎？

In order to reach a state of fighting with spiritual enlightenment, you must practice ceaselessly, and then continue to practice even more. Through the accumulation of experience, you will reach a state of natural reaction against any action. When this happens, you have reached the state of the fight of no fight. However, at the beginning of training, you must keep your Yi at a high level of alertness and awareness. Only then are you able to build up the level of sensitivity to know your opponent and responding to his incoming attacks naturally. Once you have reached the state of fighting of no fighting, then you should train to keep your spirit in a highly refined state. When this happens, the Qi can circulate smoothly and abundantly. When your spirit is high, the morale will also be high. Naturally, your alertness and awareness will be sharp and accurate.

PART X

Conclusion 終論

1. Theory of Reaching Enlightenment 通乎神明論

In the practice of Taijiquan pushing hands, Taiji circle sticking hands, and Taijiquan free fighting, etc., (you) must practice until (you) have reached a stage where there is no discrimination of the opponent. That means it is the stage where the opponent is you and you are the opponent, both are one. As a result, you know yourself and you also know your opponent. You are in an active position and the opponent's action is driven by you. (You are) able to put the opponent in your palms. When there is an intention of moving, you know immediately. When this happens, (you) have reached the stage of fighting with enlightenment. At the beginning, the keys (of training) are in listening, following, attaching, and adhering — four crucial words. If (you) are not able to use these four important keys (skillfully), then (you) will not be able to communicate with the opponent and understand the situation. Afterward, the keys (of training) are on leading, neutralizing, coiling, and turning. If (you) cannot apply these four keys (effectively), then the coming Jins will not be neutralized and dissolved (by you) and thus (you) will not be able to control (your) opponent in your palms. If (you) are able to reach the above (eight words), then the techniques such as Cai (i.e., pluck), Lie (i.e., split), Zhou (i.e., elbow), Kao (i.e., bump), Ti (i.e., kicking), Da (i.e., striking), Shuai (i.e., wrestling), and Na (i.e., Chin Na), etc. can be executed as you wish.

太極拳推手、太極圈纏手、太極拳自由散手等練習須練到敵我不分。亦即敵即是我，我即是敵之境界。如此，我知我，我亦知敵，我為主動，敵為我所使。置敵於掌中，稍有動意，即為我所知。如此可通乎神明。起初，竅在於聽、隨、粘、黏四字。不能運用此四訣，則無法溝通敵情。之後，竅在於引、化、纏、轉四字。不能運用此四訣，則來勁無法化解，不能置敵於掌中。能夠如此，採、挒、肘、靠、踢、打、摔、拿等任我所便。

When you practice Taijiquan skills to a high level and have reached a state of 'fight of no fight' (i.e., regulating without regulating), then every action is ultimately natural, comfortable, skillful, and effective. This is the stage of 'fighting with enlightenment.' In this stage, you know yourself and you also know your opponent. You are the one who controls the entire fighting situation.

The keys to reaching this stage of training are in the eight crucial practices. At the beginning, you must practice listening (i.e., feeling), following, attaching, and adhering until you become proficient. If you can do so, you will be able to communicate with your opponent easily. Only then can you perform the skills of leading, neutralizing, coiling, and turning effectively. In fact, these eight key words are the crucial secrets of executing all of the Taijiquan fighting techniques successfully.

> *In beginning of your training, the focus is on regulating the body, and then on regulating the breathing, regulating the Xin (i.e., emotional mind), regulating the Qi, and then regulating the spirit. Its final stage is to regulate the spirit until no regulating is necessary. This is the stage of regulating without regulating. If (you) really are able to reach this level, your enlightened spirit will be focused on it fully. This is the Dao of reaching enlightenment.*

其練習程次，開始在於調身，再於調息、調心、調氣、調神著手。其最終之境界，在於調神而至調而不調，不調而自調之境界。果達此境地，神明貫注焉。此乃通乎神明之道。

In order to reach the final stage of enlightenment, you must regulate your body, and then your breathing, mind, Qi, and finally spirit. Once you are able to reach a stage at which your whole spirit is in the actions without any effort, then you have reached the stage of enlightenment. This is the level of action without action.

> *Generally speaking, to reach enlightenment is to comprehend the meaning of physical life, to cherish all living things, to know the mandate of heaven, and to fulfill the will of heaven. That means, during the training process of killing and surviving in Taijiquan practice, to comprehend the reasons for human life, to cherish the value of millions of living things, to search for the rules of heaven Dao, and finally to achieve the great Dao of heaven and human's unification. This is the original meaning of Taijiquan's creation by the Daoist family in Wudang mountain.*

廣義而言，通乎神明者，在悟生理，在惜生靈，在知天命，在達天意。亦即在練習太極生殺之理中，去悟解人生之道理，去珍惜萬物生命之可貴，去尋求天道之理，並臻天人合一之大道也。此乃武當道家創太極拳之本意。

Taijiquan was created at the Daoist monasteries on Wudang mountain. The final goal of Daoist spiritual cultivation is to reunite the human spirit with the heaven's (i.e., natural) spirit. To reach this goal, first we must comprehend the meaning of our lives, cherish all living things, search for the mandate of nature, and finally fulfill this mandate. From this, we can see that, though Taijiquan was created as a martial art, it does not mean to destroy or to kill life. On the contrary, it is the tool for us to understand life. From self-understanding and discipline, we learn how to control ourselves and to appreciate life everywhere. Only then can we have a pure and kind heart to understand nature and its mandate. All of these are the required procedures for the unification of human and heaven's spirit.

2. Discussing the Song of Taijiquan's Real Meaning 論太極真義歌

The Song of Taiji's Real Meaning says: "No shape, no shadow. Entire body transparent and empty." This means that (you) have reached "the stage of forgetting self" and have attained "the level of Wuji state." No shape and no shadow means that (you) have forgotten the existence of the self's physical body. (If you) are able to be relaxed, soft, reach extreme calmness, and can transport your Qi anywhere without stagnation, then the physical body will gradually disappear. This is the feeling of transparency of the entire physical body and this means that (you) have reached the highest Wuji stage of the body's regulating.

太極真義歌云：〝無形無象。全身透空。〞 此乃達乎「忘我之境」歸乎「無極之地」也。無行無象者，忘我物理之存在也。能極鬆軟。能極靜，氣無不行。物理之體，漸趨無形。此即為全身透空，歸於最高調身無極之境界。

When you have reached the final stage of regulating the body, the body is extremely relaxed and the mind is in a deep and profound meditative state. When this occurs, the Qi is ultimately smooth and can circulate and radiate anywhere in the body without the slightest stagnation. As a result, you will feel that your physical body has disappeared. In order to reach this stage, your mind must be in the center of your physical body (i.e., Real Dan Tian), which is located in the physical center of gravity. Since this physical center is also the residence of our original Qi, this is the state of Wuji.

The Song of Taiji's Real Meaning also says: "Forget (your) surroundings and be natural. Like a stone chime suspended from West Mountain." This implies that you should "do as (you) wish in the heart" and "the sea is broad and the sky is vast." There also exists the concept of 'controlling in the profound meditative stage.' Forget (your) surroundings and be natural refers to the natural state of regulating without regulating. In this case, you may fulfill the wish in your heart and (the spirit) will be able to travel anywhere (in the universe). However, there must be control (of this spirit). If there is no control, then the spirit will gallop, cannot be restrained, and will become wild and untamed. Like a stone chime suspended from West Mountain implies there is control during the profound meditative state: free but not uncontrolled, forget yourself but restrained. This is the highest cultivative stage of regulating the mind in meditation.

又云：〝忘物自然。西山懸磬。〞此蘊意之「隨心所
欲」，「海闊天空」，但存乎「冥中有宰」也。忘物自
然者，不調而調之自然境界也。如此，則能隨心所欲，
無所不行。然而，其中必有主宰。無宰，則神馳而不斂，
性野而不馴。西山懸磬者，冥中之宰也。逍遙而不放，
忘我而束然。此為靜修最高調心之境界。

After you have reached the stage of feeling transparent in your physical body, then gradually you will reach a stage of forgetting your surroundings. You are in a semi-sleeping state, comfortable and so natural. This is the state of regulating without regulating. When this happens, your mind and spirit are able to travel anywhere in the universe and are not restricted by time. Even then there is a control that always connects your spirit in residence to your spirit aloft.

The Song of Taiji's Real Meaning also says: "Tigers roaring, monkeys screeching. Clear fountain, peaceful water." This tells you "to find calmness within movements and to find Yin within Yang." Tigers roaring, monkeys screeching describes the releasing of the Xin and Yi's action and the raising of the Yang spirit. Clear fountain and peaceful water means the Yi's restraining and the Xin's convergence, and this implies the Xin is peaceful and the spirit is clear. This is the stage of regulating the Xin and entering the stage of regulating the spirit.

又云：〝虎吼猿鳴。泉清水靜。〞乃指「動中求靜，陽
中覓陰」之謂也。虎吼猿鳴，乃心意放動與陽神上提之
意。泉清水靜，乃意收而心斂，心平神清之意。此為由
調心而至調神之境界。

In Taijiquan, even if you are in a physically active Yang state, you must always seek the peaceful and calm Yin mind. From this, you are able to maintain your spiritual center while in action. From this training, you are able to raise up your spirit, and also still be able to control it. This is the coordination of the emotional mind and the spirit.

The Song of Taiji's Real Meaning also says: "Turbulent river, stormy ocean. With (your) whole being, develop (your) life." Turbulent river and stormy ocean is to understand the meaning of life. Understanding the meaning of life, then leads to the goal of knowing the meaning of heaven (i.e., nature). From knowing the meaning of heaven, (you) are able to end (your) human nature and return it to its origin. This is the root and foundation of life. If you know the meaning of death, then you know the value of life. From appreciating the value of life, you comprehend (your) human nature. From knowing (your) human nature, you understand the meaning of nature. From knowing the meaning of nature, (you) are able to end your human nature and finally reach the goal of regulating the spirit—the unification of heaven and human.

又云：〝翻江鬧海。盡性立命。〞翻江鬧海者，悟命也。由命之悟而知達天命。由知達天命，了性返本。此為立命之根基。知死而知生，由知生而悟性，由悟性而知天命，由知天命而了吾性並終臻於天人合一最高之調神境界。

All human cultures have experienced four stages of spiritual evolution. These four stages are: self-recognition (Zi Shi, 自識), self-awareness (Zi Jue, 自覺), self-awakening (Zi Xing, Zi Wu, 自醒·自悟), and finally self-liberation from spiritual bondage (Jie Tuo, 解脫). From the ugliness of humanity's history of death and destruction (i.e., turbulent river and stormy ocean), we recognize how low our spirit can be and how vile we can become. From this self-recognition, we can enter the stage of self-awareness. From this self-awareness, we learn to understand each other and our environment. Then, we can come to a stage of awakening. From this awakening, we comprehend that the truth of nature is that we must love each other and harmonize with each other. Without love and harmony, we will destroy each other completely. If we continue this pursuit, we will be able to free ourselves from all spiritual bondage such as glory, jealousy, dignity, pride, etc. These spiritual bonds were set up in the past to fulfill personal desires. Only if we are able to set ourselves free from these bonds (i.e., to end our human nature) can we reunite our spirit with the spirit of great nature. Without this evolutionary process, we will not be able to exist and harmonize with other spiritual beings from beyond this earth.

References

1. 《性命圭旨全書 · 魂魄圖說》："陽神曰魂，陰神曰魄。"

2. 《性命圭旨全書 · 魂魄圖說》："魂者氣之神，有清有濁。…魄者精之神，有虛有實。" 為肝主魂，魂為肝之神；肺藏魄，魄為肺之神。

3. 《龍虎返丹訣頌 · 谷神子注》："地魄天魂是虎龍。天陽為魂，龍也。地陰為魄，虎也。"

4. 《諸真聖胎神用訣 · 陳希夷胎息訣》："神通萬變，謂之曰靈。"

5. *Chinese Qigong Dictionary* (中國氣功辭典), by Lu, Guang-Rong (呂光榮), 人民衛生出版社, Beijing, 1988.

6. *Chinese Traditional Qigong Study Dictionary* (中國傳統氣功學辭典), by Zhang, Wen-Jiang and Chang, Jin (張文江，常近主編), 山西人民出版社, Shanxi Province (山西省), 1989.

7. *Complex and Hidden Brain in the Gut Makes Stomachaches and Butterflies*, by Sandra Blakeslee, The New York Times, Science, January 23, 1996.

8. *The Second Brain: The Scientific Basis of Gut Instinct and a Groundbreaking New Understanding of Nervous Disorders of the Stomach and Intestine*, Michael D. Gershon, New York: Harper Collins Publications, 1998.

9. 太極拳論："有不得機得勢處，身便散亂。其病必於腰腿求之。"

10. 李清菴云："調息要調無息息。"

11. 太極拳論："有上即有下，有前即有後，有左即有右。"

12. 十三勢行功心解（武禹襄）："牽動往來氣貼背，而練入脊骨。"

13. 武禹襄："意氣須換得靈，乃有圓活之妙，所謂變轉虛實也。"

14. 武禹襄："一身五弓備蓄發，敷蓋對吞仔細研。"

15. 王宗岳："蓄勁如張弓，發勁如放箭。"

16. 王宗岳："力由脊發，步隨身換。"

17. 武禹襄："行氣如九曲珠，無微不到。運勁如百鍊鋼，無堅不摧。"

18. 武禹襄："極柔軟，然後極堅剛。能呼吸，然後能靈活。"

19. 王宗岳："精神能提得起，則無遲重之虞，所謂頂頭懸也。"

20. 王宗岳：〝全身意在精神，不在氣。〞

21. 李亦畬曰：〝五曰神聚。上四者俱備，總歸神聚，神聚則一氣鼓
    鑄，練氣歸神，氣勢騰挪，精神貫注，開合有致，虛實清楚…〞

22. 〝拿住丹田練內功，哼哈二氣妙無窮，動分靜合屈伸就，緩應急
    隨理貫通。〞

23. 李亦畬：〝虛中隨機變，妙在圓中求。〞

24. 孫子：〝知彼知己，百戰不殆。〞

25. 十三勢行功心解（武禹襄）：〝敵不動，我不動。敵微動，我先
    動。〞

Translation and Glossary of Chinese Terms

Abraham Liu 劉振寰

One of Cheng, Man-Ching's disciples, who currently resides in California, United States.

An 按

Means "pressing or stamping." One of the eight basic moving or Jin patterns of Taijiquan. These eight moving patterns are called "Ba Men" (八門) which means "eight doors." When An is done, first relax the wrist and when the hand has reached the opponent's body, immediately settle down the wrist. This action is called "Zuo Wan" (坐腕) in Taijiquan practice.

An Jin 按勁

The martial power generated from the An moving pattern of Taijiquan.

Bagua (Ba Kua) 八卦

Literally, "Eight Divinations." Also called the Eight Trigrams. In Chinese philosophy, the eight basic variations; shown in the *Yi Jing* (易經) (*Book of Change*) as groups of single and broken lines.

Ba Men Wu Bu 八門五步

Means "eight doors and five steppings." The art of Taijiquan is built from eight basic moving or Jin patterns and five basic steppings. The eight basic moving or Jin patterns that can be used to handle the eight directions are called the "eight doors" (Ba Men, 八門) and the five stepping actions are called the "five steppings" (Wu Bu, 五步).

Bai He 白鶴

White Crane. A style of Chinese martial arts.

Bai Yuan 白猿

White Ape. A style of Chinese martial arts.

Baihui (Gv-20) 百會

Hundred Meetings. Name of an acupuncture cavity which belongs to the Governing Vessel. Baihui is located on the crown of the head.

Bao-Xi (2852-2737 B.C.) 包義

Also named Fu Xi (伏羲). The first important and unifying ancestor of the Chinese Han race (漢族).

Bi Xi 鼻息

Nose breathing.

Bu 步

Stepping.

Cai 採

Plucking.

Cai Jin 採勁

The martial power of plucking.

Can Si Jin Chan Shou Lian Xi 纏絲勁纏手練習

Silk reeling Jin coiling training. One of the important basic trainings in Taijiquan.

Chan 纏

To wrap or to coil. A common Chinese martial arts technique.

Chan Jin 纏勁

The martial power of wrapping or coiling.

Chan Si Jin 纏絲勁

Means "Silk Reeling Jin."

Chang 長

Long.

Chang Chuan (Changquan) 長拳

Means "long range fist or long sequence." Chang Chuan includes all northern Chinese long range martial styles. Taijiquan is also called Chang Chuan simply because its sequence is long.

Chang Jin 長勁

Long Jins. The Jins that reach the long fighting range.

Chang Ju 長距

Means "long range or long distance."

Changqiang (Gv-1) 長強

Long strength. Name of an acupuncture cavity which belongs to the Governing Vessel.

Changquan (Chang Chuan) 長拳

Means "long range fist or long sequence." Chang Chuan includes all northern Chinese long range martial styles. Taijiquan is also called Chang Chuan simply because its sequence is long.

Chen Shi 辰時

The time period from 7 to 9 A.M.

Chen, Yan-Lin 陳炎林

A well-known Taijiquan master in China during the 1940's who wrote a book entitled: *Tai Chi Chuan: Saber, Sword, Staff, and Sparring,* (太極拳，刀、劍、桿、散手合編), Reprinted in Taipei, Taiwan, 1943.

Cheng, Gin-Gsao (1911-1976 A.D.) 曾金灶

Dr. Yang, Jwing-Ming's White Crane master.

Cheng, Man-Ching 鄭曼清

A well-known Chinese Taijiquan master in America during the 1960's.

Chi (Qi) 氣

The energy pervading the universe, including the energy circulating in the human body.

Chi Kung (Qigong) 氣功

The Gongfu of Qi, which means the study of Qi.

Chin Na (Qin Na) 擒拿

Literally means "seize control." A component of Chinese martial arts which emphasizes grabbing techniques to control your opponent's joints, in conjunction with attacking certain acupuncture cavities.

Chong Mai 衝脈

Thrusting Vessel. One of the eight extraordinary vessels.

Da 打

Striking. Normally, to attack with the palms, fists or arms.

Da Jia 大架

Means "large posture."

Da Lu 大擴

Large Rollback. One of the common Taiji techniques.

Da Qiao 搭橋

To build a bridge. Refers to the Qigong practice of touching the roof of the mouth with the tip of the tongue to form a bridge or link between the Governing and Conception Vessels.

Da Zhou Tian 大周天

Literally, "Grand Cycle Heaven." Usually translated as "Grand Circulation." After a Nei Dan Qigong practitioner completes Small Circulation, he will circulate his Qi through the entire body or exchange the Qi with nature.

Dai Mai 帶脈

Girdle (or Belt) Vessel. One of the eight extraordinary vessels.

Dai Mai Xi 帶脈息

Girdle Vessel Breathing. A special Qigong breathing technique.

Dan Lu 丹爐

Means "elixir furnace," where the Qi (i.e., elixir) can be produced.

Dan Tian 丹田

Literally: Field of Elixir. Locations in the body which are able to store and generate Qi (elixir) in the body. The Upper, Middle, and Lower Dan Tians are located respectively between the eyebrows, at the solar plexus, and a few inches below the navel.

Dao 道

The "way," by implication the "natural way."

Dao De Jing 道德經

Morality Classic. Written by Lao Zi (老子) during the Zhou Dynasty (1122-934 B.C.) (周朝).

Dao De Jing (Tao Te Ching) 道德經

Morality Classic. Written by Lao Zi.

Dazhui (Gv-14) 大椎

Big Vertebra. Name of an acupuncture cavity that belongs to the Governing Vessel.

Deng Shan Bu 蹬山步

Climbing Mountain Stance. One of the basic fundamental stances in northern martial arts. Also called "Bow and Arrow Stance" (Gong Jian Bu, 弓箭步).

Di Hu 地戶

Ground Wicket. A martial arts term.

Di Shi 低勢

Low Stance or low posture.

Di Yi 敵意

Sense of enemy.

Dian Xue 點穴

Dian means "to point and exert pressure" and Xue means "the cavities." Dian Xue refers to those Qin Na techniques which specialize in attacking acupuncture cavities to immobilize or kill an opponent.

Dihe (M-HN-19) 地合

An acupuncture cavity located on the face.

Dong 懂

Understanding.

Dong Jin 懂勁

Understanding Jin. One of the Jins which uses the feeling of the skin to sense the opponent's energy.

Dong Mei Xi 冬眠息

Hibernation Breathing. One of the breathing techniques in Qigong practice.

Dong Mian Fa 冬眠法

Hibernation Technique. A Qigong technique that trains hibernation breathing.

Du Mai 督脈

Usually translated "Governing Vessel." One of the eight Qi vessels.

Duan 短

Short.

Duan Jin 短勁

Short Jins. Those Jins which are used for short range fighting.

Dui 兌

One of the Eight Trigrams.

Fa 法

Techniques or methods.

Fan Hu Xi (Ni Hu Xi) 反呼吸・逆呼吸

Reverse Breathing. Also commonly called "Daoist Breathing."

Fan Tong Hu Xi 返童呼吸

Back to childhood breathing. A breathing training in Nei Dan Qigong through which the practitioner tries to regain control of the muscles in the lower abdomen. Also called "abdominal breathing."

Fengfu (Gv-16) 風府

Wind's Dwelling. Name of an acupuncture cavity belonging to the Governing Vessel.

Fu Shi Hu Xi 腹式呼吸

Literally, "abdominal way of breathing." As you breathe, you use the muscles in the lower abdominal area to control the diaphragm. It is also called "back to (the) childhood breathing."

Fu Sui Xi 膚髓息

Skin and marrow breathing. Skin breathing is considered as Yang while marrow breathing is classified as Yin.

Fu Xi 腹息

Literally, "abdominal way of breathing." As you breathe, you use the muscles in the lower abdominal area to control the diaphragm. It is also called "back to (the) childhood breathing."

Fu Xi 膚息

Skin Breathing. One of the Nei Dan Qigong breathing techniques in which the Qi is led to the skin surface.

Fu Xi (2852-2737 B.C.) 伏羲

The first important and unifying ancestor of the Chinese Han race (漢族).

Gao Shi 高勢

High stance or posture.

Gen 艮

One of the Eight Trigrams which represents mountains.

Gong (Kung) 功

Energy or hard work.

Gongfu (Kung Fu) 功夫

Means "energy-time." Anything which will take time and energy to learn or to accomplish is called Gongfu.

Gu Shen 谷神

Valley Spirit.

Gu Shen 固神

Gu means to firm and solidify. An exercise for regulating the Shen in which you firm and strengthen the spirit at its residence.

Gui 鬼

Ghost. When you die, if your spirit is strong, your soul's energy will not decompose and return to nature. This soul energy is a ghost.

Gui Dao, Gui Lu 鬼道、鬼路

Ghost path. The path of death.

Gui Xi 龜息

Turtle breathing. In Chinese Qigong society, it is believed that a turtle is able to live for a long time because it knows how to breathe through its skin. Therefore, skin breathing in Qigong is called turtle breathing.

Guo Dang 裹襠

Means to wrap the groin area by turning the knee inward to protect the groin.

Ha 哈

A Yang sound that is used to manifest martial power to its highest efficiency.

Hai Di 海底

Sea Bottom. The Huiyin (Co-1) cavity or perineum.

Han Xiong Ba Bei 含胸拔背

Means to contain or draw in the chest and arc the back.

Han, Ching-Tang 韓慶堂

A well-known Chinese martial artist, especially in Taiwan in the last forty years. Master Han is also Dr. Yang Jwing-Ming's Long Fist grandmaster.

Hen 哼

A Yin Qigong sound that is the opposite of the Yang Ha sound. This sound is commonly used to lead the Qi inward and to store it in the bone marrow.

This sound can also be used for an attack when the manifestation of only partial power is desired.

Hou Tian Qi 後天氣

Post-birth Qi or post-heaven Qi. This Qi is converted from the Essence of food and air and is classified as "fire Qi" since it can make your body too Yang.

Hua 化

"To neutralize."

Hua Jin 化勁

The Jin (martial power) used to neutralize the opponent's attacking.

Huan Jing Bu Nao 還精補腦

Literally, to return the Essence to nourish the brain. A Daoist Qigong training process wherein Qi that has been converted from Essence is lead to the brain to nourish it.

Huang Ting 黃庭

Yellow yard. 1. A yard or hall in which Daoists, who often wore yellow robes, meditate together. 2. In Daoist Qigong, the place in the center of the body where Fire Qi and Water Qi are mixed to generate a spiritual embryo.

Hubei Province 湖北省

One of the provinces in southern China.

Huiyin 會陰

Perineum. An acupuncture cavity belonging to the Conception Vessel.

Hun 魂

The soul. Commonly used with the word Ling, which means spirit. Daoists believe that a human being's Hun and Po originate with his Original Qi (Yuan Qi, 元氣), and separate from the physical body at death.

Huo 火

Fire. One of the five elements in the Five Phases.

Huo Lu 火路

Fire path. One of the paths in Small Circulation meditation.

Ji 擠

Means "to squeeze" or "to press."

Ji Gong 脊弓

Spine Bow. The bow formed from the spine, which is able to store the Jin.

Ji Jin 擠勁

The martial power of pressing or squeezing.

Jia Dan Tian 假丹田

False Dan Tian. It is called Qihai (Co-6) (氣海) in acupuncture. This place is able to produce Qi. However, it cannot store Qi efficiently.

Jiaji 夾脊

Squeeze the Spine. The Daoist name of a spot on the spine in Small Circulation meditation practice. This spot is called "Lingtai" (Gv-10) (靈台) (i.e., spirit's platform) in acupuncture.

Jianjing (GB-21) 肩井

Shoulder Well. An acupuncture cavity belonging to the Gall Bladder channel.

Jianneiling (M-UE-48) 肩內陵

Shoulder's Inner Tomb. Name of an acupuncture cavity. A special point.

Jie 截

Intercepting.

Jie Jin 借勁

Borrowing Jin. One of the Jins in martial arts power manifestation.

Jie Tuo 解脫

Set the self free from spiritual and emotional bondage.

Jin 金

Metal. One of the five elements in the Five Phases.

Jin (Jing) 勁

Chinese martial power. A combination of "Li" (力) (muscular power) and "Qi" (氣).

Jin, Shao-Feng 金紹峰

Master Yang Jwing-Ming's White Crane grandmaster.

Jin-Li 勁力

Means "martial power."

Jing 靜

Calm.

Jing 經

Primary Qi Channel. Sometimes translated as "meridian." Refers to the twelve organ-related "rivers" which circulate Qi throughout the body.

Jing (Jin) 勁

Chinese martial power. A combination of "Li" (力) (muscular power) and "Qi" (氣).

Jing Qi 精氣

Essence Qi. The Qi which has been converted from Original Essence.

Jing-Shen 精神

Essence-Spirit. Often translated as the "Spirit of Vitality." Raised spirit (raised by the Qi which is converted from Essence) which is restrained by the Yi.

Jiuwei (Co-15) 鳩尾

Wild Pigeon's Tail. An acupuncture cavity belonging to the Conceptional Vessel.

Kai Di Hu 開地戶

Open the ground wicket. This means to open the opponent's lower body area for an attack.

Kai Tian Chuang 開天窗

Open the sky window. This means to open the opponent's upper body area for an attack.

Kan 坎

One of the Eight Trigrams, meaning "water." Referred to in "Kan and Li (fire)."

Kao 靠

Means "to lean or to press against." In Taijiquan, it means to bump someone off balance.

Kao Jin 靠勁

The martial power of bumping.

Kao, Tao 高濤

Dr. Yang, Jwing-Ming's first Taijiquan master.

Kong Men 空門

Empty doors. The doors you can step in to initiate an effective attack.

Kua 胯

The area on the external hip joint is called "external Kua" (Wai Kua, 外胯) whereas the area on the inner side of the hip joints (i.e., groin area) is called "internal Kua" (Nei Kua, 內胯).

Kun 坤

One of the Eight Trigrams.

Kung (Gong) 功

Means "energy" or "hard work."

Kung Fu (Gongfu) 功夫

Means "energy-time." Anything which will take time and energy to learn or to accomplish is called Kung Fu.

Lao Zi 老子

The creator of Daoism, also called Li Er (李耳). Lao Zi is also the name of the book, Dao De Jing (道德經).

Laogong (P-8) 勞宮

Labor's Palace. A cavity name. On the Pericardium Channel in the center of the palm.

Leng Jin 冷勁

Cold Jin. One of the Jins in martial arts' power manifestation.

Li 力

The power which is generated from muscular strength.

Li 理

Natural rules and principles.

Li 離

One of the Eight Trigrams, meaning "fire." Referred to in "Kan (water) and Li."

Li, Mao-Ching 李茂清

Dr. Yang, Jwing-Ming's Long Fist master.

Li-Qi 力氣

Li is muscular power, while Qi is inner energy. Li-Qi means "to manifest the inner energy into physical power," which means "Jin."

Lian 連

To connect.

Lian Jin 連勁

The martial power of connecting.

Lian Jing Hua Qi 練精化氣

To refine the Essence and convert it into Qi.

Lian Qi Hua Shen 練氣化神

To refine the Qi to nourish the spirit. Leading Qi to the head to nourish the brain and spirit.

Lian Qi Sheng Hua 練氣昇華

To train the Qi and sublimate it. A Xi Sui Jing training process by which the Qi is led to the Huang Ting or the brain.

Liang Yi 兩儀

Two Poles. It means "Yin and Yang."

Lie 挒

Means "to rend" or "to split."

Lie Jin 挒勁

The martial power of "split" or "rend."

Ling 靈

The spirit of being, which acts upon others. Ling only exists in highly spiritual animals such as humans and monkeys. It represents an emotional comprehension and understanding. When you are alive, it implies your intelligence and wisdom. When you die, it implies the spirit of the ghost. Ling also means "divine or supernatural." Ling is often used together with Shen (Ling Shen, 靈神) to mean "supernatural spirit." It is believed that Qi is the source which nourishes the Ling and is called "Ling Qi" (靈氣), meaning "supernatural energy, power, or force."

Ling Gen 靈根

The root of Ling. Means "the life or the foundation of a spiritual being."

Ling Shen 靈神

Supernatural spirit or the divine.

Lingtai (Gv-10) 靈臺

Spiritual Station. In acupuncture, a cavity on the back. In Qigong, it refers to the Upper Dan Tian. In Daoist society, the Lingtai cavity is called "Jia Ji" (夾脊).

Liu He 六合

Six Harmonies or six directions, which include north, south, east, west, up, and down. It means the universe or heaven.

Liu Shi Si Gua 六十四卦

Sixty-Four Trigrams.

Liu Yi 六藝

The six arts—consisting of writing, music, archery, chariot driving, learning rhetoric, and mathematics—which ancient Chinese scholars were required to master.

Longmen (M-CA-24) 龍門

Dragon Gate. Name of an acupuncture cavity that belongs to the Miscellaneous Points. It is the groin in the human body.

Lu 攦

Means "to rollback."

Lu Jin 攦勁

The martial power of rolling backward (rollback).

Luo 絡

The small Qi channels which branch out from the primary Qi channels and are connected to the skin and to the bone marrow.

Mi Hu 密戶

Closed Door. A special Daoist Qigong term that means the Mingmen cavity (Gv-4) (命門) in acupuncture.

Mingmen (Gv-4) 命門

Life's Door. Name of an acupuncture cavity that belongs to the Governing Vessel.

Mu 木

Wood. One of the Five Elements.

Na 拿

Means "to hold" or "to grab." However, when Na is applied in Taijiquan, it is a technique in which you use your hands to stick with the opponent's joints so as to immobilize his further action. Na is also commonly used as an abbreviation of Qin Na (擒拿) (i.e., seize and control).

Na Jin 拿勁

Controlling Jins. The Jins that are able to control the opponent through his joints or tendons.

Naohu (Gv-17) 腦戶

An acupuncture cavity belonging to the Governing vessel.

Nei Kua 內胯

The internal upper thighs near the groin area.

Nei Shen 內腎

Literally, internal kidneys. In Chinese medicine and Qigong, the real kidneys; while Wai Shen (外腎) (external kidneys) refers to the testicles.

Nei Shi 內視

Literally, internal vision. It implies feeling to the inner body. It also means "internal inspection through inner feeling."

Nei Shi Gongfu 內視功夫

Nei Shi means "to look internally," so Nei Shi Gongfu refers to the art of looking inside yourself to read the state of your health and the condition of your Qi.

Nei Wai He Yi 內外合一

Internal and external are unified as one. This means the harmonization of the internal (i.e., mind and Qi) and external (i.e., physical body).

Nei Wai Xiang He 內外相合

Unification of internal and external. This means the harmonization of the internal (i.e., mind and Qi) and external (i.e., physical body).

Neiguan (P-6) 內關

Inner Gate. An acupuncture cavity belonging to the Pericardium channel.

Ni Hu Xi (Fan Hu Xi) 逆呼吸 · 反呼吸

Reverse Breathing. Also commonly called "Daoist Breathing."

Ni Wan or Ni Wan Gong 泥丸 · 泥丸宮

Mud pill, or mud pill palace. Daoist Qigong terminology for the brain.

Nian 黏

To stick or to adhere.

Nian 念

Thoughts that stay with you and do not go away.

Nian Jin 黏勁

The martial power of adhering.

Nian Tou 念頭

Means "the initiation of the Nian (i.e., thought), that is the beginning of new thought."

Ning Shen 凝神

To condense or focus the spirit.

Peng 掤

Means "to ward off."

Peng Jin 掤勁

The martial power of warding off.

Po 魄

Vigorous life force. The Po is considered to be the inferior or animal soul. It is the animal or sentient life which is an innate part of the body which, at death, returns to the earth with the rest of the body. When someone is in high spirits and gets vigorously involved in some activity it is said he has Po Li, which means he has "vigorous strength or power."

Qi 奇

Means "surprise or change." A thought or action that is unexpected.

Qi (Chi) 氣

Chinese term for universal energy. A current popular model is that the Qi circulating in the human body is bioelectric in nature.

Qi Huo 起火

To start the fire. When you start to build up Qi at the Dan Tian.

Qi Jing Ba Mai 奇經八脈

Literally: strange channels eight vessels. Commonly translated as "extraordinary vessels" or "odd meridians." The eight vessels which store Qi and regulate the Qi in the primary channels.

Qi Xi 氣息

Qi breathing.

Qi Yan Ji Xing 氣沿脊行

Qi circulates along the spine upward.

Qi-Li 氣力

Qi is inner energy while Li is muscular power. Qi-Li means "to manifest the inner energy into physical power," which means "Jin."

Qian 乾

One of the Eight Trigrams.

Qiangjian (Gv-17) 強間

Between Strength. An acupuncture cavity on the back of the head that belongs to the Governing Vessel.

Qigong (Chi Kung) 氣功

The Gongfu of Qi, which means the study of Qi.

Qihai (Co-6) 氣海

An acupuncture cavity belonging to the Conceptional vessel.

Qin (Chin) 擒

Means "to catch" or "to seize."

Qin Na (Chin Na) 擒拿

Literally means "seize control." A component of Chinese martial arts which emphasizes grabbing techniques to control your opponent's joints, in conjunction with attacking certain acupuncture cavities.

Qing Qian Long (1736-1796 A.D.) 清乾隆

An emperor during the Chinese Qing Dynasty.

Qiu 酉

One of the twelve Terrestrial Branches (i.e., 5 to 7 P.M.).

Quchi (LI-11) 曲池

Crooked Pool. Name of an acupuncture cavity. It belongs to the Large Intestine channel.

Rang Jin 讓勁

Yielding Jin. The martial power that is used to yield to incoming force.

Ren Mai 任脈

Usually translated "Conception Vessel."

Renzhong (Gv-26) 人中

An acupuncture cavity under the nose.

Rong 戎

Ruling and martial affairs of the countries.

Ruan Jin 軟勁

Soft Jins. The manifestation of soft Jin is like the supple but sharp action of a whip.

Ruan Ying Jin 軟硬勁

Soft-hard Jins. This kind of Jin manifestation is soft at the beginning and turns into hard at the end.

San Guan 三關

Three gates. In Small Circulation training, the three cavities on the Governing Vessel which are usually obstructed and must be opened.

San Pan 三盤

Three sections. The entire body can be divided into three sections: from the knees down, from the knees to Xinkan (心坎) (or Jiuwei, Co-15) (鳩尾), and from Xinkan to the crown.

San Shi Er Gua 三十二卦

Thirty-Two Trigrams.

Shang Dan Tian 上丹田

Upper Dan Tian. Located at the third eye, it is the residence of the Shen (spirit).

Shang Dynasty 商朝

A dynasty in Chinese history during the period 1766-1122 B.C.

Shang E 上顎

The palate of the mouth.

Shaohai (H-3) 少海

Lesser Sea. Name of an acupuncture cavity belonging to the Heart channel.

Shaolin 少林

A Buddhist temple in Henan Province, famous for its martial arts.

She Gen 舌根

The root of the tongue.

Shen 神

Spirit. According to Chinese Qigong, the Shen resides at the Upper Dan Tian (the third eye).

Shen 身

Physical body.

Shen 深

Deep.

Shen Fa 身法

The body's moving skills.

Shen Gu 神谷

Spirit valley. Formed by the two lobes of the brain, with the Upper Dan Tian at the exit.

Shen Qi Xiang He 神氣相合

The Shen and the Qi combine together. The final stage of regulating the Shen.

Shen Shi 神室

The residence of the spirit.

Shen Xi 神息

Spirit breathing. The stage of Qigong training where the spirit is coordinated with the breathing.

Shen Xi Xiang Yi 神息相依

The Shen and breathing mutually rely on each other.

Shen Yi Nei Lian 神宜內斂

"Spirit should be retained internally."

Sheng Men 生門

Life Door. A Daoist term that implies the navel.

Sheng Tai 聖胎

Holy embryo. Another name for the spiritual embryo (Shen Tai).

Shenzhu (Gv-12) 身柱

Body Pillar. An acupuncture cavity that belongs to the Governing Vessel.

Shi Er Jing 十二經

Twelve Primary Qi Channels. They include the Yang primary Qi channels (The Large Intestine Channel of Hand — Yang Brightness; The Small Intestine Channel of Hand — Greater Yang; The Triple Burner Channel of Hand — Lesser Yang; The Stomach Channel of Foot — Yang Brightness; The Urinary Bladder Channel of Foot — Greater Yang; and The Gall Bladder Channel of Foot — Lesser Yang) and the Yin primary Qi channels (The Lung Channel of Hand — Greater Yin; The Heart Channel of Hand — Lesser Yin; The Pericardium Channel of Hand — Absolute Yin; The Spleen Channel of Foot — Greater Yin; The Kidney Channel of Foot — Lesser Yin; and The Liver Channel of Foot — Absolute Yin).

Shi Liu Gua 十六卦

Sixteen Trigrams.

Shi San Shi 十三勢

Thirteen Patterns. Taijiquan is also called Shi San Shi, since it is constructed from these thirteen moving or acting patterns.

Shou 手

Hands.

Shou Shen 守神

To keep the mind at the spirit. A Qigong meditation training.

Shuai 摔

Means "to stumble, to fall, or to throw down."

Shuai Jiao 摔跤

Means "wrestling."

Shuang Xiu 雙修

Double cultivation. A Qigong training method in which Qi is exchanged with a partner in order to balance the Qi in both people.

Shuang Zhong 雙重

Means "double weighting or double layering." It means when the opponent has placed a weight or pressure on you, you respond by meeting that pressure with equal or greater pressure of your own. The consequence is stagnation. When this happens, mutual resistance will be generated.

Shui 水

Water. One of the Five Elements.

Shui Lu 水路

Water Path. One of the meditation paths in which the Qi is led upward through the spinal cord (i.e., Thrusting Vessel, Chong Mai, 衝脈) to nourish the brain.

Si 祀

Religious rites or services.

Si Liang Po Qian Jin 四兩破千斤

Means to use four ounces to repel (i.e., neutralize) one thousand pounds.

Si Liu Bu 四六步

Four-Six Stance. One of the basic stances in northern styles of martial arts training.

Si Xiang 四象

Means "Four Phases," which are derived from the Two Poles.

Song Shan 嵩山

Song mountain. One of the five sacred mountains in China, located in Deng Feng county, Henan Province (河南省·登封縣). It is also called "Zhong Yue" (中嶽) and means "central mountain."

Sui 隨

Means "to follow."

Sui Jin 隨勁

Following Jin. The martial power which is used to follow the opponent's action.

Sui Qi 髓氣

The Qi circulating in the bone marrow or brain.

Sui Xi 髓息

Sui means "the marrow or brain." Therefore, Sui Xi means the Qigong breathing technique which is able to lead the Qi to the bone marrow and brain.

Sun Wu 孫武

Also named Sun Zi (孫子). A famous strategist who lived around 557 B.C. He wrote the book *Sun Zi's Fighting Strategies* (*Sun Zi Bing Fa*, 孫子兵法). This book is commonly translated as *The Art of War*.

Sun Zi 孫子

Mister Sun. Sun Wu (孫武). A famous strategist who lived around 557 B.C. He wrote a book: *Sun Zi's Fighting Strategies* (Sun Zi Bing Fa, 孫子兵法). This book is commonly translated as "The Art of War."

Sun Zi Bing Fa 孫子兵法

Sun Zi's Fighting Strategies. Name of a book which is commonly translated as *The Art of War.*

Tai Chi Chuan (Taijiquan) 太極拳

A Chinese internal martial style which is based on the theory of Taiji (grand ultimate).

Tai Xi 胎息

Embryonic Breathing. One of the final goals in regulating the breath, Embryo Breathing enables you to generate a "baby Shen" at the Huang Ting (yellow yard).

Taiji 太極

Means "grand ultimate." It is this force which generates two poles, Yin and Yang.

Taiji Quan Chan Shou Lian Xi 太極圈纏手練習

Taiji circle sticking hands training. One of the most important trainings in Yang style Taijiquan. This training is used to train listening, understanding, sticking, adhering, connecting, and following. In Chen style, it is called "Silk reeling Jin coiling training" (Chan Si Jin Chan Shou Lian Xi, 纏絲勁纏手練習).

Taijiquan (Tai Chi Chuan) 太極拳

A Chinese internal martial style which is based on the theory of Taiji (grand ultimate).

Taipei 台北

The capital city of Taiwan located in the north of Taiwan.

Taipei Xian 台北縣

A county in northern Taiwan.

Taiwan 台灣

An island to the southeast of mainland China. Also known as "Formosa."

Taiwan University 台灣大學

A well-known university located in Taipei, Taiwan.

Taizuquan 太祖拳

A style of Chinese external martial arts.

Tamkang 淡江

Name of a University in Taiwan.

Tamkang College Guoshu Club 淡江國術社

A Chinese martial arts club founded by Dr. Yang when he was studying in Tamkang College.

Tao Te Ching (Dao De Jing) 道德經

Morality Classic. The Way of Natural Virtues. Written by Lao Zi.

Ti 踢

Means "to kick."

Ti Xi 體息

Body breathing, or skin breathing. In Qigong, the exchanging of Qi with the surrounding environment through the skin.

Tian Chi 天池

Heavenly Pond. The place under the tongue where saliva is generated.

Tian Chi Shui 天池水

Heavenly water. The water generated in Tian Chi (天池) (i.e., Heavenly Pond).

Tian Chuang 天窗

Sky Window. The area above the arms. To open the opponent's upper body area for an attack is called "Kai Tian Chuan" (開天窗) (i.e., open the sky window).

Tian Ling Gai 天靈蓋

Literally, heaven spiritual cover. A person's head is considered to be heaven, and the crown is called "heaven spiritual cover" by Daoist society. This place is called Baihui (Gv-20) (百會) in acupuncture.

Tian Ren He Yi 天人合一

Literally, "Heaven and man unified as one." A high level of Qigong practice in which a Qigong practitioner, through meditation, is able to communicate his Qi with heaven's Qi.

Tian Yan 天眼

Heaven Eye. The third eye or Upper Dan Tian.

Tiantu (Co-22) 天突

Heaven's Prominence. Name of an acupuncture cavity. It belongs to the Conception Vessel.

Tiao 調

A gradual regulating process, until what is regulated has reached its harmonious state with other things.

Tiao Qi 調氣

To regulate the Qi.

Tiao Shen 調神

To regulate the spirit.

Tiao Shen 調身

To regulate the body.

Tiao Xi 調息

To regulate the breathing.

Tiao Xin 調心

To regulate the emotional mind.

Ting 聽

Listening.

Ting Jin 聽勁

Listening Jin. A special training which uses the skin to feel the opponent's energy and uses this feeling to further understand his intention.

Tong San Guan 通三關

Means "to get through the three gates." A special term used in Small Circulation.

Tui Na 推拿

Means "to push and grab." A category of Chinese massages for healing and injury treatment.

Tuo Yue 彙龠

Bellows, a tube which is used to blow up the fire in a furnace.

Wai Kua 外胯

External upper thighs near the groin area.

Wai Shen 外腎

External Kidneys. The testicles.

Wang, Zong-Yue 王宗岳

A well-known Taijiquan master during the late Qing Dynasty. Wang, Zong-Yue wrote many comprehensive Taijiquan documents and is popularly studied by Taijiquan practitioners today.

Wei Qi 衛氣

Protective Qi or Guardian Qi. The Qi at the surface of the body which generates a shield to protect the body from negative external influences such as colds.

Weilu 尾閭

Tailbone. A Daoist name. This cavity is called Changqiang (Gv-1) in acupuncture.

Wen Huo 文火

Scholar fire. Through soft and slender breathing, the Qi (i.e., fire) can be built up gently at the abdominal area.

Wilson Chen 陳威伸

Dr. Yang, Jwing-Ming's martial arts friend.

Wu 午

One of the twelve Terrestrial Branches (i.e., 11:00 A.M. to 1:00 P.M.).

Wu Bu 五步

Five steppings. They include: forward, backward, left, right, and center.

Wu Huo 武火

Martial fire. Through fast and short breathing techniques, the Qi (i.e., fire) can be built up to an abundant level for the physical manifestation in a short time. However, through this technique, though the fire can be built up in a fast way, it is hard to keep it in the body.

Wu Xin 五心

Five centers or five gates. The face, the Laogong (勞宮) cavities in both palms, and the Yongquan (湧泉) cavities on the bottoms of both feet.

Wu Xin Xi 五心息

Five-gates breathing.

Wu Xing 五行

Five Phases, including: metal (Jin, 金), wood (Mu, 木), water (Shui, 水), fire (Huo, 火), and earth (Tu, 土).

Wu Yu 五育

Five educations, which include science, art, mathematics, literature, and physical education.

Wǔ, Yu-Xiang 武禹襄

A well-known Taijiquan master during the Chinese Qing Dynasty. He is the creator of Wǔ style Taijiquan.

Wudang Mountain 武當山

Located in Hubei Province (湖北省) in China.

Wuji 無極

Means "no extremity."

Wuji Hu Xi (Wuji Xi) 無極呼吸（無極息）

Wuji Breathing. Keeping the mind at the Real Dan Tian during breathing practice.

Wushu 武術

Literally, "martial techniques."

Wuyi 武藝

Literally, "martial arts."

Xi 細

Slender.

Xi Bo Hou 西伯侯

Marquis Xi Bo, the feudal title of King Wen (Zhou Wen Wang, 周文王) before he rose in arms against emperor Zhou (紂王) during Chinese Shang Dynasty (商朝) (1154-1122 B.C.).

Xi Sui 洗髓

Washing the marrow or cleaning the brain by Qi nourishment.

Xia Dan Tian 下丹田

Lower elixir field. Located in the lower abdomen, it is believed to be the residence of water Qi (Original Qi) (Yuan Qi, 元氣). This cavity in acupuncture is called Qihai (Co-6) (氣海) which means "Qi ocean."

Xia Pan 下盤

The Chinese express the concept of root generated by the legs as the "lower disk." From the thighs to the feet is called Xia Pan (lower disk), the waist area is called "Zhong Pan" (中盤) (middle disk), while the chest and the head are "Shang Pan" (上盤) (top disk)."

Xian Tian Qi 先天氣

Pre-Birth Qi or Pre-Heaven Qi. Also called "Dan Tian Qi." The Qi which is converted from Original Essence and is stored in the Lower Tian. Considered to be "water Qi," it is able to calm the body.

Xiao Jia 小架

Small posture. It means the small circle for short range fighting purposes.

Xiao Lu 小擺

Small rollback.

Xiao Zhou Tian 小周天

Small heavenly cycle. Also called Small Circulation. The completed Qi circuit through the Conception and Governing Vessels.

Xiayin 下陰

Groin.

Xin 心

Means "heart." Xin means "the mind generated from emotional disturbance."

Xin Ling 心靈

Means "heart, soul, spirit, or mind."

Xin Yuan Yi Ma 心猿意馬

Xin-monkey and Yi-horse. Xin (i.e., heart) is related to the emotional mind, is like a monkey, and is hard to keep steady and calm. Yi is wise and logical thinking, which is like a horse that can be calm and keep still.

Xing 性

Human Nature.

Xinkan 心坎

A martial term. It is the solar plexus area and is called Jiuwei (Co-15) (鳩尾) in acupuncture.

Xinzhu Xian 新竹縣

Birthplace of Dr. Yang, Jwing-Ming in Taiwan.

Xiong Gong 胸弓

Chest bow. The bow formed from the chest, which is able to store the Jin significantly.

Xu Ling Ding Jin 虛領頂勁

An insubstantial energy leads the head upward. A secret Taijiquan phrase which helps a Taijiquan practitioner keep the head upright and the neck relaxed.

Xuan Pin 玄牝

Means "Concealed Female" or "Mysterious Female." A Daoist Qigong term originated from the *Dao De Jing* (道德經).

Xue Wei Hu Xi (Xue Wei Xi) 穴位呼吸（穴位息）

Cavity Breathing. It means while in the deep abdominal breathing, keep the mind at the Real Dan Tian. Another name of "Embryonic Breathing" (Tai Xi, 胎息).

Xun 巽

One of the Eight Trigrams which represents "wind."

Yan 眼

Eyes.

Yang 陽

Too sufficient. One of the two poles. The other is Yin.

Yang, Ban-Hou (1837-1892 A.D.) 楊班侯

Yang, Lu-Shan's second son. Also called Yang, Yu (楊鈺).

Yang, Jwing-Ming 楊俊敏

Author of this book.

Yang, Yu (1837-1892 A.D.) 楊鈺

Yang, Lu-Shan's second son. Also called Ban-Hou (班侯). A second generation practitioner of Yang style Taijiquan.

Yang-Shen 陽神

Shen (i.e., spirit) is classified as Yang, therefore, it is commonly called "Yang Shen."

Yangqiao Mai 陽蹻脈

Yang Heel Vessel. One of the eight extraordinary vessels.

Yangwei Mai 陽維脈

Yang Linking Vessel. One of the eight extraordinary vessels.

Yi 意

Wisdom mind. The mind generated from wise judgment.

Yi Jin 易筋

"Muscle/Tendon Changing." It means to change the physical body from a weak to a strong condition.

Yi Jin Jing 易筋經

Literally: *Changing Muscle/Tendon Classic*, usually called *The Muscle/Tendon Changing Classic*. Credited to Da Mo around 550 A.D., this work discusses Wai Dan Qigong training for strengthening the physical body.

Yi Jing 易經

Book of Changes. A book of divination written during the Zhou Dynasty (1122-255 B.C., 周).

Yin 陰

Deficient. One of the two poles. The other is Yang.

Yin Jin 引勁

The Jin (martial power) of leading.

Yin Jin Luo Kong 引勁落空

Means "to lead the coming Jin into emptiness." It means to neutralize the incoming force.

Yin Shui 陰水

Yin Water. The Qi stored at the Real Dan Tian is called "Yin Shui," since keeping the Qi here may keep you calm.

Ying Jin 硬勁

Hard Jins or physical Jin.

Ying Li 硬力

Hard muscular force.

Yinjiao (Co-7) 陰交

Yin's Junction. An acupuncture cavity that belongs to the Conception Vessel.

Yinqiao Mai 陰蹺脈

Yin Heel Vessel. One of the eight extraordinary vessels.

Yintang (M-HN-3) 印堂

Seal Hall. An acupuncture cavity that belongs to Miscellaneous Points.

Yinwei Mai 陰維脈

Yin Linking Vessel. One of the eight extraordinary vessels.

Yongquan (K-1) 湧泉

Bubbling Well or Gushing Spring. Name of an acupuncture cavity belonging to the Kidney Primary Qi Channel.

You 悠

Long, far, meditative, continuous, slow and soft.

Yu Huan Xue 玉環穴

Jade Ring Cavity. Another Daoist name for the Real Dan Tian.

Yuan Ji 元極

Original Extremities. It means "the beginning of life." Here it means Taiji.

Yuan Jing 元精

Original Essence. The fundamental, original substance inherited from your parents; it is converted into Original Qi.

Yuan Qi 元氣

Original Qi. Created from the Original Essence inherited from your parents.

Yun 勻

Uniform or even.

Yuzhen 玉枕

Jade pillow. One of the three gates of Small Circulation training.

Zhan 占

To occupy.

Zhan 沾

Attaching.

Zhan 輾

Half-rotating or half-turning.

Zhan 粘

Attaching or sticking.

Zhan Jin 粘勁

The martial power that is used to attack the opponent's body.

Zhang Jin 長勁

Growing Jin. One form of the martial power trained in Taijiquan.

Zhang, San-Feng 張三丰

Zhang, San-Feng is credited as the creator of Taijiquan during the Song Dynasty in China (960-1127 A.D.) (宋朝).

Zhang, Xiang-San 張祥三

A well-known martial artist in Taiwan during the 1960's.

Zhen 震

One of the Eight Trigrams which represents "thunder."

Zhen Dan Tian 真丹田

Real Dan Tian (i.e., physical center of gravity).

Zhen Xi 真息

The real breathing. Means the breathing has been regulated to a deep and profound level.

Zheng 正

Regularity, formal action or thinking.

Zheng Fu Hu Xi 正腹呼吸

Formal Abdominal Breathing. More commonly called "Buddhist Breathing."

Zheng Hu Xi 正呼吸

Formal Breathing. More commonly called "Buddhist Breathing."

Zhong Dan Tian 中丹田

Middle Dan Tian. Located in the area of the solar plexus, it is the residence of fire Qi.

Zhong Ding 中定

To firm the center.

Zhong Jia 中架

Middle-sized postures that are used for middle-range fighting.

Zhong Men 中門

Central door. In Chinese martial arts, central door means the center line between you and your opponent.

Zhong Shi 中勢

Middle high stance.

Zhou 肘

Elbow.

Zhou Jin 肘勁

The martial power generated from the elbow.

Zi 子

One of the twelve Terrestrial Branches (i.e., 11:00 P.M. to1:00 A.M.).

Zi Jue 自覺

Self-awareness.

Zi Shi 子時

Midnight. The time between 11 P.M. to 1 A.M.

Zi Shi 自識

Self-recognition.

Zi Tuo 自脫

Set yourself free from emotional or spiritual bondage.

Zi Wu 自悟

Self-awakening.

Zi Wu Liu Zhu 子午流注

Zi refers to the period around midnight (11:00 P.M. to 1:00 A.M.), and Wu refers to midday (11:00 A.M. to 1:00 P.M.). Liu Zhu means "the flowing tendency." Therefore: a schedule of the Qi circulation showing which channel has the predominant Qi flow at any particular time, and where the predominant Qi flow is in the Conception and Governing Vessels.

Zi Xing 自醒

Self-awakening.

Zou Huo Ru Mo 走火入魔

Walk into the fire and enter the demon. This means the Qi has entered the wrong path and the mind has entered a delusional state.

Zuo Wan 坐腕

Settle down the wrist.

Index

Lightning Source UK Ltd.
Milton Keynes UK
UKHW032013270121
377781UK00004B/199